Mathematical
Models in Medical
and Health Science

Innovations in Applied Mathematics

An international series devoted to the latest research in modern areas of mathematics, with significant applications in engineering, medicine, and the sciences.

Series Editor:
Larry L. Schumaker
Stevenson Professor of Mathematics
Vanderbilt University

Previously published titles include

Mathematical Methods for Curves and Surfaces (1995)

Mathematical Methods for Curves and Surfaces II (1998)

Curves and Surfaces with Applications in CAGD (1997)

Surface Fitting and Multiresolution Methods (1997)

Mathematical Models in Medical and Health Science

EDITED BY

Mary Ann Horn
Department of Mathematics
Vanderbilt University

Gieri Simonett
Department of Mathematics
Vanderbilt University

Glenn F. Webb
Department of Mathematics
Vanderbilt University

VANDERBILT UNIVERSITY PRESS
Nashville & London

First Edition 1998
98 99 00 01 02   5 4 3 2 1

This publication is made from paper that meets
the minimum requirements of ANSI/NISO Z39.48 (R 1997)
Permanence of Paper for Printed Library Materials. ⊗

Library of Congress Cataloging-in-Publication Data

Mathematical models in medical and health science / edited by Mary Ann Horn, Gieri
    Simonett, Glenn F. Webb. — 1st ed.
        p.   cm. — (Innovations in applied mathematics)
    Includes bibliographical references and index.
    ISBN 0-8265-1310-7 (cloth : alk. paper)
        1. Medical sciences—Research—Mathematical models—Miscellanea.
    2. Medicine—Research—Mathematical models—Miscellanea. I. Horn, Mary Ann,
    1965– . II. Simonett, Gieri, 1959– . III. Webb, Glenn F., 1942– . IV. Series.
    R853.M3M3747 1998
    610'.1'5118—dc21   98-38746
                                                                CIP

CONTENTS

PREFACE

The *International Conference on Mathematical Models in Medical and Health Sciences* was held at Vanderbilt University May 28-31, 1997. This conference was the thirteenth in the series of Annual Shanks Lectures held at Vanderbilt University. The Shanks Lectures are endowed by Judith Olivia Shanks Denton and Eugene Baylis Shanks, Jr. to honor the service of their parents, Baylis and Olivia Shanks, to Vanderbilt University. The support of the Shanks family and Vanderbilt University is gratefully acknowledged. The conference was attended by approximately 200 participants from 15 countries. The National Science Foundation contributed funds to support the participation of women, minority, and young researchers.

The focus of the conference was upon the development, analysis, and simulation of continuous and discrete theoretical mathematical models for the life sciences and medical sciences. The primary purpose of the conference was to bring together mathematicians, biologists, and medical researchers to a forum that promoted their interdisciplinary cooperation. The use of theoretical mathematical models to understand biological processes in medical and health sciences has seen greatly increased development in recent years. There is a recognized need to bring mathematical modeling to scientists working in these subjects. The applications of these models to fundamental research in medical and health sciences requires interdisciplinary communication and collaboration.

The Thirteenth Annual Shanks Lecture was given by Martin Nowak of Oxford University. The title of his talk was "Mathematical Models of Virus Infection and Evolution." There were 10 additional plenary lectures given by A. Aldroubi (National Institutes of Health and Vanderbilt University), E. Afenya (Elmhurst College), S. Blower (University of California at San Francisco), M. Kimmel (Rice University), M. Mackey (McGill University, Canada), S. Michelson (Roche Pharmaceuticals), R. Muira (University of British Columbia, Canada), M. Parrott (University of South Florida), S. Tucker (The University of Texas M. D. Anderson Cancer Center) and J. Velasco-Hernández (UAM-Iztapalapa, México). The conference program included contributed and special sessions. The special sessions were as follows: Epidemic Models (organized by W. Fitzgibbon), Models on Immunology and Disease (organized by D. Kirschner), Cancer Modeling (organized by J. C. Panetta), Models of Diffusive Systems in Biology (organized by W. Fitzgibbon), Cell Population Models (organized by G. Webb), Mathematical Models in Medical Imaging (organized by D. Hardin), Models of Optimization and Control (organized by M. Iannelli and H. Thieme), and Cure Models in Survival Analysis (organized by A. Yakovlev).

This volume contains articles contributed by the participants at the conference. All articles were refereed by peer review. The subjects of the contributions to this volume divide into six categories: (1) Models of cancer growth and treatment, (2) models of metabolic disease and immune system disease,

(3) models of physiological processes, (4) models of the cell cycle and cell proliferation, (5) models of epidemic populations, and (6) models of ecology and the environment.

(1) Models of Cancer Growth and Treatment:

E. Afenya analyzes and simulates models of chemotherapy and radiotherapy of leukemia and designs treatment protocols that aggressively reduce the leukemic population while maintaining the normal cell population. M. Chaplain, V. Kuznetsov, Z. James and L. Stepanova design a heterogeneous spatial model for the growth of solid tumors, such as malignant melanomas of the skin, and compare numerical simulations of their model with experimental data. P. Laub presents a model of myelosuppression of neutrophils and platelets in the blood resulting from chemotherapy and evaluates model simulations with clinical data. S. Maggelakis models the effects of angiogenic factors such as angiostatin and endostatin on tumor angiogenesis and vascularization. J. Panetta, M. Chaplain and J. Adam provide a review of dynamic models of tumor progression, angiogenesis, metastases, and heterogeneity and relate these various models to therapy and medical information. S. Tucker derives a model of tumor radiotherapy based on mechanistic assumptions regarding the distribution of cell cycle times, tumor-cell differentiation rates, and cell loss rates.

(2) Models of Metabolic Disease and Immune System Disease:

M. Berry and D. Westerman develop a cluster form analysis for a 2D color model of regions of the retina and use computer generated images to aid clinical diagnosis of diabetic retinopathy. F. Sánchez-Garduño, D. Kirschner and J. Reynolds theoretically and numerically analyze a model of disease progression in the HIV infected immune system based on interaction of viral and lymphocyte populations. W.-Y. Tan and Z. Xiang develop a stochastic model for the pathogenesis of HIV at the cellular level and compare their results to data for a HIV infected hemophilia patient.

(3) Models of Physiological Processes:

M. Ballyk and H. Smith analyze a model of competing bacterial strains in the composition of the indigenous microflora of the large intestine and discuss the influence of motility of invading organisms in stabilization and invasion of the gut. W. Fitzgibbon and J. Morgan present a reaction-diffusion model of morphogenesis in biological systems and prove the existence of a compact global attractor. J. Foweraker, D. Bashor, M. Hulliger and E. Otten construct a point-neurone model of repetitive firing for muscle sensory receptors and apply it to the control of movement. M. Parrott discusses the Hodgkin-Huxley model of nerve impulse propagation and describes recent results for models which include axon self-capacitance and self-inductance using singular perturbation analysis. B. Roth uses a model of spiral waves in cardiac tissue to explain how anisotropy of cardiac tissue influences the meandering of spiral waves.

(4) Models of the Cell Cycle and Cell Proliferation:

J. Dyson, R. Villella-Bressan and G. Webb analyze a model of cell proliferation based upon a structuring of individual cells according to cell cycle age and morphological maturity and apply their model to the distinction of normal and anemic blood cell production. R. Sennerstam and J.-O. Strömberg discuss a model of the cell cycle based upon a DNA-division cycle spanning the S phase and G2 - M phases plus a pre-S phase and use its predictions to analyze data for sister-sister, mother-daughter, and cousin cell correlations of intermitotic times. C. D. Thron develops a model of the cell division cycle which uses a saddle-node bifurcation at check points to control arrest and resumption of cycling.

(5) Models of Epidemic Populations:

V. Barbu and M. Iannelli present a nonlinear age-structured model of an infectious disease in a demographically stable population in which control of the epidemic involves intervention of vertical transmission to newborns. S. Blower, T. Porco and T. Lietman describe a model of epidemic control strategies for tuberculosis and the epidemiological consequences of reinfection, treatment delay, and the competitive dynamics between drug-sensitive and drug-resistant pathogens. Z. Feng and F. Milner analyze a deterministic epidemic model for schistosomiasis based on the life cycle of schistosome parasites and variable sizes of human host populations and intermediate snail host populations. H. Inaba analyzes a type A influenza epidemic model in which genetic or evolutionary changes in the influenza antigen are modeled by a continuous structure variable corresponding to antigenic drift in the virus strain.

(6) Models of Ecology and the Environment:

R. S. Cantrell and C. Cosner present a model of skew Brownian motion to describe diffusion in the presence of interfaces and apply their results to an ecological model with two types of habitats. K. Fister and S. Lenhart analyze a system of reaction-diffusion equations with Lotka-Volterra growth terms and apply their results to the optimal harvesting in predator-prey populations in which controls correspond to a proportion of the species being harvested. N. Handagama and S. Lenhart discuss a reaction diffusion model of a gas-phase bioreactor and characterize the optimal control for the flow rate of contaminant through metabolism of a bacteria with the objective of maximizing the amount of contaminant degraded less the cost of implementing the control. N. Navarova and H. Thieme present a model of zoo-plankton pollution interaction in a freshwater environment and prove that a relaxed feed-back control of the pollutant input drives the dynamics of model to a unique equilibrium when the environmental pollutant concentration is below a prescribed threshold.

We, the editors, would like to express our thanks to the participants of the conference and the contributors to this volume. It is our sincere hope that their efforts will encourage researchers in medical and health sciences to appreciate the value of mathematical modeling in scientific work.

Mary Ann Horn
Gieri Simonett
Glenn Webb

Nashville, Tennessee   July 15, 1998

CONTRIBUTORS

Numbers in parentheses indicate pages on which authors' contributions begin.

JOHN A. ADAM (281), *Department of Mathematics and Statistics, Old Dominion University, Norfolk, VA 23529–0077* [adam@math.odu.edu]

EVANS K. AFENYA (1), *Deptartment of Mathematics, Elmhurst College, 190 Prospect Avenue, Elmhurst, IL 60126* [evansa@elmhurst.edu]

MARY M. BALLYK (17), *Department of Mathematics, Arizona State University, Tempe, AZ 85287-1804* [mballyk@nmsu.edu]

VIOREL BARBU (29), *Department of Mathematics, "Al.I.Cuza" University, 6600 - Iasi, Romania* [barbu@uaic.ro]

D. P. BASHOR (145), *Department of Biology, University of North Carolina at Charlotte, Charlotte, NC 28223* [bashor@uncc.edu]

MICHAEL W. BERRY (35), *Department of Computer Science, University of Tennessee, Knoxville, TN 37996-1301* [berry@cs.utk.edu]

SALLY BLOWER (51), *Department of Microbiology & Immunology, University of California San Francisco, 513 Parnassus, HSE Room 420, San Francisco, CA 94143* [sally@itsa.ucsf.edu]

R. S. CANTRELL (73), *Department of Mathematics and Computer Science, University of Miami, Coral Gables, Florida 33124* [rsc@atlanta.cs.miami.edu]

MARK A. J. CHAPLAIN (79, 281), *Department of Mathematics, University of Dundee, Dundee DD1 4HN, United Kingdom* [chaplain@mcs.dundee.ac.uk]

CHRIS COSNER (73), *Department of Mathematics and Computer Science, University of Miami, Coral Gables, Florida 33124* [gcc@cs.cs.miami.edu]

JANET DYSON (99), *Mansfield College, University of Oxford, Oxford, England* [janet.dyson@mansfield.oxford.ac.uk]

ZHILAN FENG (117), *Department of Mathematics, Purdue University, West Lafayette, IN 47907-1395* [zfeng@math.purdue.edu]

K. RENEE FISTER (129), *Department of Mathematics and Statistics, Murray State University, Murray, KY 42071* [kfister@math.mursuky.edu]

WILLIAM E. FITZGIBBON (139), *Department of Mathematics, University of Houston, 4800 Calhoun, Houston, TX 77007* [fitz@math.uh.edu]

J. P. A. FOWERAKER (145), *Department of Clinical Neurosciences, Faculty of Medicine, University of Calgary, Health Sciences Building, 3330 Hospital Drive N.W., Calgary, Alberta, Canada T2N 4N1* [jonf@cns.ucalgary.ca]

FAUSTINO SÁNCHEZ GARDUÑO (161) , *Departamento de Matemáticas, Facultad de Ciencias, UNAM, Circuito Exterior, Ciudad Universitaria, México, 04510, D.F.* [faustino@servidor.unam.mx]

M. HULLIGER (145), *Department of Clinical Neurosciences, Faculty of Medicine, University of Calgary, Health Sciences Building, 3330 Hospital Drive N.W., Calgary, Alberta, Canada T2N 4N1* [manuel@cns.ucalgary.ca]

MIMMO IANNELLI (29), *Dipartimento di Matematica, Universitá di Trento, 38050 Povo (Trento), Italy* [iannelli@science.unitn.it]

Z. H. JAMES (79), *Department of Mathematical Sciences, University of Bath, Claverton Down, Bath BA2 7AY, United Kingdom*

NARESH HANDAGAMA (197), *Pellissippi State Technical Community College, University of Tennessee, Chemical Engineering Department, Knoxville, TN 37993*

HISASHI INABA (213), *Department of Mathematical Sciences, University of Tokyo, 3-8-1 Komaba Meguro-ku, Tokyo 153, Japan* [inaba@ms.u-tokyo.ac.jp]

DENISE KIRSCHNER (161), *Department of Microbiology and Immunology, 6730 Medical Science Bldg II, The University of Michigan Medical School, Ann Arbor, MI 49109-0620* [kirschne@umich.edu]

V. A. KUZNETSOV (79), *Laboratory of Experimental and Computational Biology, Division of Basic Sciences, National Cancer Institute, FCRDC, Frederic, MD 21702-120*

PAUL B. LAUB (237), *Incyte Pharmaceuticals, Inc., 3174 Porter Drive, Palo Alto, California 94304* [plaub@incyte.com]

SUZANNE LENHART (129, 197), *Department of Mathematics, University of Tennessee, Knoxville, TN 37996* [lenhart@math.utk.edu]

TOM LIETMAN (51), *F.I. Proctor Foundation, University of California San Francisco, 95 Kirkham Av., Box 0944, San Francisco, CA, 94143-0944* [tml@itsa.ucsf.edu]

SOPHIA A. MAGGELAKIS (247), *Department of Mathematics and Statistics, Rochester Institute of Technology, Rochester, NY 14623*

FABIO AUGUSTO MILNER (117), *Department of Mathematics, Purdue University, West Lafayette, IN 47907-1395* [milner@math.purdue.edu]

JEFF MORGAN (139), *Department of Mathematics, Texas A&M University, College Station, TX 77843-3368* [Jeff.Morgan@math.tamu.edu]

NATALIA NAVAROVA (267), *Department of Mathematics, Arizona State University, Tempe, AZ 85287-1804* [asnxn@acvax.inre.asu.edu]

E. OTTEN (145), *Department of Medical Physiology, University of Groningen, Bloemsingle 10, NL-9712 KZ Groningen, The Netherlands* [e.otten@med.rug.nl]

JOHN CARL PANETTA (281), *Mathematics Program, Penn State Erie, The Behrend College, Station Road, Erie, PA 16563–0203* [panetta@wagner.bd.psu.edu]

MARY E. PARROTT (311), *Department of Mathematics, University of South Florida, Tampa, FL 33620-5700* [parrott@math.usf.edu]

TRAVIS PORCO (51), *San Francisco Department of Public Health, Community Health Epidemiology Section, 25 Van Ness Avenue, Suite 710, San Francisco, CA, 94102-6033* [travis_porco@dph.sf.ca.us]

JANELLE REYNOLDS (161), *Department of Oceanography, University of North Carolina, Chapel Hill, N.C. 27599* [janelle@email.unc.edu]

BRADLEY J. ROTH (327), *Department of Physics and Astronomy, Vanderbilt University, Nashville, TN 37235* [roth@compsci.cas.vanderbilt.edu]

ROLAND SENNERSTAM (337), *Division of Cell and Molecular Analysis, Department of Oncology and Pathology, Karolinska Institute and Hospital, S-171 76 Stockholm, Sweden* [roland.sennerstam@haninge.mail.telia.com]

HAL L. SMITH (17), *Department of Mathematics, Arizona State University, Tempe, AZ 85287-1804* [halsmith@asu.edu]

L. A. STEPANOVA (79), *Laboratory of Mathematical Immunobiophysics, Institute of Biochemical Physics, Russian Academy of Sciences, Moscow, 117977, Russia*

JAN-OLOF STRÖMBERG (337), *Institute of Mathematical and Physical Sciences, University of Tromsø, Norway*

WAI-YUAN TAN (351), *Department of Mathematical Sciences, The University of Memphis, Memphis, TN 38152* [tanwy@msci.memphis.edu]

HORST R. THIEME (267), *Department of Mathematics, Arizona State University, Tempe, AZ 85287-1804* [thieme@math.la.asu.edu]

C. D. THRON (369), *5 Barrymore Road, Hanover, NH 03755* [dennis.thron@valley.net]

SUSAN L. TUCKER (381), *Department of Biomathematics, Box 237, The Univ. of Texas M. D. Anderson Cancer Center, 1515 Holcombe Blvd., Houston, Texas 77030* [tucker@odin.mdacc.tmc.edu]

ROSANNA VILLELLA-BRESSAN (99), *Dipartimento di Matematica Pura ed Applicata, Universita' di Padova, Padova, Italy* [rosannav@math.unipd.iti]

GLENN WEBB (99), *Department of Mathematics, Vanderbilt University, Nashville, TN 37240* [webbgf00@ctrvax.vanderbilt.edu]

DAX M. WESTERMAN (35), *Department of Computer Science, University of Tennessee, Knoxville, TN 37996-1301* [westerma@cs.utk.edu]

ZHIHUA XIANG (351), *Department of Mathematical Sciences, The University of Memphis, Memphis, TN 38152*

Cancer Treatment Strategies
and Mathematical Modeling

Evans K. Afenya

Abstract. A treatment regimen, which includes combinations of chemotherapy and radiotherapy, is superimposed on a simple model that describes an aggressively expanding cancer. The treatment strategy expressed by this model is then analyzed. Treatment options are studied and
investigated. Issues related to patient-specific treatment are addressed.
Achievement of massive reductions in the cancer cell population over relatively short time periods is explored. Analyses and simulations of the
model tend to support aggressive cancer treatment schemes.

§1. Introduction

Remarkable advances have been made over the years in the prevention, detection, treatment, and management of cancer. As a consequence, medical
research, which is becoming increasingly quantitative in scope and content,
is gaining a better understanding of the molecular and cellular underpinnings
of this disease. Nevertheless, despite the advances, cancer remains evasive in
most of its forms and poses enormous challenges to biomedical science. In
1996, an estimated 555,000 people in the United States died of cancer [20].
This number was up from 331,000 deaths in 1970. It is estimated that some
40 percent of Americans will eventually be stricken with the disease, and more
than 20 percent will die of it [20]. On a global scale, the World Health Organization (WHO) estimates that cancer kills roughly six million people annually
[20]. As biomedicine continues its fight against this disease, it keeps encountering and grappling with a number of problems that could be approached, in
part, through mathematical modeling. It is within this framework that our
investigative activities in this area assume relevance.

There are many types of cancers with varying degrees of lethality to the
human host. Some cancers may be benign and others may be malignant.
The malignant ones pose serious dangers to the individual if left untreated.
Cancers basically involve solid or disseminated tumors. Solid tumors that

Mathematical Models in Medical and Health Sciences
Mary Ann Horn, Gieri Simonett, and Glenn Webb (eds.), pp. 1–15.

include breast, ovarian, prostate, and lung cancers, normally grow at specific sites of the human body and have the potential of metastasizing to other parts of the body, if malignant. Disseminated tumors on the other hand, such as the leukemias, develop and grow normally in the bone marrow and eventually fill up the marrow and the blood and predispose the individual to serious fatalities. There are different types of treatment schemes that are used by medical practitioners against the cancers. The specific type of treatment scheme depends on the specific cancer in question.

In this article, we shall study and discuss certain issues pertaining to cancer treatment options and protocols by using leukemia as a focal point. Leukemia is one of the leading cancers among men and women in the United States [18]. More than 27,000 new cases of leukemia were detected in the US in 1996 and more than 21,000 patients of this disease were expected to die before the end of 1996 [18]. It is projected that forty percent of leukemia patients die within one year of diagnosis and five-year survival rates for acute myelogenous leukemia, which is common among adults, stand at 11.4% [18]. Existing data also suggest that the incidence of leukemia is increasing [21].

Leukemia is described as a disease state in which the hematopoietic system is disorganized. It is characterized by a malignant transformation of hematopoietic progenitor cells in which the malignant clone outgrows the normal hematopoietic tissue [14]. Associated with this disease are a wide variety of lesions supported by chromosomal distortions and abnormalities. The main form of treatment that is currently used for leukemia is chemotherapy, which is aimed at inducing remission and creating the necessary conditions that will make marrow transplantation possible. Chemotherapy is considered systemic treatment since the administered drugs can travel through the bloodstream and kill cells throughout the body. Radiation therapy, is another type of treatment that is used against leukemia. It involves the use of high-energy rays to destroy the leukemic cells. In this form of therapy, abnormal cells are killed through involved field irradiation or total-body irradiation [19]. Combinations of chemotherapy and radiation therapy also form part of current treatment schemes in the fight against leukemia [19].

It is significant to mention that clinicians and oncologists are always faced with choosing the best types of treatment schemes that would result in good therapeutic outcomes when treating cancer patients. This indicates that the need to find ways of improving current treatment strategies remain of paramount importance. In this regard, we shall use a mathematical model to investigate the advantages and disadvantages of administering treatment that involves combinations of chemotherapy and radiotherapy to a patient with acute leukemia (AL), which constitutes one facet of the leukemias.

A survey of the scientific literature reveals that not too much has been done in modeling the treatment of leukemia since the work of Rubinow and Lebowitz [23]. We note that in their model of leukemia therapy, it was assumed that the single administration of a drug dose resulted in the killing of a fixed fraction of all cells in S-phase, whether normal neutrophil precursors or leukemic myeloblasts. The basic aim was to maximize the killing of the leukemic cell population and minimize the killing of the normal cells. The calculations suggested that small changes in the treatment protocol could have significant effects on the result of treatment. They did not see the feasibility of aggressive treatment regimes at that time but felt it might be possible in the future. In a review of the model of Rubinow and Lebowitz [23], Eisen [9] pointed out that the trial and error method of studying different protocols by varying the drug parameters needed to be automated. This means that it is appropriate to view the issue of cancer treatment as an optimization problem and this is the approach we adopt in this article.

Even though specific mathematical modeling of the treatment of leukemia has not been addressed in the literature since the paper of Rubinow and Lebowitz, work has been going on in the general area of mathematical modeling of cancer therapy. The studies have involved optimal control models that describe drug delivery to solid tumors. For example, using the assumption of Gompertzian growth of solid tumors, Swan and Vincent [28] described the effect of an anti-cancer drug on a tumor by minimizing the cumulative drug toxicity and guiding the tumor size to a specified level at the end of the treatment period. In the work of Murray [17], the delivery of a drug to a tumor in the presence of normal cells was considered in which the drug was initially delivered at a maximum rate, followed by a rest period and then by another period of therapy. There have been a number of other studies by Costa and others [6], Martin and Teo [16], and Zietz and Nicolini [31], to mention a few. It is important to point out, though, that solid tumors, which constitute the main focus of these studies, are qualitatively different from the leukemias as we mentioned earlier.

In recent papers [1-4], we used some simple models to show that so far as leukemic cells were present in the body, normal cell growth or regrowth capabilities would be very reduced or diminished. We also pointed out that through inhibition, the space-occupying effects of a rapidly expanding leukemic clone tended to negatively alter and drive down the steady state level of the normal cells in acute leukemia. The leukemic clones essentially act to displace the normal cells from subendosteal sites where hematopoiesis is preferentially resident [3]. As a treatment-oriented follow-up to those papers, we present and study in this article, a model which highlights and addresses some issues that may arise in the administration of combinations of chemotherapy and radiotherapy for leukemia. It is important to note that medical practitioners are increasingly using such therapeutic combinations to fight a number of the leukemias [18, 19]. It is, therefore, imperative that mathematical models be used to investigate this strategy with the view to giving some insights into its merits.

§2. Model Assumptions, Formulation, and Solution

In the particular case of AL, excessive numbers of immature leukemic cells can cause severe disease via two mechanisms:

a) Migration of leukemic cells from the blood and marrow into other organs of the body which can impair venous blood flow (for example in the superior vena cava); and

b) Rapid elevation of the leukemic blast cell count in the blood, which causes clogging of small arteries and arterioles. This is associated with the invasion of the vessel walls, local anoxia, and hemorrhage with devastating consequences to the lungs and the brain.

In treatment schemes, a major aim is to restore the functioning of the bone marrow to normal by achieving maximum reductions in leukemic cell numbers throughout the body. These schemes currently involve applications of combinations of antileukemic drugs coupled with the use of radiation treatment. A few questions that may always arise and need to be constantly addressed are: How best can these schemes be carried out? Considering the toxic effects of antileukemic drugs and irradiation to normal cells, is it possible to adopt aggressive treatment schemes aimed at completely obliterating or massively reducing the leukemic population, while keeping the normal cell population at a reasonable level to guarantee their regrowth? What level of tolerance can the body of each leukemia patient have towards the insult of antileukemic drugs and radiation treatment? We must mention that antileukemic drugs and irradiation destroy leukemic as well as normal cells whenever they are administered [19, 24] and this constitutes another problem which clinicians have to deal with.

2.1. Model Assumptions

With the background information above and following ideas in [1-3], we propose the following assumptions to guide the modeling process.

1. A patient is diagnosed with leukemia and has to be hospitalized so as to receive combinations of antileukemic drugs to be delivered continuously, and also to undergo radiation treatment. The treatment includes drugs that may overcome drug-resistant strains of leukemic cells.

2. There is an extremely aggressively expanding leukemic population with negligible cell loss and a heavily dominated and suppressed normal population.

3. The leukemic population obeys the processes of Gompertzian growth while the normal cell population may be considered to be below a significantly quantifiable level.

4. Cost of treatment is proportional to the time interval of chemotherapy and to the amount of radiation energy expended during treatment.

5. Amount of radiation energy expended is in relation to the effect of the antileukemic drugs, under conditions where there is a penalty for applying unsuitable doses of drugs. It may be taken to be inversely proportional to a certain power of the concentration of the antileukemic drugs. No constraints are placed on the concentration of drugs.

We note that the cost of treatment of leukemia could depend on a number of factors. These factors may include the nature of the disease, and the age and general condition of the patient. These factors, coupled with the problems that arise in the treatment of leukemia tend to suggest that different types of model representations may exist for the cost. The choice of the best model representation for the cost of treatment of this disease may, therefore, remain a problem in itself so far as this disease remains a challenge to biomedicine. Thus, one representation for the cost may include the length of the period of chemotherapy in addition to the level of irradiation (which finds its expression in terms of the amount of radiation energy expended) to which the patient's body is exposed.

There are disadvantages associated with delivering doses of chemotherapeutic agents to a leukemia patient over a long period of time. Also, high doses of radiation administered over long time periods may not be in the interest of the patient. Within these settings, it is appropriate to consider lessening the costs related to a long chemotherapeutic period and a long period of patient exposure to radiation. It is important to mention that a relatively long treatment period may not be of benefit to the patient, both medically and financially. These points constitute some of the underlying motivations for Assumption 4. Studies of other model representations for the cost of treatment constitute part of our future studies.

It has been postulated that in combination therapy, chemotherapeutic agents may modify the response of normal and abnormal tissues to irradiation [19]. This indicates that chemotherapy may render the leukemic cells more susceptible to effective radiotherapeutic attack. It is, therefore, suggestive that the level of irradiation, which may be manifested in the amount of radiation energy expended, may have a certain relationship to the effects of the antileukemic drugs. Further, to guarantee the effectiveness of the treatment, it may be appropriate to penalize the application of drug doses that render the treatment unproductive or pose dangers to patient survival. Assumption 5 could, therefore, be viewed in these contexts.

2.2. Model Formulation and Solution

In light of the assumptions, for an extremely aggressively expanding leukemia, we have

$$\frac{dL}{dt} = gL\left(\log_e \frac{L_A}{L}\right), \tag{1}$$

$$L(0) = L_0, \tag{2}$$

where $L(t)$ represents the leukemic cell population at time t, L_A is the carrying capacity or asymptotic bound on the leukemic population, the parameter g is the leukemic growth rate, and L_0 is the leukemic population at detection. It can be observed from equation (1) that the specific growth rate, dL/Ldt, is large when L is small and is small when L approaches a large value that is bounded above by L_A. This suggests that growth retardation in the leukemic population may occur, as it becomes extremely large. From Assumption 4, an appropriate cost functional can be specified as

$$J = \int_0^R [k + \sigma E(t)]\, dt, \tag{3}$$

where k and σ are constants, R is the final time of treatment which is free, $[0, R]$ is the treatment time interval, and $E(t)$ is a measure representing the amount of radiation energy expended. From Assumption 5, we have $E(t) = pu^{-a}(t)$, where $a > 0$ and p are constants and $u(t)$ is a measure of the concentration of the combination of drugs. This implies that the amount of radiation energy expended will be very large when very low doses of drugs are used and will be relatively small with the application of extremely large drug doses. However, as we pointed out earlier, to guarantee patient safety while ensuring effectiveness of the treatment, it is important to penalize the application of inappropriate drug doses. We introduce the penalty via the constant p by letting $p = p(u(t))$, indicating a dependence on the concentration of the drug combinations. Stemming from this, we note that there could be a number of choices for the functional form of $p(u(t))$. One simple choice may be $p(u(t)) = qu^l(t)$, where $l > 0$ and q are constants. This yields $E(t) = q[u(t)]^{l-a}$, under conditions where the constant q is assumed to be adjustable. We note that this assumption is analogous to ideas propounded in [15]. Thus, within the framework of penalization of unsuitable drug doses, q may be relatively small when $l - a \geq 0$ and may be of a reasonable size if $l - a < 0$. For the sake of fixing ideas, let $k = h^2$ and let q be appropriately adjusted such that $l - a = 2$ (other cases in which $l - a$ assumes negative and positive values different from two are considered in a sequel to this article, see [5]). Then the cost functional, with $\theta = \sigma q$, becomes

$$J = \int_0^R \left[h^2 + \theta u^2(t) \right] dt. \tag{4}$$

In current clinical practice, radiotherapy of the central nervous system is used against acute lymphocytic leukemia (ALL), the most common form among children, and may be used against other types [18] during chemotherapy. Therefore, minimizing the radiation energy may be useful in lessening the harmful effects of the treatment to the acutely diminished population of normal cells. It may be especially important to minimize the length of the treatment time in the face of an extremely aggressively expanding leukemia. Consequently, the constant h could measure the relative importance of the two terms in equation (4) and could be defined as a patient-dependent parameter which is a measure of the level of tolerance the body has for the assault of the combined therapy.

Since the leukemic population is rapidly expanding, it could be supposed that at detection, the initial leukemic population is approximately equal to a certain percentage of its carrying capacity. That is, $L_0 \cong rL_A$ where $0 < r \leq 1$. Also, since the aim is to achieve maximum reductions in the leukemic population, the treatment strategy could involve the application of drugs that bind to and annihilate the expanding leukemic clones [26]. Equation (1) then becomes

$$\frac{dL}{dt} = gL\left(\log_e \frac{L_A}{L}\right) - su(t)L, \tag{5}$$

where the parameter s is measured per unit drug concentration. We therefore have the following treatment model:

$$\text{Minimize } J = \int_0^R \left[h^2 + \theta u^2(t)\right] dt, \tag{6}$$

subject to

$$\frac{dL}{dt} = gL\left(\log_e \frac{L_A}{L}\right) - su(t)L, \tag{7}$$

$$L(0) \cong rL_A \tag{8}$$

with the aim of obtaining $L(R) = w$, where w is small. Here, the leukemic population is expected to be small by the end of the treatment period. As a consequence, w could be taken to be theoretically unity. By letting

$$t^* = gt, \qquad L^* = \frac{\log_e L}{\log_e L_A}, \qquad u^* = \frac{su}{g\log_e L_A},$$

and by conveniently taking

$$h^2 = \frac{1}{2}g\varepsilon^2, \qquad \theta = \frac{s^2}{2g(\log_e L_A)^2}, \qquad T = gR, \qquad r = 1,$$

and dropping the asterisks for the sake of notational convenience, we obtain the optimal control problem,

$$\text{Minimize } J = \frac{1}{2}\int_0^T \left[\varepsilon^2 + u^2(t)\right] dt, \tag{9}$$

subject to

$$\frac{dL}{dt} = 1 - L(t) - u(t) \tag{10}$$

with

$$L(0) = 1 \quad \text{and} \quad L(T) = 0. \tag{11}$$

From these equations, we obtain a Hamiltonian of the form,

$$H = \frac{1}{2}\varepsilon^2 + \frac{1}{2}u^2(t) + \lambda(t)\left[1 - L(t) - u(t)\right], \tag{12}$$

a costate equation of the form,

$$\dot{\lambda} = -\frac{\partial H}{\partial L} = \lambda, \tag{13}$$

and an optimality condition given by,

$$0 = \frac{\partial H}{\partial u} = u - \lambda. \tag{14}$$

From equations (13) and (14) we get

$$\lambda(t) = ce^t = u(t), \tag{15}$$

where c is a constant. Since the final time T is free, transversality demands that $H(T) = 0$. Thus from equation (12), we obtain

$$H(T) = \frac{1}{2}\varepsilon^2 + \frac{1}{2}u^2(T) + \lambda(T)[1 - L(T) - u(T)] = 0. \tag{16}$$

By substituting equation (15) into equation (16), we obtain

$$(ce^T)^2 - 2ce^T - \varepsilon^2 = 0. \tag{17}$$

Ignoring the possible existence of a negative root since this may be inappropriate, we get

$$ce^T = 1 + \sqrt{1 + \varepsilon^2}. \tag{18}$$

From equation (15), substituting for $u(t)$ in equation (10) yields

$$L(t) = 1 - \frac{c}{2}e^t + be^{-t}, \tag{19}$$

where c and b are constants to be determined. By applying equations (11), we get

$$c = \frac{2}{e^T - e^{-T}} = \operatorname{csch} T \tag{20a}$$

$$\text{and } b = \frac{1}{e^T - e^{-T}} \tag{20b}$$

and substituting for c in equation (18) gives

$$e^{2T} = \frac{\sqrt{1 + \varepsilon^2} + 1}{\sqrt{1 + \varepsilon^2} - 1}. \tag{21}$$

This implies that

$$T = \frac{1}{2}\ln\left[\frac{\sqrt{1 + \varepsilon^2} + 1}{\sqrt{1 + \varepsilon^2} - 1}\right] = \coth^{-1}(\sqrt{1 + \varepsilon^2}). \tag{22}$$

From these equations we obtain $c = \varepsilon$. From equation (9), we get

$$J = \frac{1}{2}\varepsilon^2 T + \frac{\varepsilon^2}{2}\left(e^{2T} - 1\right). \tag{23}$$

§3. Results, Analysis, and Discussion

From the equations above, we get the following:

$$u(t) = \varepsilon e^t, \tag{24}$$

$$L(t) = 1 - \varepsilon \sinh t, \tag{25}$$

$$T = \coth^{-1}\left(\sqrt{1 + \varepsilon^2}\right), \tag{26}$$

$$\text{and } J = \frac{1}{2}\varepsilon^2 \coth^{-1}\left(\sqrt{1 + \varepsilon^2}\right) + \sqrt{1 + \varepsilon^2} + 1. \tag{27}$$

Analysis of the model and results arising from it, as can be observed from equations (24)-(27), indicate that the patient-dependent parameter ε plays a very important role in determining the kind of treatment strategy that is most appropriate. This means that the medical condition of the patient at the time of detection or diagnosis is very central to decisions related to treatment options. For example, equation (24) shows that the initial loading dose of drug is completely determined once ε is known. In this same vein, the time interval and the cost of treatment will be known before treatment from equations (26) and (27) respectively, once ε is specified. It can be observed that for small ε (of order $\varepsilon \ll 0.001$), which from the nondimensionalization means the patient has a low level of tolerance towards the therapy in comparison to the leukemic growth rate, equation (24) yields $u \sim 0$. From equation (26), we obtain a large final time ($T \to \infty$). Also, from equation (27) we obtain $J \sim 1$ for ε small. The strategy in this case may be to use low doses of drugs so as to avoid any further normal cell destruction or other side effects even though treatment may take a long time. In pursuance of this strategy then, negligible

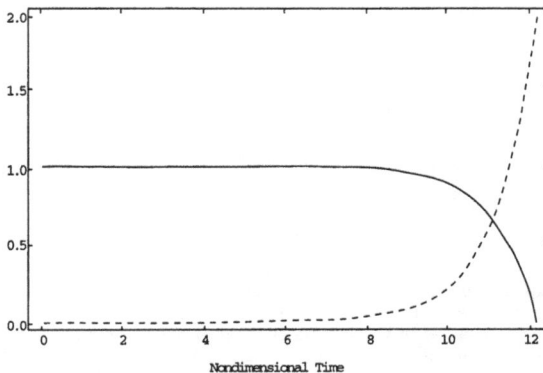

Fig. 1. Slow Decrease in the Leukemic Population for Small ε. The small value of ε yields a situation in which there is a low loading dose of drugs. This causes the concentration of drugs to increase very slowly. As a result, the reductions in the leukemic population take place over a long period of time. The dashed curve represents the nondimensional drug dose and the solid curve represents the normalized leukemic population.

amounts of radiation energy may be expended. A simulation of this case is shown in Figure 1. The parameter ε may be small among elderly patients of leukemia. However, studies have shown that there is a threshold concentration at which an anti-cancer drug ceases to have therapeutic effect [7]. Therefore, there are disadvantages associated with this strategy because the long period of treatment in Figure 1 over which the drug concentration is small will have no impact on the disease in the final analysis.

On the other hand, for large ε (of order $\varepsilon >> 0.001$), which means the patient has a high level of tolerance towards the therapy in comparison to the leukemic growth rate, equation (24) yields a large drug dose, and from equation (26) we get $T \sim 0$. Equation (27) yields $J \sim \varepsilon$. The strategy in this case may be to use heavy doses of drugs to achieve massive reductions in leukemic cell levels within a short time interval. As a consequence, reasonable amounts of radiation energy may be expended in dealing effectively with the leukemic cells over the short period of time. Most cases of leukemia in which the leukemic population is found to be rapidly expanding at the time of diagnosis may fall in this category. Also, the parameter ε may be large among children and young adults with leukemia. A simulation of this case is shown in Figure 2. In the case that yields Figure 1, a specific value of $\varepsilon = 0.00001$, yields a nondimensional final time of $T \cong 12.206$, and a cost of $J \cong 2.0$. In the case that yields Figure 2, a value of $\varepsilon = 0.8$, gives $T \cong 1.048$, and a cost of $J \cong 2.616$.

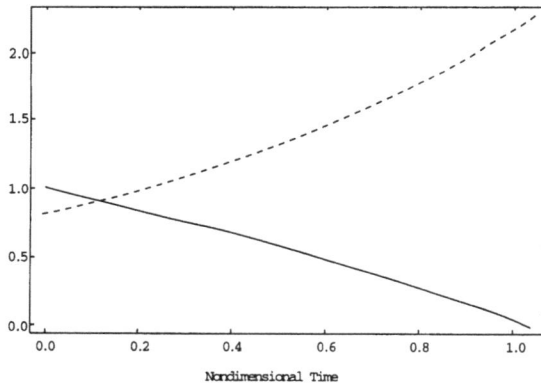

Fig. 2. Rapid Decrease in the Leukemic Population for Large ε. The large value of ε leads to a situation that yields a large loading dose of drugs. As a result, a rapid increase in the concentration of drugs occurs. Consequently, reductions in the leukemic population are achieved over a short period of time. The dashed curve represents the nondimensional drug dose and the solid curve represents the normalized leukemic population.

§4. Concluding Remarks

Results from model equations (9)-(11) indicate and highlight the importance of patient-dependent treatment protocols. It is important to mention that patients with the same disease respond to drugs differently despite similar circumstances. In this model, a measure of the severity of the therapeutic assault on the patient is expressed by the parameter ε. It can be observed from equations (24)-(27) that the loading dose, the time interval of treatment, and the cost of treatment have a dependence on this parameter. It is suggestive that when the patient's body is determined to be in a state that cannot permit aggressive treatment, ε may be small and the approach would be to start treatment with a reasonably low loading dose of drug and a negligible level of irradiation. As we have pointed out, this strategy has its drawbacks and may make its application ineffective in the long run. On the other hand, if it is determined that the patient is ready for aggressive treatment, ε may be large and the strategy will involve the delivery of a relatively large loading dose of drug and a suitable level of irradiation, all over a short span of time. The dosing and irradiation will then be continued until the leukemic population is possibly annihilated.

As shown in Figure 1, the treatment will take a relatively longer time when ε is small than when ε is large, as is depicted in Figure 2. Even though the case shown in Figure 1 yields a cheaper cost than that in Figure 2, it may not be optimal because of the amount of time it takes to achieve leukemic reduction. However, on certain medical grounds, this may be the only strategy available for treating some leukemia patients, particularly elderly patients of age 65 and above. Within the context of our model predictions, the disadvantages associated with this strategy may account for the reasons why there is a relatively low level of success in treating leukemia among the elderly [10]. The case shown in Figure 2 may be optimal since massive reductions in the leukemic population take place over a relatively short time frame even though it may be more costly than the case in Figure 1. The usefulness of this strategy (in which ε is large) may be reflected in the relatively higher level of success in treating leukemia among children and young patients [10]. It is indicative that model equations (9)-(11) can provide *apriori* estimates for the time interval of treatment, the amount of drug to be used by the end of the treatment period, the amount of radiation energy to be expended, and the cost of treatment once ε is known. However, knowledge about the value of ε will depend, most importantly, on real time estimation of the leukemic growth rate constant g in addition to measurement of the tolerance parameter h, all done possibly at the time of detection. The *apriori* estimates could give the patient and physician some insight and information about available options.

Our model predictions suggest that upon detection of malignancy, in which there is an extremely aggressively expanding leukemic population, treatment must begin and be pursued aggressively, even for the patient deemed incapable, since this will take place over a short time interval and may not predispose the patient to complications. A short treatment interval could also prevent the continued loss of normal cells. In any case, it is important to note that some leukemic cells are likely to be resistant to cytotoxic drugs because of the overexpression of P-glycoprotein or other mechanisms [30]. It is, therefore, imperative that aggressive treatment over short time scales mainly with drug combinations should include drugs, such as the cyclosporine analogue PSC-833 [10], that overcome drug-resistant leukemic cells. Barring any limitations, the model proposed in this work can predict the time to discontinue treatment and the cost of treatment once there is adequate knowledge about the state of the patient's health. The assertions of Parker and Withers [19] suggest that the state of the patient's health assumes an ever greater degree of importance when radiation therapy is also involved in the treatment process.

We must point out that our model predictions and projections may be suitable in cases involving the treatment of acute leukemia. They may not be appropriate in cases involving chronic leukemia in which there is a much gradual and possibly oscillatory progression towards an explosive state of the disease. To this end, acute lymphocytic leukemia and other types may constitute appropriate examples. Acute leukemia is a very complicated disease. Thus, the first steps in our approach to modeling it involve the use of simple models to describe some of its characteristics followed by superimposing therapeutic regimens on the models so as to arrive at certain insightful conclusions and useful suggestions about its treatment. Our future investigations will involve the construction and expansion of models that encompass more intricate characteristics of acute leukemia. It should be mentioned, though, that simple models normally give better insight into understanding the behavior of various parts of complex phenomena.

Even though our model analyses and calculations tend to support aggressive treatment schemes for acute leukemia, we do not in any way rule out the strategy of low-dose continuous infusions. It is needless to mention that the present level of development of biomedical science does demand that all types of pathways and ideas be looked at and given consideration in the treatment of diseases. Certainly, a number of questions arise as a result of adopting an aggressive treatment approach. One of the most paramount questions is whether every patient of AL can survive heavy-dosage chemotherapy combined with a suitably accelerated level of radiation treatment. In our view, aggressive treatment can be looked at as another way of fighting AL. It is important to note that a number of clinicians have actually been using this strategy. Schrier [24] and his coworkers have used this strategy and Spinolo [25] interestingly makes a strong argument for it.

Since the papers of Rubinow and Lebowitz [22, 23] and Djulbegovic and Svetina [8] on leukemia, not much has been done within a biomathematical framework to study and investigate this devastating disease. Understandably, the variable nature of the disease makes its modeling challenging. However, we believe that a lot of questions and problems associated with the disease could be addressed through the use of models that describe some of its characteristics and aid in giving insight into its treatment.

Acknowledgments. This work was supported in part by NSF grant number DMS-9710350. I would like to express my sincere gratitude to the organizers of the International Conference on Mathematical Models in the Medical and Health Sciences for inviting me to deliver a plenary address on Cancer Research. My thanks to Dr. Wilson Hartz, attending physician and consulting hematologist at Sherman Hospital in Elgin, Illinois, for making leukemia data available to me for study. I am also very grateful to him for spending his valuable time to hold fruitful discussions with me on leukemia. These greatly facilitated and enhanced my investigations. My thanks also go to the anonymous referee whose comments and suggestions aided in the revision of this manuscript.

References

1. Afenya, E. K, Acute leukemia and chemotherapy: A modeling viewpoint, Math. Biosci. **138** (1996), 79–100.

2. Afenya, E. K. and D. E. Bentil, Some perspectives on modeling leukemia, Math. Biosci., accepted for publication.

3. Afenya, E. K. and C. P. Calderón, Normal cell decline and inhibition in acute leukemia: A biomathematical modeling approach, J. Can. Det. Prev. **20**(3) (1996), 171–179.

4. Afenya, E. K. and C. P. Caldern, Diverse ideas on leukemia cell kinetics, submitted for publication (1998).

5. Afenya, E. K., Phenomenological approaches to cancer treatment regimes, to appear.

6. Costa, M. I. S., J. L. Boldrini and R. C. Bassanezi, Chemotherapeutic treatments involving drug resistance and level of normal cells as a criterion of toxicity Math. Biosci. **125** (1995), 211–228.

7. DeVita, V. T., Principles of chemotherapy, in *Cancer: Principles and Practice of Oncology*, V. T. DeVita, S. Hellman and S. A. Rosenberg (eds.), Lippincott, Philadelphia, 1985, 276–300.

8. Djulbegovic, B. and S. Svetina, Mathematical model of acute myeloblastic leukaemia: An investigation of relevant kinetic parameters, Cell Tissue Kinet. **18** (1985), 307–319.

9. Eisen M., Mathmatical models in cell biology and cancer chemotherapy, in *Lecture Notes in Biomathematics*, S. Levin (ed.), Springer-Verlag, New York, 1979.

10. Hamblin, T. J., Disappointments in treating acute leukemia in the elderly, N. Eng. J. Med. **332**(25) (1995), 1712–1713.

11. Himmelstein, K. J. and K. B. Bischoff, Models of ara-C chemotherapy of L1210 leukemia in mice, J. Pharmacokinet. Biopharm. **1** (1973), 69–81.

12. Kirk, D. E., *Optimal Control Theory: An Introduction*, Prentice-Hall, New Jersey, 1970.

13. Kreis, W., F. Chaudri, K. Chan, S. Allen, D. R. Budman, P. Schulman, L. Weiselberg, J. Freeman, M. Deere and V. Vinciguerra, Pharmacokinetics of low-dose 1-β-D-arabinofuranosylcytosine given by continuous infusion over twenty-one days, Can. Res. **45** (1985), 6498–6501.

14. Löwenberg, B., W. L. J. V. Putten, I. P. Touw, R. Delwel and V. Santini, Autonomous proliferation of leukemic cells in vitro as a determinant of prognosis in adult acute myeloid leukemia, N. Eng. J. Med. **328** (1993), 614–619.

15. Luenberger, D. G., *Optimization by Vector Space Methods*, John Wiley and Sons, Inc., New York, 1969.

16. Martin, R. and K. L. Teo, *Optimal Control of Drug Administration in Cancer Chemotherapy*, World Scientific, New Jersey, 1994.

17. Murray, J. M., Some optimal control problems in cancer chemotherapy with a toxicity limit, Math. Biosci. **100** (1990), 49–67.

18. No Authors, Twelve major cancers, Sci. Am. **275**(3) (1996), 126–132.

19. Parker, R. G. and H. R. Withers, Principles of radiation oncology, in *Cancer Treatment*, C. M. Haskell and J. S. Berek (eds), W. B. Saunders, Philadelphia, 1995, 23–31.

20. Rennie J. and R. Rusting, Making headway against cancer, Sci. Am. **275**(3) (1996), 56–59.

21. Rohatiner, A. and T. A. Lister, Acute myelogenous leukemia in adults, in *Leukemia*, E. S. Henderson, T. A. Lister and M. F. Greaves (eds), W. B. Saunders, Philadelphia 1996, 479–508.

22. Rubinow, S. I. and J. L. Lebowitz, A mathematical model of the acute myeloblastic leukemic state in man, Biophys. J. **16** (1976), 897–910.

23. Rubinow, S. I. and J. L. Lebowitz, A mathematical model of the chemotherapeutic treatment of acute myeloblastic leukemia, Biophys. J. **16** (1976), 1257–1271.

24. Schrier, S. L., The leukemias and the myeloproliferative disorders, Sci. Am. Med. Section 5, Subsection 8 (1987), 1–24.

25. Spinolo, J. A., Acute Myelogenous Leukemia, in *Current Therapy in Cancer*, J. F. Foley, J. M. Vose and J. O. Armitage (eds.), W.B. Saunders, Philadelphia, 1994, 322–326.

26. Stockdale, F. E., Cancer growth and chemotherapy, Sci. Am. Oncol. **12** (1987), 1–11.

27. Swan, G. W, Cancer chemotherapy: optimal control using the Verhulst-Pearl equation, Bull. Math. Biol. **48** (1986), 381–404.

28. Swan, G. W. and T. L. Vincent, Optimal control analysis in the chemotherapy of IgG multiple myeloma, Bull. Math. Biol. **39** (1977), 317–337.

29. Vogelzang, N. J., Continuous infusion chemotherapy: A critical review, J. Clin. Oncol. **2** (1984), 1289–1301.

30. Wood, P., R. Burgess, A. Macgregor and J. A. Y. Liu, P-glycoprotein expression on acute myeloid leukaemia blast cells at diagnosis predicts response to chemotherapy and survival, Brit. J. Haematol. **87** (1994), 509–514.

31. Zietz, S. and C. Nicolini, Mathematical approaches to optimization of cancer chemotherapy, Bull. Math. Biol. **41** (1979), 305–324.

Evans K. Afenya
Dept. of Mathematics
Elmhurst College
190 Prospect Avenue
Elmhurst, IL 60126
evansa@elmhurst.edu

A Flow Reactor with Wall Growth

Mary M. Ballyk and Hal L. Smith

Abstract. Models of competition between n bacterial strains in a plug flow reactor for a limiting nutrient incorporating wall growth are examined. Consideration of the capacity of the wall for attachment and the nature of the competition for wall sites leads to a variety of competitive situations, three extremes of which are derived. Each model consists of an $(n + 1)$-dimensional nonlinear system of parabolic partial differential equations coupled with an n-dimensional system of ordinary differential equations. It is shown that each generates a semi-dynamical system.

§1. Introduction

A fundamental problem of intestinal microecology is to identify the major mechanisms that control the composition of the indigenous microflora of the large intestine. The mammalian intestine is an example of a very stable community with a high species diversity and an even distribution of dominant species. Invading organisms have difficulty in establishing there. The term "colonization resistance" was coined by Van der Waaij et al. [14] to describe the degree of stability of the ecosystem with regard to potential new colonizers of the gut. It is a measure of the number of organisms that must contaminate the individual before colonization of the intestinal tract can occur. Lee [10] asserts that competition for limiting growth factors is the major mechanism of colonization resistance. The long retention time of the intestinal content also contributes to the stability of the system in the large intestine. Additionally, Lee indicates that motility of an invading organism could aid in its ability to colonize the gut.

Motivated by the obvious difficulties associated with investigations of the intestinal microflora involving intact animals, Freter [3, 4] made a strong case for the continuous flow culture method, or chemostat, as an appropriate in vitro model system for the mammalian large intestine. Freter and his coworkers [5, 6, 7, 8] found that wall growth was necessary to account for the variety of microorganisms comprising the microflora found there. Perhaps a tubular

Mathematical Models in Medical and Health Sciences
Mary Ann Horn, Gieri Simonett, and Glenn Webb (eds.), pp. 17–28.

reactor model, described below, provides a more reasonable approximation to the large intestine than a chemostat, provided wall growth is included.

Kung and Baltzis [9] examine a model of competition between two populations of microorganisms for a single nutrient in a tubular reactor. The reactor is externally fed by growth medium at a constant volumetric flow rate, while depleted nutrient exits at the outflow from the reactor. For reactors of equal length then, the flow rate of medium captures the retention time of the intestinal content. Kung and Baltzis assume that bacteria exhibit random motility and that the diffusion coefficient of nutrient and motility coefficients of the competing populations are equal. This model was extended in [2] by dropping this assumption, thus allowing consideration of the role of motility in the composition and stability of intestinal microflora. Among other things, sufficient conditions are given for an invading organism to establish itself in the reactor, either displacing or coexisting with the resident population. Motivated in part by the work of Freter and his coworkers [5, 6, 7, 8], the model of [2] is generalized in the present paper to incorporate the possibility that the organisms can attach to the wall of the reactor from the medium and release from the wall into the medium. Microorganisms adherent to the wall are considered immobile and do not wash out of the reactor. The result is a mathematical model of the interrelations among various mechanisms that are suspected to control intestinal flora. For a more detailed account of the development of this problem, the reader is referred to [2].

We examine competition between n bacterial strains in a plug flow reactor for a single limiting nutrient. The microorganisms may become immobilized on the wall of the reactor and are assumed to exhibit random motility in the bulk fluid. We allow the random motility coefficients to be strain-specific and to differ from the diffusion coefficient for nutrient in the growth medium. Consideration of the capacity of the wall for attachment and the form of the competition for wall sites leads to a variety of competitive situations. Three models representative of extremes are described. Each model is an $(n + 1)$-dimensional reaction-diffusion system coupled with an n-dimensional system of ordinary differential equations. We show that each generates a semi-dynamical system on an appropriate state spaces of continuous $(2n + 1)$-vector-valued functions with nonnegative components.

§2. The Models

In this section we describe generalizations of the model of microbial competition for a nutrient in a tubular reactor treated in [2]. Each model takes the form of a reaction diffusion system coupled with a system of ordinary differential equations and describes the time evolution of the volumetric density of nutrient and competing bacterial strains in the bulk liquid as well as the areal density of the wall growth associated with each strain. We begin by describing the reactor. See Table 2.1 for a summary of the mathematical notation.

Symbol	Quantity Name	Dimension
$u_i(x,t)$	Bacteria-in-solution density of population u_i	ml^{-3}
d_i	Diffusion coefficient for population u_i,	l^2/t
$w_i(x,t)$	Bacteria-on-wall density of population w_i	ml^{-2}
w_∞	Maximum bacteria-on-wall density	ml^{-2}
w_∞^i	Strain-specific maximum bacteria-on-wall density for II	ml^{-2}
$W(x,t)$	Occupation fraction $W = (\sum_{i=1}^n w_i)/w_\infty$	none
$W_i(x,t)$	Strain-specific occupation fraction for II. $W_i = w_i/w_\infty^i$	none
G_i	Fraction of offspring of population w_i which find sites on the wall. $G_i \equiv G_i(W)$ for I, $G_i \equiv G_i(W_i)$ for II, $G_i \equiv c_i$ for III	none
$S(x,t)$	Nutrient density	ml^{-3}
d_0	Diffusion coefficient for resource S	l^2/t
S^0	Input concentration of resource S	ml^{-3}
u_i^0	Input concentration of bacteria strain i	ml^{-3}
$f_{u_i}(S), f_{w_i}(S)$	Resource dependent growth rate of population u_i, w_i per unit of population u_i, w_i	t^{-1}
γ_i	Growth yield constant for strain i on resource S	none
k_{u_i}, k_{w_i}	Intrinsic death rate of population u_i, w_i	t^{-1}
α_i	Rate coefficient of attachment for population u_i	t^{-1}
β_i	Rate coefficient of detachment for population w_i	t^{-1}
L	Length of the reactor	l
A	Cross sectional area of the reactor	l^2
C	Circumference of the reactor	l
δ	The quotient C/A	l^{-1}
v	Volumetric flow rate	l/t

Table 2.1: Symbols and notation. Dimensions are defined as follows: l for length, m for mass, t for time. I, II and III refer to Models I, II and III.

Consider a very long thin tube extending along the x-axis. The reactor occupies the portion of the tube from $x = 0$ to $x = L$. It is fed with growth medium at a constant rate at $x = 0$ due to a constant laminar flow of fluid in the vessel in the direction of increasing x and at velocity v. The external feed contains all nutrients in near optimal amounts except one, denoted S, which is supplied in growth-limiting amounts and at a constant input concentration S^0. The laminar flow of medium in the tube carries medium, depleted nutrients, organisms and byproducts out of the reactor at $x = L$. Nutrient is assumed to diffuse throughout with diffusivity d_0.

We consider the tubular reactor to be inhabited by n bacterial strains that are able to attach themselves to the wall. Thus, there are $2n$ populations to consider, n in the bulk fluid and n on the wall of the reactor. The volumetric density of strain i in the bulk fluid is denoted u_i and it is assumed that the u_i exhibit random motility modeled by a diffusion coefficient d_i. We allow the possibility that the external feed contains bacterial strain i at constant concentration u_i^0. The areal density of strain i on the wall of the reactor is denoted w_i. It is assumed that the bacteria on the wall are immobile.

For any fixed $x \in [0, 1]$, nutrient is assumed to be equally available to all organisms in the fluid medium as well as on the wall. The competition for nutrient is purely exploitative; the organisms simply consume the nutrient, making it unavailable for a competitor. The function $f_{u_i}(S)$ represents the growth rate of population u_i per unit of population u_i. It is assumed that the growth rate on resource S is proportional to the rate of consumption of resource S, with corresponding growth yield constant γ_{u_i}. The intrinsic death rate of population u_i is denoted k_{u_i}. Similarly, $f_{w_i}(S)$ represents the growth rate of population w_i per unit of population w_i with corresponding growth yield constant γ_{w_i} and k_{w_i} denotes the intrinsic death rate of population w_i. We assume that, for each i, the growth yield constants for populations u_i and w_i are equal, so that $\gamma_{u_i} = \gamma_{w_i} = \gamma_i$. The experimental results of Bakke et al. [1] support such an assumption. The functions $f_{u_i}(S)$ and $f_{w_i}(S)$ are assumed to satisfy

$$f_{u_i}(0) = f_{w_i}(0) = 0, \quad f'_{u_i}(S), f'_{w_i}(S) > 0, \quad f_{u_i}, f_{w_i} \in C^1. \quad (2.1)$$

A classic example is the Monod function

$$f(S) = mS/(a + S), \quad m, \, a > 0.$$

Consideration of the capacity of the wall for attachment and the form of the competition between the w_i for wall sites leads to a variety of competitive situations. The models presented here are representative of extremes.

Model I: Finite wall capacity, strains compete for common sites

The wall of the reactor is assumed to have a finite capacity for attachment, the density of which is denoted w_∞. Thus, $W = (\sum_{i=1}^n w_i)/w_\infty$ represents the occupation fraction. In what follows, C and A denote the circumference and area, respectively, of the reactor. We define the function $G_i(W)$ to be the fraction of offspring of population w_i which find sites on the wall, a function of the occupation fraction. It is assumed to satisfy

$$G_i \in C^1[0, 1], \quad G_i(W) \in [0, 1], \quad 0 < G_i(0) = c_i \leq 1,$$
$$G_i(1) = 0, \quad G'_i(W) \leq 0. \quad (2.2)$$

Examples would be

$$G_i(W) = 1 - W \text{ or } G_i(W) = \frac{1 - W}{|1 - W| + 0.01},$$

the latter being employed by Freter et al. in [7]. Note that $(1 - G_i(W))$ is the fraction of offspring of w_i that do not find sites on the wall and become members of population u_i.

The rate of recruitment of population u_i to the wall at x is approximated by

$$A\alpha_i u_i(1 - W)dx,$$

where α_i is the rate coefficient of attachment for population u_i and the quantity $(1 - W)$ gives the fraction of unoccupied sites on the wall of the reactor. Here, dx is the length of the segment $[x, x + dx]$. The rate of detachment of population w_i from the wall of the reactor at x is approximated by

$$C\beta_i w_i dx,$$

where β_i is the rate coefficient of detachment for population w_i.

With this machinery, we can express the rate of growth of population w_i on the wall at x as

$$Cw_i f_{w_i}(S)dx,$$

while the fraction of these offspring that find unoccupied sites on the wall is

$$Cw_i f_{w_i}(S)G_i(W)dx.$$

(Clearly, the fraction $Cw_i f_{w_i}(S)(1 - G_i(W))dx$ are released into the bulk fluid and become members of population u_i at x.) Combining these, we obtain

$$C(w_i)_t dx = Cw_i f_{w_i}(S)G_i(W)dx - Ck_{w_i} w_i dx + A\alpha_i u_i(1 - W)dx - C\beta_i w_i dx.$$

Similarly,

$$A(u_i)_t dx = A[d_i(u_i)_{xx} - v(u_i)_x]dx + Au_i(f_{u_i}(S) - k_{u_i})dx$$
$$+ Cw_i f_{w_i}(S)(1 - G_i(W))dx - A\alpha_i u_i(1 - W)dx + C\beta_i w_i dx.$$

The model of exploitative competition between n bacterial strains for a single nutrient in the plug flow reactor with finite wall capacity in which all strains compete for a common set of sites on the wall is then given by

$$S_t = d_0 S_{xx} - vS_x - \sum_{i=1}^{n} \gamma_i^{-1}[u_i f_{u_i}(S) + \delta w_i f_{w_i}(S)],$$

$$(u_i)_t = d_i(u_i)_{xx} - v(u_i)_x + u_i(f_{u_i}(S) - k_{u_i}) + \delta w_i f_{w_i}(S)(1 - G_i(W))$$
$$- \alpha_i u_i(1 - W) + \delta\beta_i w_i, \qquad (2.3)$$

$$(w_i)_t = w_i f_{w_i}(S)G_i(W) - k_{w_i} w_i + \delta^{-1}\alpha_i u_i(1 - W) - \beta_i w_i,$$

where $\delta = C/A$, together with the boundary conditions

$$d_0 \frac{\partial S}{\partial x}(0, t) - vS(0, t) = -vS^0,$$

$$d_i \frac{\partial u_i}{\partial x}(0, t) - vu_i(0, t) = -vu_i^0, \qquad (2.4)$$

$$\frac{\partial S}{\partial x}(L, t) = \frac{\partial u_i}{\partial x}(L, t) = 0,$$

and the initial conditions

$$S(x,0) = S_0(x) \geq 0,$$
$$u_i(x,0) = u_{i0}(x) \geq 0, \quad 0 \leq x \leq L, \qquad (2.5)$$
$$w_i(x,0) = w_{i0}(x) \geq 0.$$

Note that there are no boundary conditions for the w_i, as they are immobilized on the wall of the reactor.

The equations can be simplified by non-dimensionalizing the parameters, dependent and independent variables. Non-dimensional quantities are indicated below with bars.

$$\bar{x} = x/L, \bar{t} = vt/L,$$
$$\bar{u}_i = u_i/(\gamma_i S^0), \bar{u}_i^0 = u_i^0/(\gamma_i S^0), \bar{S} = S/S^0,$$
$$\bar{d}_i = d_i/(Lv), \bar{k}_{u_i} = (L/v)k_{u_i}, \bar{k}_{w_i} = (L/v)k_{w_i}, \bar{\alpha}_i = (L/v)\alpha_i, \bar{\beta}_i = (L/v)\beta_i,$$
$$\bar{f}_{u_i}(\bar{S}) = (L/v)f_{u_i}(S^0\bar{S}), \bar{f}_{w_i}(\bar{S}) = (L/v)f_{w_i}(S^0\bar{S}),$$

together with

$$\bar{w}_i = \frac{w_i}{w_\infty}, \epsilon_i = \frac{\delta w_\infty}{\gamma_i S^0}, \bar{W} = \sum_{i=1}^{n} \bar{w}_i. \qquad (2.6)$$

In order to conserve notation, we drop the bars over the non-dimensional quantities, returning to the original notation. The scaled version is then

$$S_t = d_0 S_{xx} - S_x - \sum_{i=1}^{n}[u_i f_{u_i}(S) + \epsilon_i w_i f_{w_i}(S)],$$
$$(u_i)_t = d_i(u_i)_{xx} - (u_i)_x + u_i(f_{u_i}(S) - k_{u_i}) + \epsilon_i w_i f_{w_i}(S)(1 - G_i(W)) \quad (2.7)$$
$$- \alpha_i u_i(1 - W) + \epsilon_i \beta_i w_i,$$
$$(w_i)_t = w_i f_{w_i}(S)G_i(W) - k_{w_i} w_i + \epsilon_i^{-1}\alpha_i u_i(1 - W) - \beta_i w_i,$$

with boundary conditions

$$d_0 \frac{\partial S}{\partial x}(0,t) - S(0,t) = -1,$$
$$d_i \frac{\partial u_i}{\partial x}(0,t) - u_i(0,t) = -u_i^0, \qquad (2.8)$$
$$\frac{\partial S}{\partial x}(1,t) = \frac{\partial u_i}{\partial x}(1,t) = 0,$$

and initial conditions

$$S(x,0) = S_0(x) \geq 0,$$
$$u_i(x,0) = u_{i0}(x) \geq 0, \quad 0 \leq x \leq 1, \qquad (2.9)$$
$$w_i(x,0) = w_{i0}(x) \geq 0.$$

where $i = 1, \ldots, n$. We assume that the initial data S_0, u_{i0} and w_{i0} are continuous. Note that by taking $\alpha_i = 0$ in (2.7) and $w_{i0}(x) \equiv 0$ in (2.9) for $i = 1, \ldots, n$, system (2.7)-(2.9) reduces to model (2.5)-(2.7) of [2], where wall growth is not considered.

Model II: Finite Wall Capacity, strain-specific sites

In this case, the wall of the reactor is assumed to consist of evenly distributed strain-specific sites. Thus, a site will be available for attachment by a member of strain i and unavailable to any of its competitors. The capacity of the wall for attachment by strain i is finite, with corresponding density denoted w_∞^i. The strain-specific occupation fraction is then given by $W_i = w_i/w_\infty^i$. In this case, the fraction of offspring of population i which find sites on the wall is a function of the strain-specific occupation fraction, so that $G_i \equiv G_i(W_i)$. The rate of recruitment of population u_i to the wall at x is also dependent on the strain-specific occupation fraction. Note that the wall of the reactor has a finite capacity for attachment in this case, with associated density given by $w_\infty = \sum_{i=1}^n w_\infty^i$ and the corresponding occupation fraction is again $W = (\sum_{i=1}^n w_i)/w_\infty$.

The model of exploitative competition between n bacterial strains for a single nutrient in the plug flow reactor in which the wall consists of evenly distributed strain-specific sites is then given by

$$S_t = d_0 S_{xx} - v S_x - \sum_{i=1}^n \gamma_i^{-1}[u_i f_{u_i}(S) + \delta w_i f_{w_i}(S)],$$

$$(u_i)_t = d_i(u_i)_{xx} - v(u_i)_x + u_i(f_{u_i}(S) - k_{u_i}) + \delta w_i f_{w_i}(S)(1 - G_i(W_i))$$
$$- \alpha_i u_i(1 - W_i) + \delta \beta_i w_i, \tag{2.10}$$

$$(w_i)_t = w_i f_{w_i}(S) G_i(W_i) - k_{w_i} w_i + \delta^{-1}\alpha_i u_i(1 - W_i) - \beta_i w_i,$$

together with the boundary and initial conditions (2.4) and (2.5). Applying the scaling of Model I with appropriate modifications to (2.6), that is

$$\bar{w}_i = \frac{w_i}{w_\infty^i}, \epsilon_i = \frac{\delta w_\infty^i}{\gamma_i S^0}, \bar{W}_i = \bar{w}_i, \tag{2.11}$$

we obtain

$$S_t = d_0 S_{xx} - S_x - \sum_{i=1}^n [u_i f_{u_i}(S) + \epsilon_i w_i f_{w_i}(S)],$$

$$(u_i)_t = d_i(u_i)_{xx} - (u_i)_x + u_i(f_{u_i}(S) - k_{u_i}) + \epsilon_i w_i f_{w_i}(S)(1 - G_i(W_i))$$
$$- \alpha_i u_i(1 - W_i) + \epsilon_i \beta_i w_i, \tag{2.12}$$

$$(w_i)_t = w_i f_{w_i}(S) G_i(W_i) - k_{w_i} w_i + \epsilon_i^{-1}\alpha_i u_i(1 - W_i) - \beta_i w_i,$$

together with the boundary conditions (2.8) and initial conditions (2.9).

Model III: Infinite Wall Capacity

The model to be described can be obtained from Model I by taking $w_\infty = \infty$ or from Model II by taking $w_\infty^i = \infty$ for $i = 1, \ldots, n$. Thus, the wall of the reactor has infinite capacity for attachment. In either event, the (strain-specific) occupation fraction is identically zero, so that $G_i \equiv c_i$.

The model of exploitative competition between n bacterial strains for a single nutrient in the plug flow reactor in which the wall has infinite capacity for attachment is then given by

$$
\begin{aligned}
S_t &= d_0 S_{xx} - v S_x - \sum_{i=1}^{n} \gamma_i^{-1}[u_i f_{u_i}(S) + \delta w_i f_{w_i}(S)], \\
(u_i)_t &= d_i(u_i)_{xx} - v(u_i)_x + u_i(f_{u_i}(S) - k_{u_i}) + \delta w_i f_{w_i}(S)(1 - c_i) \\
&\quad - \alpha_i u_i + \delta \beta_i w_i, \\
(w_i)_t &= w_i f_{w_i}(S) c_i - k_{w_i} w_i + \delta^{-1} \alpha_i u_i - \beta_i w_i,
\end{aligned}
\tag{2.13}
$$

together with the boundary and initial conditions (2.4) and (2.5). Applying the scaling of Model I with appropriate modifications to (2.6), that is

$$
\bar{w}_i = \frac{\delta w_i}{\gamma_i S^0},
\tag{2.14}
$$

we obtain

$$
\begin{aligned}
S_t &= d_0 S_{xx} - S_x - \sum_{i=1}^{n}[u_i f_{u_i}(S) + w_i f_{w_i}(S)], \\
(u_i)_t &= d_i(u_i)_{xx} - (u_i)_x + u_i(f_{u_i}(S) - k_{u_i}) + w_i f_{w_i}(S)(1 - c_i) \\
&\quad - \alpha_i u_i + \beta_i w_i, \\
(w_i)_t &= w_i f_{w_i}(S) c_i - k_{w_i} w_i + \alpha_i u_i - \beta_i w_i,
\end{aligned}
\tag{2.15}
$$

together with boundary conditions (2.8) and initial conditions (2.9).

§3. Global Existence of Solutions

In this section we show that each of equations (2.7), (2.12), and (2.15), together with the boundary conditions (2.8) and initial conditions (2.9), generates a semi-dynamical system on an appropriate state space of continuous functions with nonnegative components. We give details in the case of Model II, and indicate appropriate modifications to the argument for Models I and III.

In order to simplify the notation, it will be convenient to introduce the vector $v = (v_0, \ldots, v_{2n})$, where

$$
v_i = \begin{cases}
S, & i = 0, \\
u_i, & i = 1, \ldots, n, \\
w_{i-n}, & i = n+1, \ldots, 2n.
\end{cases}
$$

Further, v^0 will denote the $(2n+1)$-dimensional vector of initial conditions in (3.3). Equations (2.12), (2.8), and (2.9) can now be written as

$$
(v_i)_t = \begin{cases}
d_i(v_i)_{xx} - (v_i)_x + f_i(v), & i = 0, \ldots, n, \\
f_i(v), & i = n+1, \ldots, 2n,
\end{cases}
\tag{3.1}
$$

with boundary conditions

$$d_0^{-1} v_0(0,t) - \frac{\partial v_0}{\partial x}(0,t) = d_0^{-1},$$

$$d_i^{-1} v_i(0,t) - \frac{\partial v_i}{\partial x}(0,t) = d_i^{-1} u_i^0, \quad i = 1, \ldots, n, \tag{3.2}$$

$$\frac{\partial v_i}{\partial x}(1,t) = 0, \quad i = 0, \ldots, n,$$

and nonnegative initial conditions

$$v_i(x,0) = v_i^0(x), \quad i = 0, \ldots, 2n. \tag{3.3}$$

The nonlinearities $f_i : \mathbf{R}^{2n+1} \longrightarrow \mathbf{R}$, obtained from (2.12), are continuously differentiable by (2.1) and (2.2). They also satisfy, by (2.1), (2.2), and (2.12),

$$\begin{aligned} &\text{(a)} \quad f_i(v) \geq 0 \quad \text{whenever} \quad v_i = 0, \quad i = 0, \ldots, 2n, \\ &\text{(b)} \quad f_i(v) < 0 \quad \text{whenever} \quad v_i = 1, \quad i = n+1, \ldots, 2n. \end{aligned} \tag{3.4}$$

System (3.1)-(3.3) is biologically relevant in the region

$$\Lambda = \{v \in \mathbf{R}^{2n+1} : v_i \geq 0, i = 0, \ldots, 2n; v_i \leq 1, i = n+1, \ldots, 2n\}.$$

Let $\mathbf{X}$ denote the Banach space $C([0,1], \mathbf{R}^{2n+1})$ of continuous functions on $[0,1]$ taking values in $\mathbf{R}^{2n+1}$ with the usual supremum norm and $\mathbf{X}_\Lambda$ the convex subset of $\mathbf{X}$ consisting of functions taking values in the set Λ. We assume that the initial data $v^0 \in \mathbf{X}_\Lambda$. We show that the map $\Phi_t : \mathbf{X}_\Lambda \longrightarrow \mathbf{X}_\Lambda$ defined by $\Phi_t(v^0) = v(t)$, where $v(t) = (v_i(\bullet, t))_0^{2n}$ is the solution of (3.1)-(3.3) at time t corresponding to v^0, generates a semi-dynamical system on $\mathbf{X}_\Lambda$.

Proposition 3.1. *For each $v^0 \in \mathbf{X}_\Lambda$ there is a unique global (mild) solution $v(\bullet, t) \in \mathbf{X}_\Lambda$ of (3.1)-(3.3). This solution satisfies (3.1)-(3.3) in the classical sense for $t > 0$.*

Proof: The result follows the pattern of Theorem 1 and Remark 1.2 of Martin and Smith [12] using Theorem 2 of [12]. Our semigroup, described below, satisfies all of the properties needed to conclude the results of Theorem 1 of [12] for our system. The notation used herein reflects that of Martin and Smith. We provide some details. Consider the linear parabolic system obtained from (3.1)-(3.3) by taking $f_i(v) = 0$, $i = 0, \ldots, 2n$, with homogeneous Robin boundary conditions, that is

$$(v_i)_t = \begin{cases} d_i(v_i)_{xx} - (v_i)_x, & i = 0, \ldots, n, \\ 0, & i = n+1, \ldots, 2n, \end{cases} \tag{3.5}$$

$$d_i^{-1} v_i(0,t) - \frac{\partial v_i}{\partial x}(0,t) = \frac{\partial v_i}{\partial x}(1,t) = 0, \quad i = 0, \ldots, n,$$

$$v_i(x,0) = v_i^0(x) \quad i = 0, \ldots, 2n.$$

Define the family of operators $T(t) = (T_i(t))_0^{2n}$ on $\mathbf{X}$ as follows: $T_i(t)v_i^0 = v_i(\bullet, t)$ with $v_i(\bullet, t)$ the solution of (3.5). Note that $T_i(t)v_i^0 = v_i^0$ for $i = n+1, \ldots, 2n$. It is well-known that $T_i(t)$ is a positive analytic semigroup on $C([0,1], \mathbf{R})$ (see Stewart [13]). If $\phi = (\phi_i)_0^{2n} \in \mathbf{X}_\Lambda$, then $T(t)\phi = (T_i(t)\phi_i)_0^{2n}$ satisfies $T_i(t)\phi_i \geq 0$, $i = 0, \ldots, 2n$, since $T(t)$ is positive. By the definition of $T(t)$, $T_i(t)\phi_i \leq 1$, $i = n+1, \ldots, 2n$. Therefore, $T(t)\mathbf{X}_\Lambda \subset \mathbf{X}_\Lambda$.

To incorporate the nonhomogeneous boundary condition in (3.2), consider the system

$$(v_i)_t = \begin{cases} d_i(v_i)_{xx} - (v_i)_x, & i = 0, \ldots, n, \\ 0, & i = n+1, \ldots, 2n, \end{cases} \quad t > s \geq 0, \qquad (3.6)$$

$$\begin{cases} d_0^{-1}v_i(0,t) - \dfrac{\partial v_i}{\partial x}(0,t) = d_0^{-1}, \\ d_i^{-1}v_i(0,t) - \dfrac{\partial v_i}{\partial x}(0,t) = d_i^{-1}u_i^0, & i = 1, \ldots, n, \quad t \geq s \geq 0, \\ \dfrac{\partial v_i}{\partial x}(1,t) = 0, & i = 0, \ldots, n, \end{cases}$$

$$v_i(x,s) = v_i^0(x) \quad i = 0, \ldots, 2n.$$

Define the family of operators $S(t,s) = (S_i(t,s))_0^{2n}$ on $\mathbf{X}$ as follows:

$$S(t,s)v^0 = (S_i(t,s)v_i^0)_0^{2n},$$

where $S_i(t,s)v_i^0 = v_i(\bullet, t)$ with $v_i(\bullet, t)$ the solution of (3.6). Note that

$$S_i(t,s)v_i^0 = v_i^0 \quad \text{for } i = n+1, \ldots, 2n.$$

The form of the boundary conditions in (3.6), together with the maximum principle, imply that if $\phi = (\phi_i)_0^{2n} \in \mathbf{X}_\Lambda$, then $S(t,s)\phi = (S_i(t,s)\phi_i)_0^{2n}$ satisfies $S_i(t,s)\phi_i \geq 0$, $i = 0, \ldots, 2n$. By the definition of $S(t,s)$, $S_i(t,s)\phi_i \leq 1$, $i = n+1, \ldots, 2n$. Therefore, $S(t,s)\mathbf{X}_\Lambda \subset \mathbf{X}_\Lambda$. See Remark 1.2 of [12]. As equation (3.6) and its boundary conditions are independent of time, the operator $S(t,s)$ depends only on the parameter $t-s$, that is, $S(t,s) = S(t-s)$.

The other condition which must be satisfied is that

$$\lim_{h \longrightarrow 0+} h^{-1}\text{dist}(\Lambda; \xi + hf(\xi)) = 0 \qquad (3.7)$$

for all $\xi \in \Lambda$, where $f(\xi) = (f_i(\xi))_0^{2n}$ for $\xi \in \Lambda$. But this follows from Remark 1.2 of [12] and (3.4).

After noting that f is Lipschitz on bounded subsets of Λ and $T(t)$ is analytic, one can conclude that $v(\bullet, t)$ exists locally, i.e. for $0 \leq t < b(v^0)$. It remains to show that solutions can be extended to $t \geq 0$.

First note that, for any $v^0 \in \mathbf{X}_\Lambda$, $v_i(\bullet, t) \leq 1$ for $i = n+1, \ldots, 2n$. Since $f_0(v) \leq 0$, $z(x,t) = v_0(x,t) - 1$ satisfies

$$z_t \leq d_0 z_{xx} - z_x, \quad 0 = z_x(0,t) - d_0^{-1}z(0,t) = z_x(1,t).$$

As established in Proposition 2.1 of [2], the principle eigenvalue λ_0 of the eigenvalue problem corresponding to the above inequality is negative. Let z_0 denote the positive eigenfunction corresponding to λ_0, normalized so that its integral over $[0,1]$ is one. Then $Z(x,t) = Cz_0(x)e^{\lambda_0 t}$ is a solution of the linear parabolic equation corresponding to the above inequality. Letting $C > 0$ be the minimal constant such that $z(x,0) \leq Cz_0(x)$, a standard comparison result implies that $z(x,t) \leq Z(x,t)$ for $x \in [0,1]$ and $t \geq 0$. Thus, v_0 is bounded.

For each $i \in \{1,\ldots,n\}$ we note that

$$(v_i)_t \leq d_i(v_i)_{xx} - (v_i)_x + L_i v_i + M_i$$

for some L_i, M_i since v_i is bounded for $i = 0, n+1, \ldots, 2n$. It follows from a standard comparison theorem that $v_i(x,t) \leq V_i(x,t)$, where V_i is the solution of the partial differential equation corresponding to the above inequality with boundary and initial equations as in (3.2) and (3.3). Since $V_i(x,t)$ exists for all $t \geq 0$, we conclude that solutions of (3.1)-(3.3) can be extended to $t \geq 0$. □

Remarks:

1. In the case of Model I,

$$\Lambda = \{v \in \mathbf{R}^{2n+1} : v_i \geq 0, i = 0, \ldots, 2n; \sum_{i=n+1}^{2n} v_i \leq 1\}.$$

The conditions $T(t)\mathbf{X}_\Lambda \subset \mathbf{X}_\Lambda$ and $S(t,s)\mathbf{X}_\Lambda \subset \mathbf{X}_\Lambda$ are established as for Model II. Here, (3.4)(b) is replaced by

$$f_i(v) < 0 \text{ whenever } \sum_{n+1}^{2n} v_i \leq 1,$$

and is used to show that condition (3.7) holds in Λ. The proof that solutions can be extended to $t \geq 0$ is as for Model II.

2. In the case of Model III,

$$\Lambda = \{v \in \mathbf{R}^{2n+1} : v_i \geq 0, i = 0, \ldots, 2n\}.$$

Here again, the conditions $T(t)\mathbf{X}_\Lambda \subset \mathbf{X}_\Lambda$ and $S(t,s)\mathbf{X}_\Lambda \subset \mathbf{X}_\Lambda$ are established as for Model II. Condition (3.4)(a) is used to show that condition (3.7) holds in Λ. The proof that v_0 is bounded is as for Model II. Then (3.1) is bounded by a quasimonotone linear system. By Corollary 5 of [12] it then follows that solutions of (3.1)-(3.3) can be extended to $t \geq 0$.

Acknowledgments. Mary M. Ballyk gratefully acknowledges the support of the Natural Sciences and Engineering Research Council of Canada. This author's contribution is dedicated to Lillian M. Ballyk. Hal L. Smith is supported in part by NSF grant DMS-9700910.

References

1. Bakke, R., M. G. Trulear, J. A. Robinson and W.G. Characklis, Activity of *Pseudomonas aeruginosa* in Biofilms: Steady state, Biotech. Bioeng. **26** (1984), 1418–1424.

2. Ballyk, M., Le Dung, D. Jones and H. Smith, Effects of Random Motility on Microbial Growth and Competition in a Flow Reactor, SIAM J. Appl. Math., to appear.

3. Freter, R., Mechanisms that control the microflora in the large intestine, in *Human Intestinal Microflora in Health and Disease*, D. Hentges (ed.), Academic Press, New York, 1983.

4. Freter, R., Interdependence of mechanisms that control bacterial colonization of the large intestine, Microecology and Therapy **14** (1984), 89–96.

5. Freter, R., E. Stauffer, D. Cleven, L. V. Holdeman and W. E. C. Moore, Continuous-flow cultures as in vitro models of the ecology of large intestinal flora, Infect. Immun. **39** (1983), 666–675.

6. Freter, R., H. Brickner, M. Botney, D. Cleven and A. Aranki, Mechanisms that control bacterial populations in continuous-flow culture models of mouse large intestinal flora, Infect. Immun. **39** (1983), 676–685.

7. Freter, R., H. Brickner, J. Fekete, M. M. Vickerman and K.E. Carley, Survival and implantation of *Escheridia coli* in the intestinal tract, Infect. Immun. **39** (1983), 686–703.

8. Freter, R., H. Brickner and S. J. Temme, An understanding of colonization resistance of the mammalian large intestine requires mathematical analysis, Microecology and Therapy **16** (1986), 147–155.

9. Kung, C.-M. and Baltzis, The growth of pure and simple microbial competitors in a moving distributed medium, Math. Biosc. **111** (1992), 295–313.

10. Lee, A., Neglected niches. The microbial ecology of the gastrointestinal tract, in *Advances in Microbial Ecology*, K.C. Marshall (ed.), Plenum Press, New York, 1985.

11. Martin, R. H., *Nonlinear Operators and Differential Equations in Banach Spaces*, Wiley & Sons, New York, 1976.

12. Martin, R. H. and H. L. Smith, Abstract functional differential equations and reaction diffusion systems, Trans. Amer. Math. Soc. **321** (1990), 1–44.

13. Stewart, H. B., Generation of analytic semigroups by strongly elliptic operators under general boundary conditions, Trans. Amer. Math. Soc. **259** (1980), 299–310.

14. Van der Waaij, D., J. M. Berghuis-de Vries and J. E. C. Lekkerkerk-van der Wees, Colonization resistance of the digestive tract in conventional and antibiotic-treated mice, J. Hyg. **69** (1971), 405–413.

Controlling the S-I-S Age-Structured Epidemics

Viorel Barbu and Mimmo Iannelli

Abstract. A general method to approach control problems for non-linear age-structured populations is presented and an application to a model in the field of age structured epidemics is given. Conditions for existence and uniqueness of an optimal controller are given, together with equations giving an implicit description of the control.

§1. Introduction

In this paper we provide a brief description of a general approach to optimal control problems for non-linear age-structured population models, and give an application in the field of age structured epidemics. Actually, we consider such a typical example as the well known S-I-S age-structured epidemic model in order to illustrate the main features of the method. Thus we will not discuss the biological implications of the model. Furthermore, we will not give full technical details of the proofs, but will sketch the main ideas that will be exposed in more detail elsewhere, in the general context of non-linear age-structured population problems. We think that this method, though rather abstract and general, nevertheless provides a setting to analyze more specific problems of interest in the field of disease control.

§2. The S-I-S Epidemics

The age-structured S-I-S epidemics, through a stable population, is usually described by the following problem (see for instance [4])

$$y_t + y_a + \gamma(a)y = \lambda(a, t; y)(1 - y),$$
$$y(0, t) = \int_0^{a_t} m(a)y(a, t)da,$$
$$y(a, 0) = y_0(a),$$
$$0 \le y(a, t) \le 1,$$

$$(2.1)$$

Mathematical Models in Medical and Health Sciences
Mary Ann Horn, Gieri Simonett, and Glenn Webb (eds.), pp. 29–34.
Copyright © 1998 by Vanderbilt University Press, Nashville, TN.
ISBN 0-8265-1310-7.

where $y(a,t) = \dfrac{i(a,t)}{p_\infty(a)}$ is the normalization of the infective people distribution $i(a,t)$ to the total population distribution in the stable state, denoted by $p_\infty(a)$ (a denotes age and ranges in the interval $[0, a_\dagger]$).

Actually, if $\beta(\cdot)$ and $\mu(\cdot)$, respectively, are the natural fertility and mortality rates of the population, and the following condition is satisfied

$$\int_0^{a_\dagger} \beta(a) e^{-\int_0^a \mu(\sigma)d\sigma} da = 1, \tag{2.2}$$

then the population has a demographic stable state p_∞ given by

$$p_\infty(a) = b_0 e^{\int_0^a \mu(\sigma)d\sigma}. \tag{2.3}$$

Thus if we suppose that the population has attained its stable demographic state, then problem (2.1) describes the evolution of a typical non-immunizing disease through the population.

In (2.1), $\gamma(\cdot)$ denotes the recovery rate and $m(a) = q\beta(a)p_\infty(a)$ is the specific reproductive rate of the infection, where $q \in [0, 1]$ is the vertical transmission coefficient. Finally, $\lambda(a, t; y)$ is the so called force of infection and is usually given the constitutive form,

$$\lambda(a, t; y) = \int_0^{a_\dagger} K(a, \sigma) y(\sigma, t) d\sigma. \tag{2.4}$$

This describes the mechanism of transmission from the infectives to the susceptible part of the population.

Problem (2.1) has been extensively studied and the behavior of the age-structured S-I-S epidemics is well known. In this paper we are interested in determining a control strategy for the disease described by (2.1); namely we assume that an intervention on the vertical transmission of the disease is possible trough a reduction of the parameter q. Thus we consider the following problem

$$y_t + y_a + \gamma(a)y = \lambda(a, t; y)(1 - y),$$

$$y(0, t) = (1 - u(t)) \int_0^{a_\dagger} m(a) y(a, t) da, \tag{2.5}$$

$$y(a, 0) = y_0(a),$$

where $u(\cdot)$ belongs to the set of controls

$$\mathcal{U} \equiv \{u(\cdot) \in L^\infty[0, T]; \ \ 0 \le u(t) \le 1 \quad a.e. \ in \ \ [0, T]\}. \tag{2.6}$$

Denoting by $y^u(a, t)$ the solution to (2.5), relative to u, we are concerned with the optimal control problem of minimizing the following functional

$$\int_0^T \int_0^{a_\dagger} y^u(a, t) da\, dt + \frac{\rho}{2} \int_0^T u^2(t) dt, \tag{2.7}$$

where $u(\cdot) \in \mathcal{U}$; that is, we try to minimize, in a given interval $[0, T]$, the total number of infectives plus the "cost" of the intervention.

Actually, before going through this problem we must provide precise statements for existence of a solution to problem (2.1); in fact we can rely on the following result which can be proved with the typical methods of age-structured population problems (see for instance [1, 3, 4]).

Theorem 2.1. *For any* $u \in \mathcal{U}$ *there exists one and only one solution* $y^u(\cdot, \cdot) \in$ $L^\infty([0, a_\dagger] \times [0, T])$ *to problem* (2.5). *Moreover this solution has the following properties:*

$$0 \leq y^u(a, t) \leq 1 \quad a.e. \ on \quad [0, a_\dagger] \times [0, T], \tag{2.8}$$

$$|y^u(\cdot, t) - y^v(\cdot, t)|_{L^1} \leq \int_0^t |u(s) - v(s)| ds. \tag{2.9}$$

By a solution of (2.5) we mean a function $y(a, t)$ which is absolutely continuous along the lines $t + a = constant$ so that the directional derivative $\dfrac{\delta}{\delta t} + \dfrac{\delta}{\delta a}$ does exist. We can then interpret the conditions in (2.5) as follows:

$$y(0, t) = \lim_{h \to 0+} y(h, t + h), \quad y(a, 0) = \lim_{h \to 0+} y(a + h, h).$$

§3. The Optimality Conditions

In order to provide a precise formulation to the problem introduced in the previous section, we embed it in the space $E = L^1[0, T]$ by defining

$$\phi(u) = \begin{cases} \displaystyle\int_0^T \int_0^{a_\dagger} y^u(a, t) da dt + \frac{\rho}{2} \int_0^T u^2(t) dt & if \quad u \in \mathcal{U}, \\ \\ +\infty & if \quad u \notin \mathcal{U}. \end{cases} \tag{3.1}$$

Then we consider the problem of finding an optimal controller, that is $u^* \in \mathcal{U}$ such that

$$\phi(u^*) = \min_{u \in \mathcal{U}} \phi(u). \tag{3.2}$$

First we have the following property of $\phi(\cdot)$.

Proposition 3.1. *The functional* ϕ *is lower semi-continuous on* E.

The proof of this proposition follows with standard arguments and depends on (2.8)-(2.9). Then we can prove the following necessary condition of optimality:

Theorem 3.1. *Let* u^* *be an optimal controller satisfying* (3.2). *Then*

$$u^*(t) = \mathcal{L}\left(\frac{1}{\rho} q^{u^*}(0, t) \int_0^{a_\dagger} m(a) y^{u^*}(a, t) da\right) \quad a.e. \ in \quad [0, T], \tag{3.3}$$

where

$$\mathcal{L}(x) = \begin{cases} 0 & for \quad x \in (-\infty, 0), \\ x & for \quad x \in [0, 1], \\ 1 & for \quad x \in (1, +\infty), \end{cases} \tag{3.4}$$

and $q^u(a,t)$ is the solution of the following "dual" problem:

$$q_t + q_a + (1 - u(t))m(a)q(0,t) - \gamma(a)q$$
$$= \lambda(a,t;y^u)q - \Lambda(a,t,y^u,q) + 1,$$
$$q(a,T) = 0 \quad a.e. \ in \ \ [0,a_\dagger],$$
$$q(a_\dagger,t) = 0 \quad a.e. \ in \ \ [0,T],$$
$$(3.5)$$

where $u \in \mathcal{U}$ and

$$\Lambda(a,t,y^u,q) = \int_0^{a_\dagger} (1 - y^u(\sigma,t))K(\sigma,a)q(\sigma,t)d\sigma. \qquad (3.6)$$

We note that for problem (3.5) we can again prove the following result:

Proposition 3.2. *Let* $u \in \mathcal{U}$. *Then problem (3.5) has one and only one solution* $q^u(\cdot,\cdot) \in L^\infty([0,a_\dagger] \times [0,T])$ *such that*

$$|q^u - q^v|_\infty \le CT|u - v|_\infty, \qquad (3.7)$$

where C *is a constant which is independent of* u *and* v.

By a solution of (3.5), we again mean a function $q(a,t)$ which is absolutely continuous along the lines $t + a = constant$ and we interpret the conditions in (3.5) as

$$q(a_\dagger,t) = \lim_{h \to 0^-} q(a_\dagger + h, t + h), \quad q(a,T) = \lim_{h \to 0^-} q(a + h, T + h).$$

In order to prove the theorem we must also consider the following auxiliary problem

$$z_t + z_a + \gamma(a)z + \lambda(a,t;y^u) - (1 - y^u(a,t))\lambda(a,t;z) = 0,$$
$$z(0,t) = (1 - u(t)) \int_0^{a_\dagger} m(a)z(a,t)da - v(t) \int_0^{a_\dagger} m(a)y^u(a,t)da, \qquad (3.8)$$
$$z(a,0) = 0,$$

where $u(\cdot) \in \mathcal{U}$ and $v(\cdot) \in L^\infty(0,T)$. For this problem, by the same methods used for (2.5) and (3.5), the following proposition holds.

Proposition 3.3. *Let* $u \in \mathcal{U}$ *and* $v \in L^\infty(0,T)$, *then problem (3.8) has one and only one solution* $z \in L^\infty([0,a_\dagger] \times [0,T])$.

Actually, problem (3.8) is obtained by differentiating problem (2.1). In fact, denoting by $T_\mathcal{U}(u^*)$ the tangent cone to $\mathcal{U}$ at u^* (see [2]), we have

Proposition 3.4. *Let $u \in \mathcal{U}$ and $v \in T_\mathcal{U}(u^*)$. Then*

$$z(a,t) = \lim_{h \to 0+} \frac{1}{h}[y^{u+hv} - y^u]$$

exists in $L^\infty([0, a_\dagger] \times [0, T])$ and z satisfies problem (3.8).

We are now able to prove Theorem 3.1.

Proof: Let $u^* \in \mathcal{U}$ be an optimal controller and $v \in T_\mathcal{U}(u^*)$. Then for $h > 0$,

$$\frac{1}{h}[\phi(u^* + hv) - \phi(u^*)] \geq 0, \tag{3.9}$$

so that by Proposition 3.4 we have

$$\int_0^T \int_0^{a_\dagger} z^*(a,t)dadt + \rho \int_0^T u^*(t)v(t)dt \geq 0,$$

where z^* is the solution of problem (3.8) with $u(\cdot)$ replaced by u^* and $v(\cdot) \in T_\mathcal{U}(u^*)$.

Now let $q^*(\cdot,\cdot)$ be the solution of problem (3.5) at u^*, then multiplying the first equation in (3.8) by q^* and integrating by parts we get

$$\int_0^T \int_0^{a_\dagger} z^*(a,t)dadt = \int_0^T \int_0^{a_\dagger} m(a)y^{u^*}(a,t)q^*(0,t)v(t)dadt, \tag{3.10}$$

so that from (3.13) we have $\forall v \in T_\mathcal{U}(u^*)$,

$$\int_0^T \left[\rho u^*(t) + q^{u^*}(0,t) \int_0^{a_\dagger} m(a)y^{u^*}(a,t)da\right] v(t)dt \geq 0. \tag{3.11}$$

This implies that the square bracket belongs to the normal cone $N_\mathcal{U}(u^*)$ of $\mathcal{U}$ at u^* and (3.3) follows. $\square$

§4. Existence of an Optimal Controller

As it is claimed in Proposition 3.1, the functional ϕ is strongly lower semi-continuous, but not weakly lower semi-continuous. Thus we are obliged to build suitable minimizing sequences, which are strongly convergent. In order to do this we will use Ekeland's principle (see [2]); namely applying this principle we have that

$$\begin{cases} \forall \epsilon > 0 \quad \text{there exists} \quad u_\epsilon \in L(0,T) \quad \text{such that} \\ i) \quad \phi(u_\epsilon) < \inf_{u \in \mathcal{U}} \phi(u) + \epsilon, \\ ii) \quad \phi(u_\epsilon) = \min\left\{\phi(u) + \sqrt{\epsilon}|u - u_\epsilon|_{L^1}, \quad u \in \mathcal{U}\right\}. \end{cases} \tag{4.1}$$

Actually, (4.1.ii) says that the approximating functional,

$$\phi_\epsilon(u) = \phi(u) + \sqrt{\epsilon}|u - u_\epsilon|_{L^1},$$

attains its minimum at u_ϵ, thus the same argument as in Theorem 3.1 shows that

$$u_\epsilon(t) = \mathcal{L}\left(\frac{1}{\rho}q^{u_\epsilon}(0,t) \int_0^{a_\dagger} y^{u_\epsilon}(a,t)da + \frac{\epsilon}{\rho}\vartheta_\epsilon(t)\right), \tag{4.2}$$

where $\vartheta_\epsilon(\cdot)$ belongs to $L_\infty(0,T)$ and $|\vartheta_\epsilon|_\infty \leq 1$. This allows us to prove our next theorem.

Theorem 4.1. *If* $\dfrac{T}{\rho}$ *is sufficiently small then there exists one and only one optimal controller* $u^* \in \mathcal{U}$ *satisfying (3.2).*

Proof: First we prove uniqueness which follows from Theorem 3.1 and from the estimates (2.9), (3.7). In fact, we define the mapping $\mathcal{T} : \mathcal{U} \subset L^\infty \to \mathcal{U}$ by setting

$$\mathcal{T}(u)(t) \equiv \mathcal{L}\left(\frac{1}{\rho}q^u(0,t)\int_0^{a_\dagger} m(a)y^u(a,t)da\right). \tag{4.3}$$

Then we have

$$|\mathcal{T}(u) - \mathcal{T}(v)|_{L^\infty} \le \frac{CT}{\rho}|u - v|_{L^\infty}, \tag{4.4}$$

where C is a constant. Thus if $\dfrac{CT}{\rho} < 1$ there is one and only one fixed point u^* of $\mathcal{T}$. This means that the possible optimal controller is unique because it coincides with this fixed point.

In order to see that this fixed point is actually an optimal controller, we use the sequence u_ϵ. In fact, from (4.2) and (4.3) we have:

$$\left|\mathcal{T}(u_\epsilon)(t) - \mathcal{L}\left(\frac{1}{\rho}q^{u_\epsilon}(0,t)\int_0^{a_\dagger} m(a)q^{u_\epsilon}(a,t)da + \frac{\epsilon}{\rho}\vartheta_\epsilon\right)\right|_{L^\infty} \le \frac{\epsilon}{\rho}$$

and

$$|u^* - u_\epsilon|_{L^\infty} \le |\mathcal{T}(u^*) - \mathcal{T}(u_\epsilon)|_{L^\infty} + \frac{\epsilon}{\rho} \le \frac{CT}{\rho}|u^* - u_\epsilon|_{L^\infty} + \frac{\epsilon}{\rho}.$$

This gives

$$|u^* - u_\epsilon|_{L^\infty} \le \frac{1}{\rho - CT}\epsilon.$$

Thus $u_\epsilon \to u^*$ in L_∞ and, by (4.1.i),

$$\phi(u^*) \le \inf_{u \in \mathcal{U}} \phi(u). \quad \square$$

Concluding this paper we note that the main result that we obtain, together with existence and uniqueness of an optimal controller, is formula (3.3) which implicitly provides u^* via problems (2.5) and (3.5). Thus the study of these problems should give information on the optimal controller itself.

References

1. Anita, S., M. Iannelli, M. Y. Kim and E. J. Park, Optimal harvesting for periodic age-dependent population dynamics, SIAM J. Appl. Anal., to appear.

2. Barbu, V., *Mathematical Methods in Optimization of Differential Systems*, Kluwer Publishing, 1995.

3. Brokate M., Pontryagin principle for control problems in age dependent population dynamics, J. Math. Biol. **23** (1985), 75–101.

4. Iannelli, M., *Mathematical Theory of Age-Structured Population Dynamics*, Applied Mathematics Monographs C.N.R., Vol. 7, Giardini, Pisa, 1995.

Cluster Form Analysis Techniques
for Diabetic Retinopathy

Michael W. Berry and Dax M. Westerman

Abstract. In diabetic retinopathy, the detection of blood and lipid deposits in critical regions of the retina can reflect the early stages of diabetes and potential blindness. Using cluster form analysis for 2D color images of the retina, computer-generated statistics of the cluster properties such as size, number, radius of gyration, and ellipsoidal eccentricity can be used to classify both obvious and subtle abnormalities in the macula (back of the retina). Different neighborhood rules (e.g., 4-node von Neumann and Moore neighborhoods) can be used to identify, quantify and index clusters of retinal features from large databases of retina images. As part of an integrated software environment for image analysis, such an automated approach for classifying retina images should prove to be an important decision-support tool for the clinical diagnosis of diabetes and other diseases detectable from retina images.

§1. Introduction

The eye condition referred to as *diabetic retinopathy* is one of the most common complications associated with diabetes, and is considered to be the leading cause of blindness among working-age Americans [10]. Patients with diabetes mellitus suffer from improper use and storage of sugar in the body. Elevated blood sugar levels can cause severe damage to the blood vessels in the eyes and consequently diabetic retinopathy. To be more specific, damaged retinal blood vessels can leak fluid (lipids) or simply bleed. Associated swelling of the retina (layer of nerves inside the eye which converts light into signals for brain interpretation) results in the formation of yellowish deposits (lipids) called *exudates* [9].

Although there is no noticeable change in vision with the presence of exudates (referred to as nonproliferative or background retinopathy), the early detection of lipid deposits and blood leakage can (through treatment) prevent the onset of a more serious forms of retinopathy: *Proliferative retinopathy* [2, 9]. In this stage, the *macula* of the retina (i.e., the center 10% of the retina)

Mathematical Models in Medical and Health Sciences
Mary Ann Horn, Gieri Simonett, and Glenn Webb (eds.), pp. 35–50.
Copyright © 1998 by Vanderbilt University Press, Nashville, TN.
ISBN 0-8265-1310-7.

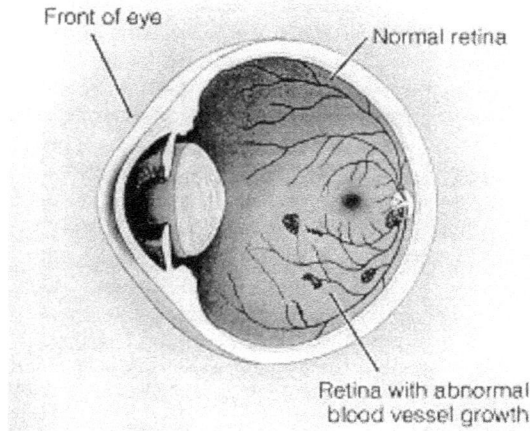

Fig. 1. Abnormal blood vessel growth associated with diabetic retinopathy.

can become filled with fluid (macular edema) so that fine detail vision (e.g., reading) is blurred. The growth of fragile (fine hair-like) blood vessels on the surface of the retina (neovascularization) can lead to serious vision loss (see Figure 1). If these tiny blood vessels break, they may subsequently bleed into the vitreous (center of the eye) which is normally a clear gel. A clouded (blood filled) vitreous prevents the passage of light to the retina causing blurred vision. If scar tissue develops on the surface of retina (from neovascularization), the retina may detach from the back of the eye (see Figure 2). Without treatment, retinal detachment can lead to total blindness in the eye. Abnormal blood vessel growth in other regions of the eye (e.g, the iris) can lead to other serious eye diseases such as glaucoma [10].

The primary treatment for diabetic retinopathy is laser surgery. By focusing laser light onto the retina, the target area can be treated while leaving the surrounding tissues untouched. The absorbed energy heats, or *photocoagulates*, the retina, creating a microscopic spot. The leaking vessels causing macular edema can be sealed by the laser (focal or grid photocoagulation). Newly formed vessels in the eye with associated with proliferative retinopathy can often be eliminated with *panretinal* photocoagulation [4].

As with most serious diseases, early detection can substantially improve the odds of a successful prognosis. In the context of diabetic retinopathy, the *identification* and *classification* of exudates (whether lipid or blood) and neovascularization are two of the primary tasks in the analysis of retinal images. In order to relieve the physician of repetitive and tedious procedures in comparing volumes of retinal images, computer software environments are now being designed to function as decision support systems. The STARE (STructured Analysis of the REtina) system [6], in particular, has been designed to fully automate the diagnosis of diabetic retinopathy. STARE uses a framework for measuring the similarity of images based on a layer of *primitives* for

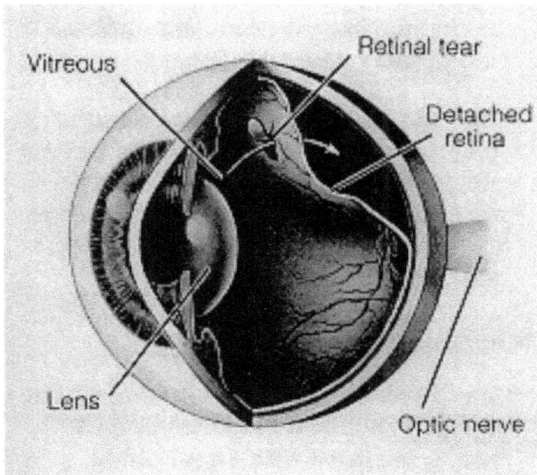

Fig. 2. Retinal detachment in proliferative retinopathy.

color, composition, texture, and structure [6]. Determining the best metrics for measuring these primitives is an open question in computer vision and visual information retrieval.

The focus of this work is on the use of techniques from cluster form analysis [1,7] to automate the identification of exudates and the tiny hair-like blood vessels associated with neovascularization in the retina. Cluster identification and geometry can be used to further image understanding and provide a consistent framework for the comparison of accumulating volumes (or more precisely computer disks) of archived retinal images. In the context of content-based retrieval frameworks such as STARE [6], cluster geometries can be used as metrics for the structure (or shape) primitive for comparing images.

In section 2, the identification of clusters by neighborhood rules and a few cluster shape characterizations are discussed followed by a description of a promising algorithm, the Enhanced Hoshen Kopelman (EHK) algorithm, for both cluster identification and geometry in section 3. Specific applications of alternative neighborhood rules to identify exudates and neovascularization from a few sample images are presented in section 4 followed by a statistical-based categorization of retinal *clusters* using computed cluster properties in section 5. A summary and brief discussion of future work are provided in section 6.

§2. Neighborhood Rules and Cluster Shape

Since clustering is determine by the adjacency of cells, a *nearest-neighbor* rule is usually employed to identify all clusters of a given resource type.

Four–Node von Neumann   Four–Node Moore

Twelve–Node

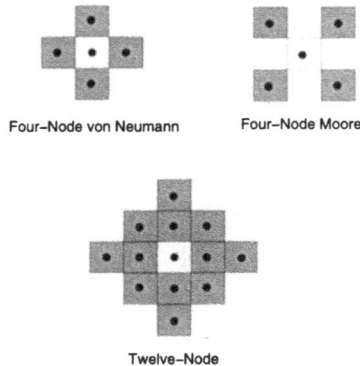

Fig. 3. Three possible nearest-neighborhood rules for cluster identification with 2D maps or grids.

2.1 Neighborhood Rules

As discussed in [1], the four-nearest-neighbor rule (see Figure 3) or *von Neumann neighborhood* [11] has been widely used for landscape ecology applications utilizing 2D grids or maps. In these applications, clusters usually represent habitat type or vegetation cover in the study of landscape heterogeneity [1]. The four-nearest neighborhood rule based on the von Neumann neighborhood is sometimes referred to as the North-East-West-South (or NEWS) neighborhood rule [1].

As discussed in [12], other neighborhood rules for cluster identification in lattices or 2D images are possible: the 8-node nearest-neighbor rule or Moore neighborhood [11] or the 12-node nearest-neighbor rule (see Figure 3). There are numerous neighborhood rules than can be used in cluster form analysis including those which are *asymmetrical*. Asymmetrical rules, in particular, have been used in landscape ecology applications [12] to simulate fire starts in windy conditions. Such rules are typically sensitive to the starting position (cell) in the cluster identification process (discussed in more detail in section 3). In this work, only symmetrical neighborhood rules such as those pictured in Figure 3 are considered for the identification of exudates and neovascularization.

Figure 4 illustrates the differences in cluster assignments for the 4-node NEWS and Moore neighborhood rules. The 11 occupied cells of the 5×5 grid form either 3 or 4 clusters depending on the neighborhood rule used. If the grids in Figure 4 represent encoded images, the shape or geometries of objects (clusters) determined by a particular neighborhood rule can be very different from those derived by an alternative rule. Exploiting alternative neighborhood rules so that clusters may better conform to features such as exudates (lipids or blood) and neovascularization is illustrated in section 4.

$$
\begin{array}{ccccc}
0 & 1 & 0 & 0 & 0 \\
1 & 1 & 0 & 0 & 0 \\
0 & 1 & 0 & 0 & 0 \\
2 & 0 & 3 & 3 & 0 \\
2 & 2 & 0 & 3 & 3
\end{array}
\qquad
\begin{array}{ccccc}
0 & 1 & 0 & 0 & 0 \\
1 & 2 & 0 & 0 & 0 \\
0 & 1 & 0 & 0 & 0 \\
1 & 0 & 1 & 4 & 0 \\
3 & 1 & 0 & 1 & 4
\end{array}
$$

NEWS   Moore

Fig. 4. Clustering by NEWS and Moore neighborhood rules for a 5 × 5 grid.

2.2 Cluster Shape

As mentioned in section 1, cluster geometries are potential metrics that can be used in shape primitives for image comparisons. The squared *radius of gyration*, R_s, is an important shape quantity [3, 14] that can be used in cluster classification. that can be used in cluster classification. Specifically, define

$$
R_s^2 = \frac{1}{2s^2} \sum_i \sum_j |\mathbf{r_i} - \mathbf{r_j}|^2, \tag{1}
$$

where s is the size of the cluster, r_i and r_j denote the positions of sites (cells) i and j, respectively. Here, the double summation involves all i and j sites of the cluster of interest. The summation over the distances in Eq. (1) can also be rewritten [7] as

$$
|\mathbf{r_i} - \mathbf{r_j}|^2 = \sum_{\mu=1}^{d} (x_{i,\mu} - x_{j,\mu})^2, \tag{2}
$$

where $x_{i,\mu}$ and $x_{j,\mu}$ denote the μth coordinates of sites i and j, respectively, in d dimensions ($d = 2$ for retinal images, of course).

Since each dimension μ can be treated independently in Eq. (2), the summation in Eq. (1) can be reduced [7] for each μ to

$$
\sum_i \sum_j (x_{i,\mu} - x_{j,\mu})^2 = 2s \sum_i x_{i,\mu}^2 - 2 \left(\sum_i x_{i,\mu} \right)^2 = 2 \left[sX_\mu^{(2)} - (X_\mu^{(1)})^2 \right], \tag{3}
$$

where

$$
X_\mu^{(1)} = \sum_i x_{i,\mu} \text{ and } X_\mu^{(2)} = \sum_i x_{i,\mu}^2
$$

are referred to as the first and second spatial moments [13], respectively, for the given cluster and μ^{th} coordinate. Using Eqs. (1)-(3) it follows that

$$
R_s^2 = \frac{1}{s^2} \sum_{\mu=1}^{d} \left[sX_\mu^{(2)} - \left(X_\mu^{(1)} \right)^2 \right]. \tag{4}
$$

Borrowing concepts from mechanics, cluster shapes can also be characterized using the *moment of inertia*. Assume that each pixel reflects a point unity mass so that the *mass* of the cluster of interest is the cluster size, s. Also, assume that any nearest neighbor pixel is 1 unit distance away to yield a mass density (mass per unit area) of 1. It can be shown that the moment of inertia, I, perpendicular to the X-Y plane which passes through the cluster's center of mass is given by

$$I = sR_s^2.$$

Now, consider the superposition of an ellipse with major axis a and minor axis b whose center is at the cluster's center of mass. If the ellipse has the same area (mass) and moment of inertia as the cluster, then the area of the ellipse is $s = \pi ab$. The moment of inertia through the center of the ellipse and perpendicular to the X-Y plane is then

$$I = (s/4)(a^2 + b^2),$$

where $a = (\xi + \phi)/2$, $b = (\xi - \phi)/2$, $\xi = \sqrt{4I/s + 2s/\pi}$, and $\phi = \sqrt{4I/s - 2s/\pi}$. The effective eccentricity e of the ellipse defined by

$$e = (\sqrt{a^2 - b^2})/a \qquad (5)$$

can then be used to characterize the shape of the ellipse/cluster. That is, small values of e near 0 specify more circular clusters while values of e near 1 reflect more elongated clusters. Figure 5 illustrates the extremes of eccentricity for two clusters having the same size (2025 pixels). Here, $R_s^2 = 322.277$ and $e = 0$ for the circular cluster while $R_s^2 = 2834.077$ and $e = 0.998$ for the elongated cluster.

Both the squared radius of gyration R_s^2 (Eq. (4)) and ellipsoidal eccentricity e (Eq. (5)) are candidate metrics for any shape primitive used to compare clusters (or retinal image features). Fortunately, an enhanced version [7] of the original Hoshen Kopelman algorithm [1, 3, 8] for cluster identification can derive both metrics using only one pass (covering all pixels) of the image.

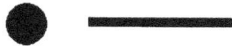

Fig. 5. Extreme cases for eccentricity of best-fit ellipse.

§3. Enhanced Hoshen-Kopelman (EHK) Algorithm

The Hoshen-Kopelman (HK) algorithm [8] is a one-pass approach to cluster identification that utilizes two working arrays, `matrix` and `csize`, to store image data. As previously demonstrated in applications such as landscape ecology [1, 3], image data can be is read into a holding buffer, filtered, and then transferred into the `matrix` array for cluster identification and characterization. This three-step process constitutes pre-processing for the HK algorithm.

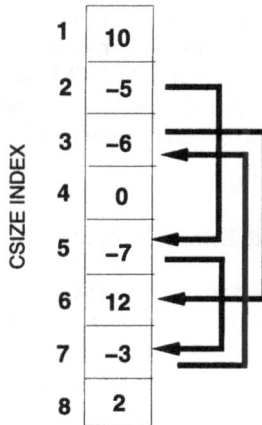

Fig. 6. Sample `csize` working array used in the Hoshen-Kopelman algorithm.

3.1 Original Design

The HK algorithm traverses an image from left to right, and then from top to bottom, assigning a temporary cluster label (integer) to each non-zero pixel and recording any pixel label or cluster membership changes in the two working arrays. Temporary label assignment is a function of the current neighborhood rule (see section 2.1) and the algorithm implementation. Matrix is a two-dimensional integer array of size $(n + 1) \times (m + 1)$, where n is the height (rows) and m is the width (columns) of the image in pixels. The dimensions n and m are increased by 1 to accommodate boundary columns and rows, containing unique boundary integer values. Pointers are used to both index and traverse the `matrix` array and to minimize the overhead of base-plus-offset array indexing.

Integer storage (32 bits per pixel) is required because the `matrix` array serves a dual purpose: it holds the post-processed map data, and also serves as a working array for the pixels' temporary cluster label. If the entire `matrix` array cannot be stored in memory, a *divide-and-conquer* approach can be implemented whereby cluster identification is performed by partitioning the map along row boundaries and merging the results of each partition [3]. Each partition is of size $k \times m$ where k is the number of rows in each partition.

An integer array (`csize`) is typically used to store either the running total of cluster size or an index value for another entry in the `csize` array. If the stored value is positive, it represents the current number of pixels in that cluster. If it is negative, the absolute value of the stored number is treated as an index to the true cluster label. Negative indexes may follow a non-circular, recursive path for a finite number of steps.

Figure 6 illustrates a `csize` working array having positive or negative entries for each index. Temporary cluster 1 has a total of 10 pixels whereas temporary cluster 2 is the beginning of a 5-step pointer path $(2 \rightarrow 5 \rightarrow 7 \rightarrow$

$3 \rightarrow 6$) pointing to temporary cluster 6 which contains 12 pixels. The existence of the path represents the fact that the temporary cluster at the beginning of the path (i.e., array index 2) had been previously merged into the temporary cluster at the end of the path (i.e., array index 6). Compression of this path is significant to the overall efficiency of Hoshen-Kopelman algorithm [3, 8].

3.2 Implementation and Enhancement

As each row of an image is traversed in the HK algorithm (using the NEWS neighborhood rule), the value of the current pixel is compared to the value of the previous pixel in that row (west neighbor) and the pixel value in the same column of the previous row (north neighbor). If all pixels are in the same cluster, the smallest cluster label is assigned to all three pixels and any changes in the status of the west and north neighbors are recorded in the working arrays. The smallest of the two values is chosen to reduce the memory requirements of the csize array where the maximum size is a function of the pixel density and clustering patterns. When the algorithm completes, each index in the csize array holds one of three values: a zero, the number of pixels in the cluster identified by the csize index value, or a pointer to another csize index. The last two values are differentiated by the arithmetic sign of the value – positive represents the pixel count in the indexed cluster whereas negative represents a pointer to another csize array index. De-referencing the pointer, which could follow a non-circular, multi-step path, is accomplished by indexing into the csize array using the absolute value of the pointer. The HK algorithm does not guarantee a properly labeled map; however, relabeling, or adjusting pixel values to accurately reflect cluster membership can be accomplished in linear time using the working array produced by the HK algorithm. Figure 7 illustrates the results of the working array csize after merging the temporary cluster labeled 3 from the top row into the temporary cluster labeled 1.

Before the merge, temporary cluster 1 contained 7 pixels, and temporary cluster 3 contained 2 pixels. After the addition of the current pixel (1 pixel) and the pixels from temporary cluster 3 (2 pixels), temporary cluster 1 now contains 10 pixels $(7 + 2 + 1)$, and temporary cluster 3 shows a pointer to temporary cluster 1 in the csize working array. As shown in [3], it is possible to process large images in linear time using a divide-and-conquer approach to cluster identification since (at any step) the algorithm only requires access to the working array csize, the current pixel, the north neighboring pixel, and the pixel value of the west neighbor.

Using a finite state machine to reduce redundant integer comparisons [3], cluster identification on a single processor/machine can be as much as twice as fast as the original HK serial implementation in [1]. As shown in [7], metrics such as the radius of gyration defined by Eq. (4) (and hence the ellipsoidal eccentricity given in Eq. (5)) can be accumulated as partial sums during the one-pass cluster identification phase. This feature which now defines the *Enhanced* HK algorithm which avoids the $\mathcal{O}(n^2)$ comparisons

MATRIX Array

0	1	1	1	0	3	3	0
0	1	1	1	1	-1	-1	0

CSIZE Array

1	7
2	0
3	2
4	0

1	10
2	0
3	-1
4	0

Before   **After**

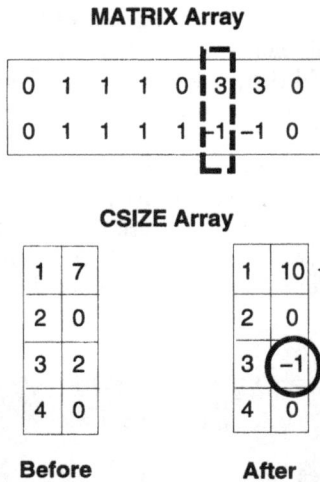

Fig. 7. Effect of merging operation on `csize` and `matrix` working arrays.

which would normally be required to compute most cluster properties (e.g., spatial moments) of a pre-processed $n \times n$ cluster-labeled image.

§4. Identification of Retinal Features

In order to identify features found in both a healthy and a non-healthy (diabetic) eye, a series of preprocessing steps are needed to generate the `matrix` array used by the EHK algorithm. This preprocessing begins with the transformation of the color image into an array of appropriate size with 1 byte per entry. Each element in the image (pixel) is then averaged using the RGB (red, green and blue) components, ranging from 0 to 255 each, and the result is stored in the corresponding location in the array. This approach is somewhat different from that taken by the STARE project which only analyzes the green and blue components of retinal images [5].

Once the entire image had been averaged in such a manner, the resulting array can be treated as an intensity image, again with values ranging from 0 to 255, though viewed as levels of grey instead of color. It must noted here that these intensity images are not *enhanced* save for adjusting the average values in the image such that each element in the image is incremented by a constant. As a result of subtracting the largest averaged value from 255, this constant provides some standardization without altering basic information in the image.

Once the intensity map has been created, filters can then be applied to this array in order to isolate what areas of the image are of interest. It is important to note that the original images and the resulting overlays of identified clusters were in color. In order to present results here, the images had to be translated into grey-scale images then enhanced manually to facilitate the observation of anomalies. A small amount of background noise has been generated as a result of this enhancement, though it does not impede interpretation of the images. In addition, unless specified otherwise, the images shown below have been analyzed using the Four-Node von Neumann neighborhood rule (see Figure 3).

For images of the eye, certain objects exist in a fairly well-defined range of intensities, thus making their identification more intuitive. Certain objects which are easier to isolate in an image are the macula and the optic nerve (Figure 8). This can be accredited to the fairly constant ranges of intensities in which these objects are found (usually 75 to 100 and 200 to 255, respectively).

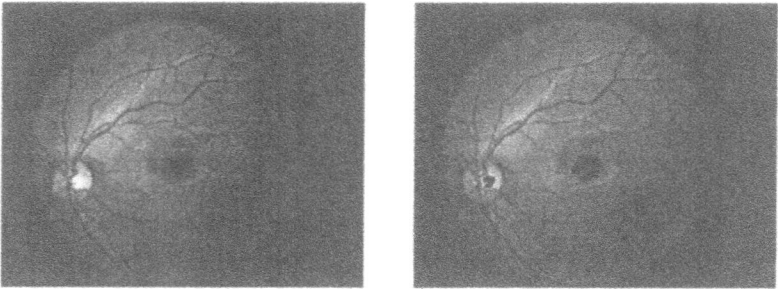

Fig. 8. The identification of the optic nerve and macula.

The presence of lipids (exudates) is relatively easy to identify by a range of intensities. Such objects are by far the easiest aberations (Figure 9) to detect using the EHK algorithm.

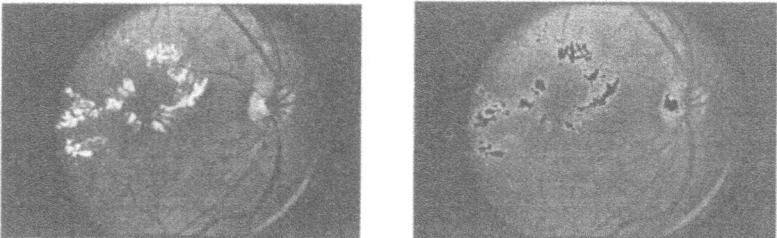

Fig. 9. The identification of lipids.

Some of the more difficult objects to extract from a retinal image include microaneurysms and blood vessels. The difficulty can be attributed to a *single range* of intensities (see Figure 10) which span both sets of objects (with additional background noise).

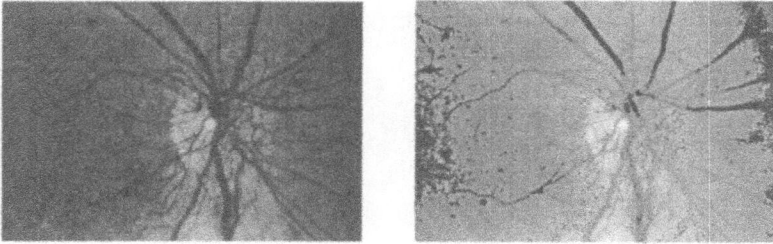

Fig. 10. The identification of microaneurysms and blood vessels.

The effects of using different neighborhood rules on the identification of retinal features (normal or abnormal) can vary with the target object (cluster). One result of using the 4-node Moore neighborhood rule (see Figure 3) and other *symmetric* rules is the detection of several disjoint clusters in a region where a more *compact* rule (NEWS, 8-node, or 12-node) would identify a single cluster. Although the more compact rules (NEWS, 8-node, and 12-node rules) performed well for most of the images considered in this study, there was a noticeable tendency to gather too much information into a very small amount of clusters (specifically the 8-node and 12-node rules) which ultimately led to a loss of fine detail in some retinal features (lipid clusters and tiny blood vessels). As discussed in section 5, an approach which uses different neighborhood rules along with different metrics for cluster evaluation can be quite effective for the characterization of clusters/objects in retinal images.

§5. Feature Classification by Cluster Statistics

In the classification of objects from retinal images, cluster statistics such as radius of gyration, size, and the eccentricity of a best-fit ellipse can be used to characterize and classify objects (clusters). Comparing the values of several metrics can be helpful in determining the nature of a cluster. Using only one determining metric, such as the eccentricity, may only be useful in a few extreme cases (Figure 5). As illustrated in Figure 11, a graph of the eccentricity e of an ellipse (Eq. (5)), as the length of the semi-minor axis (b) ranges from 0 to the length of the semi-major axis (a), does not rapidly deviate from the extremes.

The difficulty in using a single metric to exclusively determine/identify clusters of lipids (Figure 12) is illustrated in Table 1. From the range of intensity levels (200 to 255) and location in the image, these clusters are resolved as lipids since the only other object associated the same intensity levels is the optic nerve. It can be seen, however, that the more elongated lipid deposit (left image, Figure 12), corresponding to the first entry in Table 1, has a larger eccentricity than any of the clusters in the second image of Figure 12. The three clusters of the right image of Figure 12 are clearly more compact than the larger (elongated) cluster.

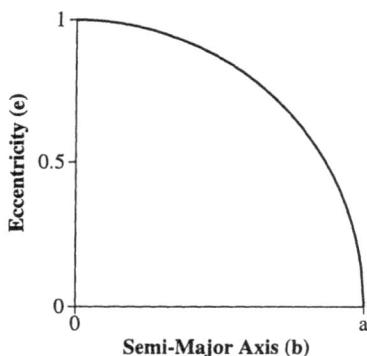

Fig. 11. The graph of the eccentricity of an ellipse, $0 \leq b \leq a$.

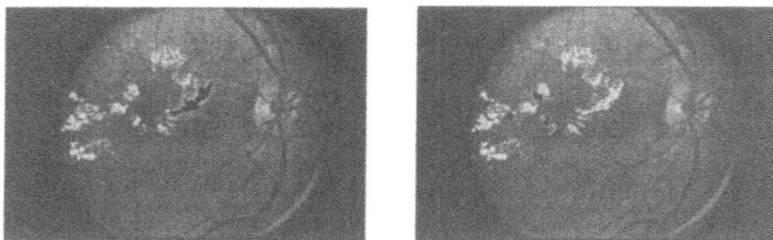

Fig. 12. Clusters of same type (lipids) located with different eccentricities.

R_s^2	Size	Eccentricity
830.793	1734	0.985
58.552	241	0.927
48.109	248	0.852
47.135	229	0.880

Tab. 1. Examples of cluster statistics from Figure 12.

Another illustration of the variations in ellipsoidal eccentricity among several lipid clusters (Figure 13) is given in Table 2. Here, the ten-largest (dark shaded) clusters of the image in Figure 13 are ranked according to size (number of pixels).

As noted earlier, the detection of microaneurysms can be problematic since these objects are often found in the same range of intensities as larger blood vessels. To further complicate the problem, the intensity levels of these objects may overlap with intensities associated with *noise* in the image. In using a combination of metrics to assist in the analysis of an image, one may be able to circumvent some of these issues. The left image of Figure 14 demonstrates (with dark-shaded clusters) all the objects found in the range

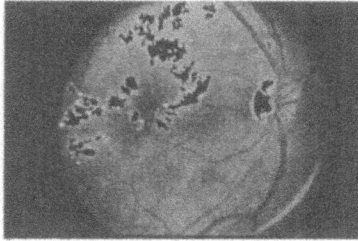

Fig. 13. All lipids with cluster sizes greater than 50.

Rank	R_s^2	Size	Eccentricity
1	745.959	2932	0.936
2	830.793	1734	0.985
3	260.050	1375	0.837
4	335.715	1295	0.939
5	323.317	991	0.965
6	138.629	676	0.879
7	145.452	649	0.909
8	231.460	556	0.980
9	94.675	544	0.759
10	112.679	494	0.913

Tab. 2. Statistics for the ten-largest clusters of Figure 13.

of intensity levels associated with blood vessels and microaneurysms. The right image of Figure 14, on the other hand, shows a filtered image with clusters depicted for extreme values of the radius of gyration R_s^2 or ellipsoidal eccentricity e (see Table 3).

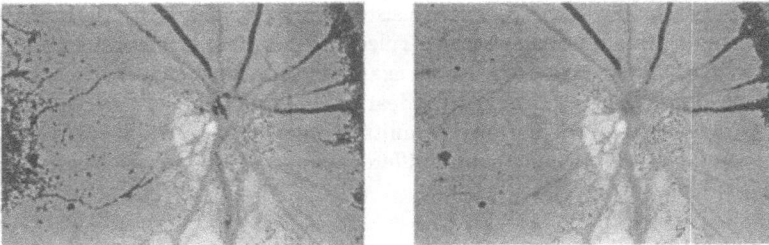

Fig. 14. Specific examples of microaneurysms and blood vessels.

Cluster	R_s^2	Size	Eccentricity
1	4.352	25	0.759
2	4.998	25	0.868
3	8.352	25	0.967
4	5.227	30	0.760
5	7.139	35	0.877
6	12.191	35	0.970
7	13.735	77	0.788
8	28.134	147	0.845
9	93.659	472	0.864
10	3622.997	1286	0.999
11	3602.741	2048	0.998
12	1971.145	4193	0.984
13	7489.689	9495	0.994

Tab. 3. Comparison of metrics between clusters (microaneurysms and blood vessels).

One approach for differentiation among objects found in the same range of intensities involves the use of different neighborhood rules over the same region of an image and a subsequent comparison of *shape* metrics generated by each rule. Such an approach can be applied to differentiate features such as an isolated blood spot and blood vessel from Figure 14. For this example, two neighborhood rules were used for cluster characterization. First, the NEWS rule was used to locate the objects in a specified range of intensity. Next, a second rule, the 4-node Moore neighborhood rule, was used over the same region of the image. As illustrated in Table 4, comparing the values for R_s^2 and eccentricity e generated by both rules reveals a significant increase in e for clusters associated with the blood spot (microaneurysm) of interest. Although the value of e does not exceed .992 for the 4-node Moore neighborhood rule, the rapid change in e is more apparent than that for the more elongated clusters representing the blood vessel. Hence, a rapid change in eccentricity e when using the 4-node Moore neighborhood rule (in contrast to the NEWS rule) may be a stronger indication of compactness. Empirical data suggests that this trend in larger values of e is consistent for rules other than the NEWS, 8-node, and 12-node neighborhood rules. When comparing values for the squared radius of gyration R_s^2 in this example, compactness versus elongation becomes much easier to quantify. Clearly, size and shape characterizations of clusters may require the use of multiple metrics and neighborhood rules to resolve both obvious and subtle differences among objects detected within similar intensity ranges.

§6. Summary and Future Work

Developing a computational framework for the identification and character-ization of clusters from retinal images is an important part of any decision

	R_s^2	Size	Eccentricity
Microaneurysm			
NEWS	23.257	141	0.644
Moore Neighborhood	23.913	36	0.992
	22.256	35	0.991
	23.020	35	0.992
	23.157	35	0.992
Blood vessel			
NEWS	1628.585	1257	0.998
Moore Neighborhood	670.026	232	0.999
	1772.563	317	0.999
	1721.986	315	0.999
	1544.404	313	0.999

Tab. 4. Cluster statistics resulting from different neighborhood rules.

support system for the diagnosis of diabetic retinopathy. This research has demonstrated the use of different neighborhood rules and metrics which can be used to assess the size and shape of features such as exudates (lipids) and neovascularization. The implementation of the Enhanced Hoshen-Kopelman (EHK) algorithm is completely general and can be applied in other image processing applications.

Future software development involves the creation of a graphical user interface (GUI) which will facilitate the use of the EHK algorithm and cluster *shape* metrics. The archival and retrieval of cluster information (metrics) stored in a database is another feature which can accessed by the GUI. The underlying goal of this work is not to produce a software package to replace medical knowledge and intuition; rather the primary focus is augmenting the abilities/expertise of a clinical examiner by providing a method of comparison based on consistent (repeatable) computational data.

Acknowledgments. The authors would like to thank Leonard Goldschmidt, M.D., Ph.D. (Pleasanton, CA) and Joseph (Yosi) Hoshen, Ph.D. (Napierville, IL) for their help in the acquisition and interpretation of the retinal images used in this work. The retinal diagrams shown in Figures 1 and 2 are courtesy of the American Academy of Opthalmology.

References

1. Berry, M., E. Comiskey and K. Minser, Parallel Analysis of Clusters in Landscape Ecology, IEEE Computational Science and Engineering **1**(2) (1994), 24–38.

2. Bresnick, G. H., Diabetic Retinopathy, in *Principles and Practice of Clinical Electro-physiology of Vision*, J. R. Heckenlively and G. B. Arden (eds.), St. Louis: Mosby Year Book, 1991.

3. Constantin, J. M., M. W. Berry and B. T. Vander Zanden, Parallelization of the Hoshen-Kopelman Algorithm Using a Finite State Machine, J. of Super. Applic. and High Perf. Comput. **11**(1) (1997), 31–45.

4. Favard C., C. Guyot-Argenton, M. Assouline, C. Marie-Lescure, and Y. Pouliquen, Full Panretinal Photocoagulation and Early Vitrectomy Improve Prognosis of Florid Diabetic Retinopathy, Opthal. **103** (1996), 561–574.

5. Goldbaum, M., S. Moezzi, A. Taylor, S. Chatterjee, E. Hunter and R. Jain, Automated Diagnosis and Image Understanding with Object Extraction, Object Classification, and Inferencing in Retinal Images, IEEE International Conference on Image Processing, Vol. ICIP-96, 1996.

6. Gupta, A., S. Moezzi, A. Taylor, S. Chatterjee, R. Jain, S. Burgess and M. Goldbaum, Content-Based Retrieval of Opthalmological Images, IEEE International Conference on Image Processing, Vol. ICIP-96, 1996.

7. Hoshen, J., M. W. Berry and K. S. Minser, Percolation and Cluster Structure Parameters. II. The Enhanced Hoshen-Kopelman Algorithm, Physical Review E **56**(2) (1997), 1455-1460.

8. Hoshen, J. and R. Kopelman, Percolation and Cluster Distribution. I. Cluster Multiple Labeling Technique and Critical Concentration Algorithm, Physical Review B **14** (1976), 3438-3445.

9. Murphy, R. P., Management of Diabetic Retinopathy, American Family Physician **51**(4) (1995), 785–796.

10. Olk, R. W. and C. M. Lee, *Diabetic Retinopathy: Practical Management*, J. B. Lippincott Company, Philadelphia, 1993.

11. Packard, N. H. and S. Wolfram, Two-Dimensional Cellular Automata, J. Statistical Physics **38** (1985), 901–946.

12. Plotnick, R. E. and R. H. Gardner, Lattices and Landscapes, American Mathematical Society Series: *Lectures on Mathematics in the Life Sciences* **23** (1993), 129–17.

13. Pratt, W. K., *Digital Image Processing*, Second Edition, John Wiley, New York, 1991.

14. Stauffer, D. and A. Aharony, *Introduction to Percolation Theory*, Taylor & Francis Ltd, London, 1991.

Tuberculosis: The Evolution of Antibiotic Resistance and the Design of Epidemic Control Strategies

Sally Blower, Travis Porco and Tom Lietman

Abstract. Epidemic control strategies alter the competitive dynamics between drug-sensitive and drug-resistant pathogens. In this paper, we describe and discuss a mathematical model that can be used to understand, and to predict, the effects of epidemic control strategies on both drug-sensitive and drug-resistant *Mycobacterium tuberculosis*. We begin by briefly reviewing the structure of the model. We then present new analytical results, and show how these results can be used: (i) to predict the epidemiological outcomes of epidemic control strategies and (ii) to design epidemic control strategies. We also include two new factors in our epidemic control models (reinfection and treatment delay); we discuss the epidemiological consequences of these two factors in the design of control strategies. Finally, we conclude with a brief discussion of the implications of our theoretical results for tuberculosis control in light of recently reported results from the WHO's Global Project on Anti-tuberculosis Drug Resistance Surveillance.

§1. Introduction

A third of the world's population has been infected with *Mycobacterium tuberculosis* [3]. Tuberculosis accounts for more deaths among adults than all other infectious diseases combined. Recently, the World Health Organization (WHO) has estimated that over 30 million adults will die from tuberculosis in the next decade unless effective global control programs are successfully implemented. Effective treatment of patients with active tuberculosis requires a multiple drug regimen for as long as 6 to 12 months. Treatment is highly effective (with a 95% cure rate) if the patient harbors drug-sensitive pathogens and is compliant with the treatment regimen [1]. Treatment cures drug-sensitive cases, but inadequate treatment can generate drug resistance. Acquired drug

Mathematical Models in Medical and Health Sciences
Mary Ann Horn, Gieri Simonett, and Glenn Webb (eds.), pp. 51–72.
Copyright © 1998 by Vanderbilt University Press, Nashville, TN.
ISBN 0-8265-1310-7.

resistance may quickly emerge if patients are noncompliant, or if they receive ineffective or inappropriate treatment. Tuberculosis patients who develop acquired drug resistance can then generate primary drug resistance by transmitting drug-resistant *M.tuberculosis* to susceptible individuals. Hence, the design of effective tuberculosis control strategies is a complex problem, because treatment can produce opposing effects at the epidemic-level. Indeed, the emergence of drug resistance has created a significant problem for tuberculosis control programs in both developing and developed countries [11]. The WHO has recently estimated that up to 50 million people worldwide may already carry drug-resistant strains [27]. In this paper, we show how transmission models can be used as health policy tools to design new and effective tuberculosis control strategies based upon a theoretical understanding of the underlying epidemic dynamics.

A transmission model consists of a series of equations that are formulated based upon specific biological assumptions about the transmission processes, the treatment regimens and the pathogenic mechanisms of any specified pathogen. Such models contain explicit mechanisms that translate the risk behavior of an individual into a population-level outcome such as incidence (number of new infections or cases per unit time) or prevalence (number of infections or cases at any specified time). Hence, transmission models can be used as health policy tools to understand and to predict the epidemiological consequences of medical or behavioral interventions. Previously, transmission models (that assume that all pathogens are drug-sensitive) have been used to suggest rational epidemic control strategies for many infectious diseases; for a review see [2], and for specific examples see [5,6,9]. Only very few epidemic control models have been formulated that include the dynamics of drug-resistant pathogens [9,10,13,17,20].

The first mathematical model of a tuberculosis epidemic was published by Waaler, Geser and Andersen in 1962 [26], but the first transmission model that included the dynamics of both drug-sensitive and drug-resistant tuberculosis was not published until 34 years later by Blower, Small and Hopewell [9]. Blower et al. have developed a series of transmission models that can be used for understanding, predicting and controlling tuberculosis epidemics [9,4,7,18,21,22]. In their earliest studies they focused on formulating mathematical models of untreated tuberculosis epidemics; they analyzed these models in order to provide new understanding of the historical epidemiology of tuberculosis [7,18,21,22]. They have analyzed these models in order to derive the epidemic doubling time, calculate the probable length of a tuberculosis epidemic (which was found to be approximately 100 years), estimate the value of the basic reproduction number, and quantitatively assess how three linked time-lagged sub-epidemics (that are the result of progressive primary disease, endogeneous reactivation and relapse tuberculosis) combine to produce a single epidemic cycle [7,18,21,22]. They have also assessed the effect that tuberculosis epidemics may have had in the historical decline of leprosy epidemics [18].

Tab. 1. Parameter Definitions.

Symbol	Definition
Π	Recruitment rate of susceptibles
$1/\mu$	Average life expectancy
p	Proportion of new infections that directly progress to disease
v	Average per capita progression rate to disease (for latently infected individuals)
σ	Per capita effective chemoprophylaxis rate
μ_T	Average per capita mortality rate due to tuberculosis
ϕ	Per capita effective treatment rate
δ	Relative treatment efficacy

Blower et al. have also used their tuberculosis transmission models as a basis for designing a series of new epidemic control models [4,9]. One of these models can be used to understand, and to predict, the epidemic-level effects of control strategies on both drug-sensitive and drug-resistant *M.tuberculosis* [4,9]. In this paper, we briefly review the structure of this model (section 2). We then present new analytical results from this model, and show how these results can be used: (i) to predict the epidemiological outcomes of control strategies (section 3) and (ii) to design epidemic control strategies (section 4). We also include two new factors in our epidemic control models (reinfection (section 5) and treatment delay (section 6)); we discuss the epidemiological consequences of these two factors in the design of control strategies. Finally, we conclude with a brief discussion of the implications of our theoretical results for tuberculosis control in light of recently reported results from the WHO's Global Project on Anti-tuberculosis Drug Resistance Surveillance (section 7).

§2. Transmission Dynamics of Drug-sensitive and Drug-resistant M.tuberculosis: An Epidemic Control Model

Blower et al. have previously formulated a transmission model that links the transmission dynamics of both drug-sensitive and drug-resistant pathogens [4,9]. In this epidemic control model, both the drug-sensitive and the drug-resistant epidemics are driven by their own transmission dynamics. However, the epidemics are also linked, because a drug-sensitive case can be transformed into a drug-resistant case when (for whatever reason) treatment fails and acquired resistance develops. The epidemic control model consists of eight ordinary differential equations; susceptibles (X), latently infecteds (L), latently infecteds who have received effective chemoprophylaxis (C_S), infectious cases (T), and effectively treated cases (E), where the subscript defines whether the pathogen is drug-sensitive (S) or drug-resistant (R). All parameters are defined in Table 1.

$$\frac{dX}{dt} = \Pi - X(\beta_S T_S + \beta_R T_R) - \mu X, \tag{1}$$

$$\frac{dL_S}{dt} = (1-p)\beta_S T_S X - (v + \mu + \sigma)L_S, \tag{2}$$

$$\frac{dL_R}{dt} = (1-p)\beta_R T_R X - (v + \mu)L_R, \tag{3}$$

$$\frac{dC_S}{dt} = \sigma L_S - \mu C_S, \tag{4}$$

$$\frac{dT_S}{dt} = p\beta_S T_S X + v L_S - (\mu + \mu_T + \phi)T_S, \tag{5}$$

$$\frac{dT_R}{dt} = p\beta_R T_R X + v L_R + \phi r T_S - (\mu + \mu_T + \delta\phi)T_R, \tag{6}$$

$$\frac{dE_S}{dt} = \phi(1-r)T_S - \mu E_S, \tag{7}$$

$$\frac{dE_R}{dt} = \delta\phi T_R - \mu E_R. \tag{8}$$

The size of the susceptible subgroup (X) increases as individuals enter the community (at rate Π) and decreases as individuals: (i) die (at a per capita background rate μ); (ii) become infected with either drug-sensitive tuberculosis (at rate $X\beta_S T_S$); or (iii) drug-resistant tuberculosis (at rate $X\beta_R T_R$); β_S represents the transmission coefficient for the drug-sensitive pathogen, and β_R represents the transmission coefficient for the drug-resistant pathogen. We have assumed that genetic mutations resulting in drug resistance impose a "fitness cost" which is expressed in terms of a reduction in transmissibility (i.e., infectivity) relative to drug-sensitive strains [4,9]; thus $\beta_R = \alpha\beta_S$, where α specifies the relative transmissibility. This "fitness cost" has been observed *in vivo* by experiments in which monkeys were infected with either isoniazid-sensitive or isoniazid-resistant bacilli [23]. The degree to which β_R is less than β_S (i.e., the value of α) determines how much more transmissible the drug-sensitive strains will be than the drug-resistant strains.

A proportion $(1-p)$ of the newly infected will become latently infected; such latently-infected individuals are non-infectious. Individuals who are latently infected with drug-sensitive tuberculosis (L_S) will either: (i) progress to active disease (at a per capita rate v); (ii) die (at a per capita background rate μ); or (iii) receive effective chemoprophylaxis, which will prevent progression to disease (at a per capita rate σ). Individuals latently infected with drug-resistant tuberculosis (L_R) will either: (i) progress to active disease (at a per capita rate v) or (ii) die (at a per capita background rate μ); chemoprophylaxis is ineffective in preventing disease progression in these individuals. The number of drug-sensitive tuberculosis cases (T_S) will increase due: (i) to newly infected individuals developing primary progressive disease (at rate $p\beta_S T_S X$; where p represents the probability that a newly infected individual will develop primary progressive disease) and (ii) to latently infected individuals developing disease due to endogeneous reactivation (at rate vL_S). Individuals who have drug-sensitive tuberculosis (T_S) experience three competing exponential risks: (i) effective treatment, at per capita rate ϕ; (ii) death due to tuberculosis, at per capita rate μ_T; and (iii) death due to other causes, at a per capita rate μ. Thus, the residence times in the T_S state are exponentially distributed with mean $1/(\mu + \mu_T + \phi)$, and the probability that an individual in the T_S state will undergo effective treatment (instead of dying before treatment) is $\phi/(\mu + \mu_T + \phi) = F_T$, the fraction treated. Since $\phi = F_T(\mu + \mu_T)/(1 - F_T)$, as the fraction treated approaches one, the mean residence time in the T_S state (i.e., the time infectious) approaches zero.

The parameter r specifies the probability that treatment fails (due to the development of antibiotic resistance) and that acquired drug resistance develops during the treatment of a drug-sensitive case. Treatment of a drug-sensitive case can therefore result in one of three outcomes: (i) treatment can cure the patient (cases are removed from the T_S state at a rate equal to $\phi(1-r)$); (ii) treatment can fail and the patient acquires drug resistance (cases are removed from the T_S state at a rate equal to ϕr, and enter the T_R state); or (iii) treatment can fail and the patient remains infected with drug-sensitive tuberculosis (such treated cases remain in the T_S state). The number of drug-resistant tuberculosis cases (T_R) increases as a result of primary drug resistance due: (i) to newly infected individuals developing primary progressive disease (at rate $p\beta_R T_R X$) and (ii) to latently infected individuals developing tuberculosis due to endogeneous reactivation (at rate vL_R). The number of drug-resistant tuberculosis cases (T_R) also increases due to acquired drug resistance at rate $\phi r T_S$. It is assumed that drug-resistant cases can be treated, but less effectively than drug-sensitive cases; the relative treatment efficacy of drug-resistant cases (in comparison with treatment of drug-sensitive cases) is denoted by the parameter δ. Hence, drug-resistant cases are untreatable (and/or untreated) if $\delta = 0$, drug-resistant and drug-sensitive cases are treated with equal effectiveness if $\delta = 1$, and drug-resistant cases are only partially effectively treated if $0 < \delta < 1$. Hence, the model includes the possibility that treatment of a drug-resistant case can result in one of two outcomes: (i) treatment can cure the patient (cases are removed from the T_R state at a rate equal to $\delta\phi$) or (ii) treatment failure occurs (treated cases remain in the T_R state). Hence, the number of drug-resistant cases (T_R) decreases as individuals die (at a per capita background rate μ or due to tuberculosis at a per capita rate μ_T) or are treated (at a per capita rate $\delta\phi$).

2.1. Single versus multiple drug resistance

The structure of the epidemic control model (specified by equations (1-8)) may be used for understanding and predicting the emergence of strains of *M. tuberculosis* that are resistant to either single and multiple drug regimens. In order to model the emergence of single versus multiple drug resistance, it is necessary to vary only the values of two of the parameters: r (the probability that treatment failure occurs due to the development of antibiotic resistance during a particular drug regimen) and δ (the relative treatment efficacy of drug-resistant cases). In practice with monotherapy, acquired drug resistance develops quickly with a very high probability; for example, if patients are treated with a single drug, such as only isoniazid (INH), then 71% develop drug resistance within three months [19]. Cases that are resistant to only a single drug (such as INH) are usually curable if at least two other active drugs are included in their regimen. Infections with *M.tuberculosis* strains that are resistant to both isoniazid and rifampin (termed multidrug-resistant, or MDR) arise less frequently than those which are resistant to a single drug, but such cases are more difficult to treat; cure rates of MDR tuberculosis can be as low as 56% [15] compared with cure rates of almost 95% for drug-sensitive cases [14]. The model can be used to understand and to predict the emergence of single drug resistance in a developed country (where multiple drug regimens are readily available and single drug resistance is usually cured), in which case r and δ are both relatively high. In order to understand and to predict the emergence of single drug resistance in some developing countries, a high value for r should be used, but δ should be set to almost zero (because even cases that are only resistant to a single drug will not receive effective treatment). The model can also be used to understand and to predict the emergence of MDR *M.tuberculosis* by using an extremely low value for r and either a moderate value for δ (to model the situation in developed countries) or a low value for δ (to model the situation in developed countries).

2.2. Endemic equilibria

The epidemic control model (specified by equations (1-8)) can be solved under equilibrium conditions; the endemic equilibria are given in equations (9-16).

$$\hat{X} = \frac{\Pi}{\mu R_S}, \tag{9}$$

$$\hat{L}_S = \frac{(1-p)\beta_S \hat{X} \hat{T}_S}{\sigma + v + \mu}, \tag{10}$$

$$\hat{L}_R = \frac{(1-p)\beta_R \hat{X} \hat{T}_R}{v + \mu}, \tag{11}$$

$$\hat{C}_S = \frac{\sigma \hat{L}_S}{\mu}, \tag{12}$$

$$\hat{T}_S = \frac{(R_S - 1)\mu}{\left[\beta_S + \frac{\beta_R \phi r}{(\mu + \mu_T + e\phi)(1 - R_{DR})} \right]}, \tag{13}$$

$$\hat{T}_R = \frac{\phi r \hat{T}_S}{(\mu + \mu_T + e\phi)(1 - R_{DR})}, \tag{14}$$

$$\hat{E}_S = \frac{\phi(1-r)\hat{T}_S}{\mu}, \tag{15}$$

$$\hat{E}_R = \frac{\delta \phi \hat{T}_R}{\mu}. \tag{16}$$

Rearrangement of equation (14) reveals the mathematical relationship shown in equation (17), which illuminates the biological relationship (at equilibrium) between the drug-sensitive and the drug-resistant pathogens. Equation (17) shows that the number of drug-resistant cases (at equilibrium) can be decomposed into two sources; one source is due to the generation of acquired drug resistance (the first component on the right hand side of the equation) and the other source is due to the generation of primary drug resistance (which is specified by the second component on the right hand side of the equation):

$$\hat{T}_R = \frac{\phi r \hat{T}_S}{\mu + \mu_T + e\phi} + \hat{T}_R R_{DR}, \quad \text{where } R_{DR} = \frac{R_R}{R_S},$$

$$R_R = \left(\frac{\beta_R \Pi}{\mu}\right)\left(\frac{1}{\delta\phi + \mu + \mu_T}\right)\left(p + \frac{(1-p)v}{v + \mu}\right),$$

$$R_S = \left(\frac{\beta_S \Pi}{\mu}\right)\left(\frac{1}{\phi + \mu + \mu_T}\right)\left(p + \frac{(1-p)v}{\sigma + v + \mu}\right).$$

$\qquad(17)$

R_{DR} is defined as the average number of secondary infectious cases of primary drug resistance that are produced by one drug-resistant case when drug-sensitive tuberculosis is at equilibrium [4,9]; consequently, R_{DR} is also a measure of the relative fitness of drug-resistant pathogens relative to drug-sensitive pathogens in the presence of a control program. R_S and R_R specify the effective reproduction number for drug-sensitive and drug-resistant tuberculosis respectively, where the effective reproduction number is defined as the average number of secondary infectious cases that are produced when one infectious case is introduced into a disease-free population in which a control program is in place [9]. In the absence of treatment ($\phi = 0$) and chemoprophylaxis ($\sigma = 0$), the effective reproduction number reduces to the basic reproduction number (R_0) (see [7]). In the absence of any control efforts (i.e., when $\phi = 0$ and $\sigma = 0$) then the relative fitness R_{DR} is equivalent to the relative transmissibility of the drug-resistant strains in relation to the drug-sensitive strains (i.e., $R_{DR} = \beta_R/\beta_S = \alpha$), since all the other parameters are the same for the drug-sensitive and the drug-resistant strains.

§3. Predicting the Outcomes of Epidemic Control Strategies

Epidemic control strategies alter the competitive dynamics between the drug-sensitive and the drug-resistant pathogen. Our epidemic control model (described in section 1) can be used to predict both the long-term (equilibrium) epidemiological outcomes, and the short-term (transient dynamics) of control strategies. Any epidemic control strategy can be defined simply by specifying particular values for the three control parameters in the model: the per capita effective treatment rate for active tuberculosis cases (ϕ), the probability of acquired resistance emerging during treatment (r), and the relative treatment efficacy of drug-resistant cases (δ). The parameter ϕ specifies the per capita effective treatment rate for drug-sensitive cases, and hence ϕ is calculated as the product of the actual treatment rate and the efficacy of treatment for these cases. The effect of any specified control strategy (as defined by the three treatment parameters: ϕ, r and δ) on the long-term (equilibrium) epidemiological outcome can be predicted by calculating the value of the fitness (as specified by the effective reproduction number, R) of both drug-sensitive (R_S) and drug-resistant (R_R) tuberculosis. If acquired drug resistance can emerge (i.e., $r > 0$), then only three equilibrium epidemiological outcomes are possible: (i) eradication of both drug-sensitive and drug-resistant tuberculosis if $R_S < 1$ and $R_R < 1$; (ii) persistence of only drug-resistant tuberculosis (i.e., eradication of only drug-sensitive tuberculosis) if $R_R > 1$ and $R_R > R_S$; or (iii) persistence of both drug-sensitive and drug-resistant tuberculosis (i.e., co-existence) if $R_S > 1$ and $R_S > R_R$ [4]. Whenever treatment occurs and $r > 0$, drug-resistant tuberculosis will always be present, unless tuberculosis is eradicated entirely. The endemic prevalence (or incidence) of infection and/or disease that will occur as the result of the specified control strategy can then be predicted by using equations (9-16).

The long-term epidemiological outcomes of a variety of different control strategies that were chosen to reflect treatment conditions in a hypothetical developing country are shown graphically in Figure 1. The baseline control strategy was defined to be $F_T = 0.5$, $r = 0.2$, and $\delta = 0.0$; it was assumed that $\alpha = 0.25$, see the figure legend for the other parameter values. Figure 1A shows the effect on the reproductive number of varying only the treatment rate (in terms of the fraction of cases that receive treatment (F_T)), Figure 1B shows the effect of varying only the probability of acquired drug resistance developing during treatment (r), Figure 1C shows the effect of varying only the relative efficacy of treatment of drug-resistant cases (δ) and Figure 1D shows the effect of the relative transmissibility of drug-resistance (α). Depending upon the treatment rate, two long-term epidemiological outcomes are possible: If treatment rates are low to fairly high, then both drug-resistant and drug-sensitive pathogens will co-exist, but if treatment rates are very high, then ultimately only drug-resistant tuberculosis will remain (Figure 1A). The relative transmissibility (α) of drug-resistant strains is also extremely important in determining the long-term epidemiological outcomes of control strategies (Figure 1D). If the relative transmissibility of the drug-resistant strain is low to moderate ($\alpha < 0.5$), then both drug-resistant and drug-sensitive pathogens will co-exist, but if the relative transmissibility is moderate to high ($\alpha > 0.5$), then control strategies will enable drug-resistant tuberculosis to eventually out-compete drug-sensitive tuberculosis (Figure 1D). However, both the value of the probability of acquired drug resistance developing during treatment (r) and the value of the relative efficacy of treatment of drug-resistant cases (δ) do not affect the long-term epidemiological outcomes; for all values of r and δ shown in Figure 1B and 1C both drug-sensitive and drug-resistant pathogens will co-exist.

The epidemic control strategies that are illustrated in Figure 1 will have a wide variety of effects on the endemic prevalence of disease; these effects were predicted by using equations (9-16), and the results are shown graphically in Figure 2. Figure 2 illustrates how the endemic prevalence of disease varies as a function of: The treatment rate (in terms of the fraction of cases that receive treatment (F_T)) (Figure 2A), the probability of acquired drug resistance developing during treatment (r) (Figure 2B), the relative efficacy of treatment of

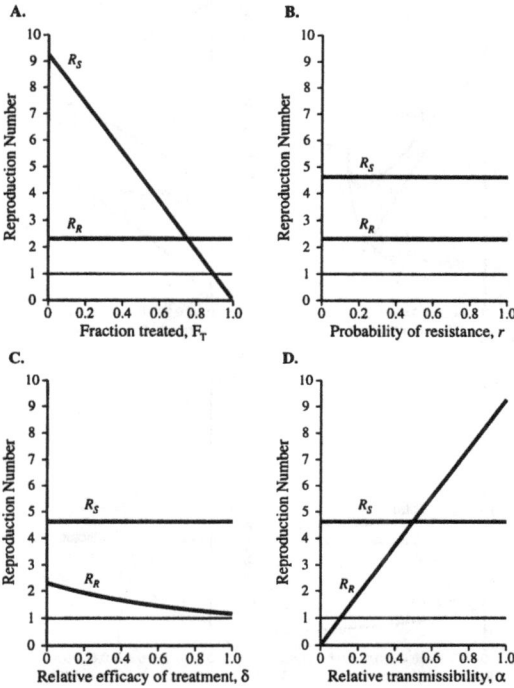

Fig. 1. The reproduction numbers of drug-sensitive (R_S) and drug-resistant (R_R) tuberculosis under conditions in a hypothetical devloping country: $\beta = 0.0001$ persons/year, $\Pi = 2200$ persons/year, $\mu = 0.022$/year, $\mu_T = 0.139$/year, $v = 0.00256$/year, $p = 0.05$. A) The fraction of cases that receive treatment, F_T, is varied. B) The probability of acquired resistance developing during treatment, r, is varied. C) The relative efficacy of treatment of drug-resistant tuberculosis, δ, is varied. D) The relative transmissibility of drug-resistant strains, α, is varied. Baseline treatment and drug resistance parameters are: $F_T = 0.50$, $r = 0.20$, $\delta = 0.0$ and $\alpha = 0.25$.

drug-resistant cases (δ) (Figure 2C) and the relative transmissibility of drug-resistance (α) (Figure 2D). Figure 2A concurs with our previous result, that increasing treatment rates can sometimes produce a perverse outcome [4,9]. Increasing the treatment rate will decrease the overall endemic prevalence of disease (when drug-sensitive and drug-resistant strains co-exist); however, once the treatment rate is high enough to switch the competitive balance between the drug-resistant and the drug-sensitive strains, then increasing the treatment rate can increase the overall endemic prevalence of disease (Figure 2A). The probability that acquired drug resistance will emerge during treatment, r, has a significant effect on the endemic prevalence of disease;

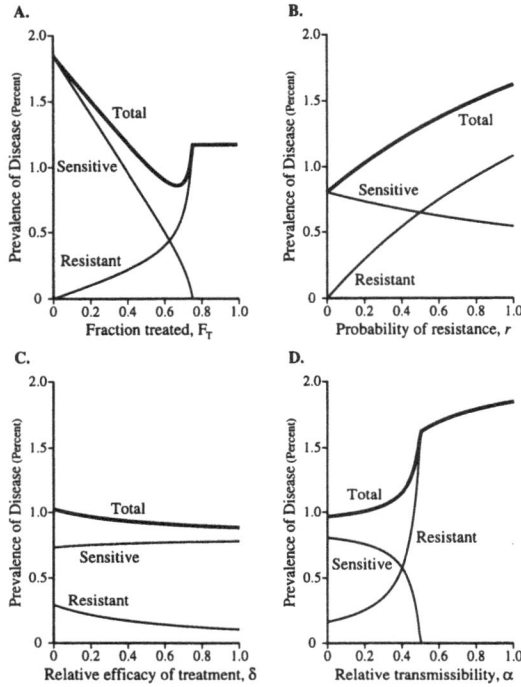

Fig. 2. The (equilibrium) prevalence of tuberculosis, plotted for drug-sensitive, drug-resistant and total (drug-sensitive plus drug-resistant) strains. The same parameters are used as for Figure 1. A) The fraction of cases that receive treatment, F_T, is varied. B) The probability of acquired resistance developing during treatment, r, is varied. C) The relative efficacy of treatment of drug-resistant tuberculosis, δ, is varied. D) The relative transmissibility of drug-resistant strains, α, is varied.

a high value of r will generate a high endemic prevalence of disease, even if treatment rates are moderately high (Figure 2B). Conversely, increasing the efficacy with which drug-resistant cases are treated (i.e., increasing the value of δ) will always decrease the overall endemic prevalence of disease (Figure 2C). The endemic prevalence of disease that will occur as the result of any particular control strategy will be highly dependent upon the transmissibility of drug resistance; drug-resistant strains that are moderate to highly transmissible will significantly increase the burden of disease (Figure 2D). If drug-resistant strains emerge that are more transmissible than drug-sensitive strains (i.e., $\beta_R > \beta_S$), then the drug-resistant strains will eventually outcompete the drug-sensitive strains and finally all cases of tuberculosis will be drug-resistant.

Tuberculosis epidemics rise and fall over a period of many decades or even hundreds of years [7,21]; hence, tuberculosis epidemic dynamics are very slow in comparison to the epidemic dynamics of many other infectious diseases. Previously we have shown that these slow dynamics ensure that it can take many decades for both drug-sensitive and drug-resistant tuberculosis to reach the endemic equilibrium [4]. Consequently, when predicting the epidemiological outcomes of control strategies it is very important to also assess the transient dynamics. Our epidemic control model can also be used to assess the short-term (transient dynamics) of the effects of control strategies through scenario analyses (as we have done previously [4]) or by uncertainty and sensitivity analyses based upon Latin Hypercube Sampling (as we have done previously in order to quantify the intrinsic transmission dynamics of tuberculosis epidemics [7] and to predict the emergence of antiviral resistance [8]).

§4. Designing Epidemic Control Strategies

Our epidemic control model can be used to design both eradicating and non-eradicating tuberculosis control strategies. In order to eradicate tuberculosis in the absence of drug-resistance, it is only necessary to specify the critical value of the treatment rate (ϕ_c) that will ensure that $R_S = 1$ [9]. However, in order to design control strategies that will result in disease eradication in the presence of drug-resistance, since both drug-sensitive and drug-resistant strains need to be eradicated, the eradication criteria are that $R_S < 1$ and $R_R < 1$ [4]. As is apparent from equation (14), only two of the three control parameters in our model affect this eradication criteria: The per capita effective treatment rate for active tuberculosis cases (ϕ) and the relative treatment efficacy of drug-resistant cases (δ). Although r (the value of the probability of acquired drug resistance emerging during treatment) significantly affects the level of the endemic prevalence of disease (Figure 2C), it does not affect the eradication conditions.

The critical (minimum) values of ϕ and δ (i.e., ϕ_c and δ_c) that will ensure disease eradication in the presence of drug resistance can be caluculated by setting the expressions for R_S and R_R, given in equation (14), to unity and then simultaneously solving for ϕ_c and δ_c. An example of such calculations is shown in the four graphs in Figure 3, where the only parameter that is varied is the relative transmissibility of drug-resistance (α) (see the figure legend for parameter values). In each graph, ϕ_c and δ_c are plotted separately for drug-sensitive and drug-resistant tuberculosis, hence, the two plotted functions represent $R_S = 1$ and $R_R = 1$, respectively. The area that is bounded by both these functions delimits the parameter space that will ensure disease eradication ($R_S < 1$ and $R_R < 1$); these regions are shaded in Figure 3. To eradicate tuberculosis, it is necessary to treat a high fraction ($F_T = 0.9$) of the drug-sensitive cases (Figure 3); this fraction is independent of the value of δ and α. It is also necessary to treat a high fraction of the drug-resistant cases (Figure 3); however, this fraction depends upon both the relative transmissibility of drug resistance (α) and the relative efficacy of treatment of

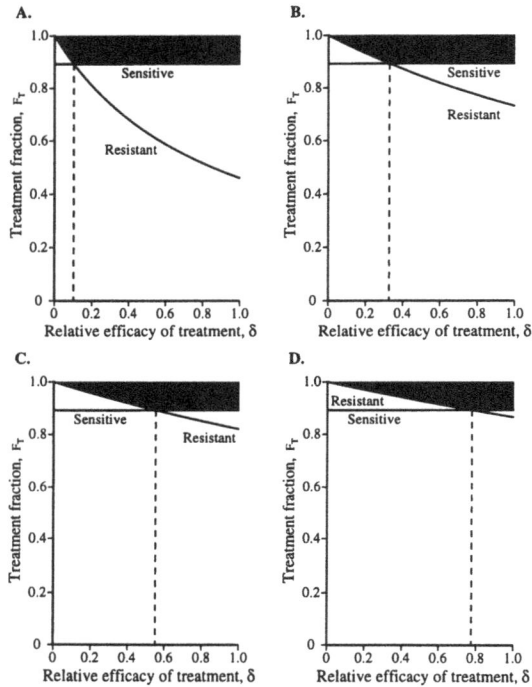

Fig. 3. Combinations or treatment fraction, F_T, and relative efficacy of treatment of drug-resistance (δ) that will result in the eradication of drug-resistant and drug-sensitive strains are plotted. Drug-sensitive strains and drug-resistant strains will be eradicated with combinations of F_T and δ above the curves labeled "sensitive" and "resistant," respectively. Tuberculosis, i.e., both drug-sensitive and drug-resistant strains, will be eradicated in the shaded areas. The relative transmissibility of drug-resistant strains, α, is taken to be: A) $\alpha = 0.2$, B) $\alpha = 0.4$, C) $\alpha = 0.6$ and D) $\alpha = 0.8$.

drug-resistant cases (δ). More transmissible drug-resistant strains have to be treated with a greater relative efficacy of treatment in order to achieve eradication (compare Figures 3A, 3B, 3C and 3D). Obviously, as many cases of both drug-sensitive and drug-resistant cases should be treated with as great an efficacy of treatment as possible. If a high treatment rate of drug-resistant cases is coupled with a high efficacy of treatment such that the actual values of ϕ and δ become greater than the calculated critical (minimum) eradication values of ϕ_c and δ_c (plotted in Figure 3), then disease eradication will progress at an even faster rate.

Our model can also be used to design non-eradicating control strategies for a variety of different epidemiological goals [4]. For example, if the specified epidemiological goal was a particular endemic prevalence of disease, then a control strategy could be specified by using equations (9-17) to calculate prevalence, assuming different values for r and δ, and then solving for ϕ under these conditions. To decide upon the appropriate treatment rate that is necessary to achieve the desired goal, ϕ could then be used to calculate the proportion of tuberculosis cases that would need to receive effective treatment per unit time [9].

§5. Reinfection and the Design of Epidemic Control Strategies

In our previous studies of tuberculosis transmission models, we did not include the possibility that individuals who are latently infected with *M.tuberculosis* could become reinfected; this process is known as exogeneous reinfection. The significance of the role of exogeneous reinfection in the epidemiology of tuberculosis is controversial. There are both animal and clinical data from which it can be inferred that it is much more difficult to reinfect than to infect, except when there is immune compromise; consequently, we did not initially include the process of exogeneous reinfection in our original analyses of tuberculosis epidemics in immunocompetent populations. In order to quantify the role of exogeneous reinfection in the transmission of *M.tuberculosis*, and to assess the implications of this process for the design of control strategies, we have now included the process of exogeneous reinfection in the original model specified in section 1. In order to aid clarity in the analysis, we set $r = 0$, and $\sigma = 0$; consequently, this reinfection model is specified by the following equations:

$$\frac{dX}{dt} = \Pi - X\beta T - \mu X, \tag{18}$$

$$\frac{dL}{dt} = (1-p)\beta TX - (v + \mu + p\theta\beta T)L, \tag{19}$$

$$\frac{dT}{dt} = p\beta TX + (v + p\theta\beta T)L - (\mu + \mu_T + \phi)T, \tag{20}$$

$$\frac{dE}{dt} = \phi T - \mu E. \tag{21}$$

The number of cases of infectious tuberculosis (T) increases due: (i) to newly infected individuals developing primary progressive disease (at rate $p\beta TX$); (ii) to latently infected individuals developing disease due to endogeneous reactivation (at rate vL_S); and (iii) to latently infected individuals developing disease due to exogeneous reinfection (at rate $p\theta\beta TL$, where θ reflects the susceptibility to reinfection, i.e., the per individual degree of naturally induced immunity against reinfection). A latently infected individual is as susceptible to reinfection as a susceptible individual is to fast progression with an initial infection with *M.tuberculosis* if $\theta = 1$, a latently infected individual is partially protected against reinfection if $0 < \theta < 1$, and a latently infected individual is immune to reinfection if $\theta = 0$ (in this case the reinfection model reduces to

our previously published model without reinfection [9]). The contribution of
exogeneous reinfection (CER) to the transmission of tuberculosis at any given
can be calculated from equation (22):

$$CER = \frac{p\theta\beta T(t)L(t)}{I(t)},\tag{22}$$

where $I(t) = p\beta T(t)X(t) + vL(t) + p\theta\beta T(t)L(t)$ is the total incidence of disease at time t. The contribution of exogeneous reinfection to the transmission
of tuberculosis during an epidemic is time-dependent; clearly exogeneous reinfection can play a significant role in tuberculosis transmission if $\theta > 0$ and
when there is a high prevalence of latent infection (Figure 4A).

We assessed the epidemiological implications of exogeneous reinfection for
the design of control strategies. The expressions for the basic reproduction
number (R_0) and the effective reproduction number (R) for the reinfection
model, specified by equations (18-21), are identical to our previously derived
R_0 and R for our previous tuberculosis transmission models that did not
include the process of exogeneous reinfection [4,9,7,21,22]. The degree to
which a latently infected individual is susceptible to reinfection (θ) does not
affect the invasion condition, because when $M.tuberculosis$ initially invades
there are no latently infected individuals present to be reinfected. Exogeneous
reinfection (i.e., $\theta > 0$) does not change the value of R_0 or R, but it does
change the endemic equilibria. For any specified value of R_0, as the value
of θ increases, both the prevalence of infection and the prevalence of disease
will increase (Figure 4B); the more severe the epidemic (as measured by R_0),
the more dramatic the effect of reinfection will be in increasing the prevalence
(Figure 4B). Exogeneous reinfection also "inflates" the incidence rate (when
the prevalence of latent infection is high); hence, the value of R_0 that is
necessary to generate a specified incidence rate decreases as the value of θ
increases (Figure 4C). Therefore a high incidence rate can be the result of
the severity of the epidemic (i.e., due to a high R_0) or simply due to the fact
that latently infected individuals have a high susceptibility to reinfection (i.e.,
due to a low/moderate R_0 coupled with a high θ). For example, an R_0 of 6.0
would generate an equilibrium disease incidence rate of 262 cases/100,000/year
if latently infected individuals were completely protected against exogeneous
reinfection $(\theta = 0)$), but if exogeneous reinfection could occur (and $\theta = 0.5$)
an R_0 of only 2.9 would generate the same incidence rate (Figure 4C).

For any particular (endemic equilibrium) incidence rate, the higher the
susceptibility to reinfection the easier it will be to achieve eradication (Figure 4C and 4D). For example, if susceptibility to reinfection is high ($\theta = 0.5$,
hence $R_0 = 2.9$), then only 71% of the cases need to be treated to achieve
eradication, but if reinfection cannot occur ($\theta = 0$, hence $R_0 = 6.0$), then 86%
of the cases need to be treated to eradicate tuberculosis (Figure 4C). This
effect occurs because, for a given equilibrium incidence: (i) the R_0 (for the
epidemic where $\theta \gg 0$) is less than the R_0 (for the epidemic where $\theta \sim 0$), and
(ii) the critical treatment rate that is necessary to eradicate tuberculosis (ϕ_c)
only depends on the value of R_0 (see [9] for previously calculated treatment

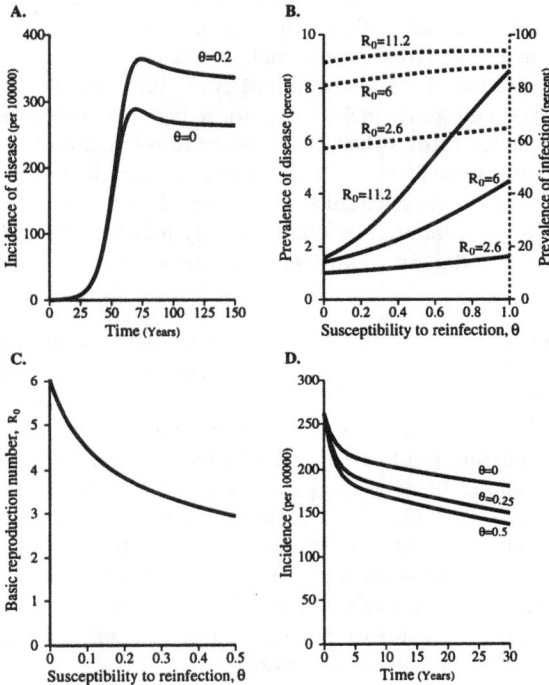

Fig. 4. Incidence (per 100,000 individuals per year) of disease is shown for two different assumptions concerning the degree of susceptibility to reinfection: $\theta = 0.20$ (i.e., reinfection is possible, but the individual is less susceptible than to the initial infection), and $\theta = 0.0$ (i.e., no reinfection is possible). For this figure, we added reinfection to the detailed tuberculosis model described in detail elsewhere [7]; this detailed model includes: (i) the possibility of recovery without treatment and; (ii) the development of noninfectious tuberculosis. One infectious case is introduced at time zero. The following parameters are used: $p = 0.05$, $\beta = 0.00007$, $\pi = 1333.33$, $f = 0.7$, $\mu = 0.013333$, $q = 0.85$, $v = 0.0026$, $c = 0.0575$, $\omega = 0.005$, and $\mu_T = 0.1386$. B) The relationship between the equilibrium prevalence of infection (dotted line) and disease (solid line) with the susceptibillity to reinfection (θ) is plotted, as θ increases from zero to one. Three different values of the basic reproduction number are shown; to plot this figure, we only varied β, all other parameters were held constant at the values used in Figure A. C) Values of the basic reproduction number calculated from the value of the β necessary to produce the same equilibrium incidence rate of disease for a given value of θ are shown; as the susceptibility to reinfection increases, β decreases, all other parameters are the same as in Figure A. D) Scenarios illustrating the decline in disease incidence following the introduction of a control program at time zero. All three scenarios begin at a constant incidence rate (as in Figure C) for each specified value of θ, the value of β is calculated to produce the constant incidence rate. All parameters are the same as in Figure A; the fraction treated (F_T) is 0.7.

rates for tuberculosis eradication). The transient dynamics of treatment are illustrated in three scenarios shown in Figure 4D; in these scenarios treatment is begun at time zero. These three scenarios have the same equilibrium disease incidence rate (when treatment is begun), but because these three epidemics have different θ's and different R_0's, they decline at different rates (Figure 4D). For any given incidence rate, it becomes progressively easier to reduce the incidence rate as the susceptibility to reinfection (θ) increases (Figure 4D). The disease incidence rate declines more rapidly when the reinfection susceptibility is the highest (Figure 4D). This effect of exogenous reinfection occurs, because the pool of individuals latently infected with $M.tuberculosis$ is progressively eliminated by treatment, and hence gradually ceases to "inflate" the incidence rate.

Our results illustrate that in order to design the appropriate control strategy it is extremely important to understand the causal transmission processes that are generating the incidence rate. In developed countries, where the prevalence of latent infection is low and treatment levels are at eradication levels [9], exogenous reinfection is a relatively minor component in tuberculosis transmission. In developing countries, where the prevalence of latent infection can be 50-70% [21] and treatment levels are low to moderate [9], exogeneous reinfection can play an important role in tuberculosis transmission. The effect of exogenous reinfection on the control of tuberculosis will depend not only on the treatment levels, the severity of the epidemic (i.e., the value of R_0), but also upon the value of θ; a high value of θ will facilitate eradication under the circumstances detailed above.

The role of exogenous reinfection in tuberculosis transmission remains controversial. At the population-level, the significance of exogenous reinfection can be determined simply by the proportion of tuberculosis cases that are due to reinfection at any given time; however, this proportion (and hence the significance) will vary with time (Figure 4A). Sutherland and Svandova have estimated the contribution of exogenous reinfection to the transmission of tuberculosis in the Netherlands over a twenty-five year period (1952-1967) [24]. Their analysis showed that the role of exogenous reinfection declined dramatically over this time period, as the prevalence of latent infection decreased. In order to quantify the role of exogenous reinfection to tuberculosis transmission the central question that needs to be answered is: What is the value of θ? Unfortunately, very few studies have been conducted that allow measurement of this parameter; Sutherland and Svandova stratified their data by gender and estimated that the probability of reinfection was 0.37 for men and 0.19 for women [24]. Recently molecular epidemiological studies have shown that reinfection with $M.tuberculosis$ in HIV-infected individuals may occur more frequently than reinfection in immunocompetent individuals; unfortunately, the sample sizes in these studies are too small to allow the estimation of θ. Futher empirical studies using molecular epidemiological techniques are necessary to estimate the value of θ in order to resolve the controversy of the role of reinfection in tuberculosis epidemiology.

§6. Treatment Delays and the Design of Epidemic Control Strategies

Previously we have used our tuberculosis transmission models to calculate the treatment rates that would lead to tuberculosis eradication, and to predict the effects of non-eradicating treatment levels on tuberculosis morbidity [4,9]. In these analyses, we modelled the residence time in the T_S state as being exponential, with the mean time given by the reciprocal of the total rate of removal $(\mu + \mu_T + \phi)$. Thus, increasing treatment rates continuously reduced transmission by reducing the average duration of infectiousness; as F_T approaches one, the average duration of infectiousness approaches zero. In practice, however, patients do not present for treatment as soon as they become infectious, and even if $F_T = 1$, individuals would still be expected to spend some time in the infectious state. Hence, we extended our basic model to allow a more general relationship between the treatment rate and the fraction treated. We modified the model specified by equations (1-8) (setting $r = 0$ for clarity) as follows. We let τ denote the minimum time to treatment (or treatment delay), so that whenever an individual becomes infectious, he or she will not be available for treatment until time τ has elapsed; let $T^{(0)}$ denote the number of such individuals. After time τ, those individuals (the fraction $e^{-(\mu+\mu_T)\tau}$) who survive the (competing) risks of death due to tuberculosis and due to other causes will then be subject to the constant per capita treatment rate ϕ as before; let $T^{(1)}$ denote the number of such individuals (hence, the total number of infectious cases, $T = T^{(0)} + T^{(1)}$). Thus no matter how high ϕ is, an individual will spend at least time τ in an infectious state. Consequently, in this model the rate of change of the number of infectious cases is specified by the following three equations:

$$\frac{dT^{(0)}}{dt} = I(t) - (\mu + \mu_T)T^{(0)}(t) - e^{-(\mu+\mu_T)\tau}I(t - \tau), \qquad (23)$$

$$\frac{dT^{(1)}}{dt} = e^{-(\mu+\mu_T)\tau}I(t - \tau) - (\mu + \mu_T + \phi)T^{(1)}(t), \qquad (24)$$

$$I(t) = p\beta_S X(t)\left(T_S^{(0)}(t) + T_S^{(1)}(t)\right) + vL_S(t). \qquad (25)$$

Including a treatment delay (τ) in the model changes the effective reproduction number, R. R for the model specified by equations (23-25) is given in equation (26):

$$R = \left(\frac{\beta\Pi}{\mu}\right)\left(\frac{1}{\mu + \mu_T} - \frac{e^{-(\mu+\mu_T)\tau}}{\mu + \mu_T} + \frac{e^{-(\mu+\mu_T)\tau}}{\phi + \mu + \mu_T}\right)\left(p + \frac{(1-p)v}{\sigma + v + \mu}\right) \quad (26)$$

When designing an epidemic control strategy, it is not only necessary to specify how many cases should be treated (i.e., the value of ϕ), but also how quickly they should be treated (i.e., how small should τ be) (Figure 5A). Both ϕ and τ are components of case-finding (i.e., they both determine how many cases of tuberculosis are effectively treated); the value of τ determines the minimum duration of infectiousness before treatment is possible, and the value of

ϕ determines the rate at which cases are found and effectively treated (once treatment is possible). This treatment delay model can be used to evaluate the explicit tradeoff, when designing control strategies, between ϕ and τ; i.e., as the length of the treatment delay (τ) increases, the treatment rate (ϕ) has to increase in order to achieve the same epidemic control effect. The tradeoff between ϕ and τ that ensures that $R = 1$ is shown in Figure 5B; hence, this figure shows the values of ϕ and τ that are necessary to eradicate tuberculosis. When the treatment delay is sufficiently large, no level of treatment (ϕ) directed at $T_S^{(1)}$ is capable of eradicating tuberculosis (Figure 5B). When drug resistance is included in the treatment delay model ($r > 0$), and treatment delays are included for both drug-sensitive and drug-resistant tuberculosis the situation becomes even more complex.

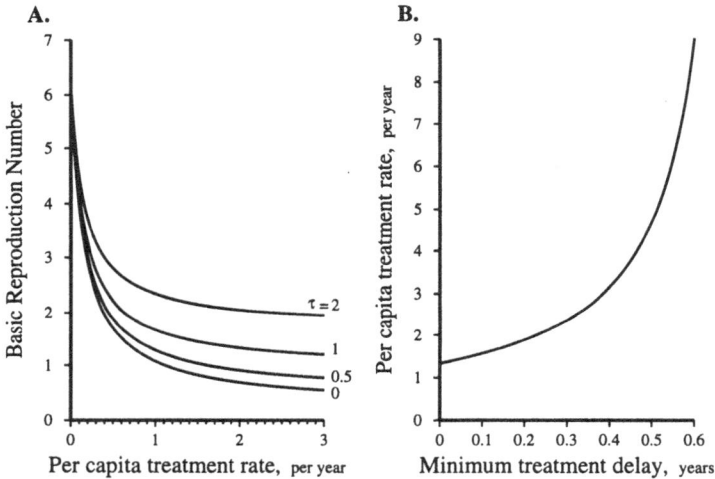

Fig. 5. A) The relationship between the average duration of infectiousness and the per capita treatment rate (ϕ) is displayed for treatment delays (τ) of 0, 0.5, 1 and 2 years. B) The relationship between the treatment delay (τ) and the per capita treatment rate (ϕ) necessary to eradicate tuberculosis. Combinations of τ and ϕ above the line will result in the eradication of tuberculosis.

Treatment delay can have two important effects on epidemic dynamics, treatment delay can: (i) increase the death rate (as individuals can die before they receive treatment) and (ii) increase the transmission of tuberculosis (as individuals are infectious until treated). Currently, almost nothing is known about the actual length of treatment delays. It is likely that in developed countries the treatment delay may be only a few months, but in some areas in certain developing countries the treatment delay may be several years. Our results suggest that it is essential: (i) to collect empirical data to determine the length of treatment delays throughout the world, and (ii) to increase active case-finding and community surveillance to reduce treatment delays.

§7. WHO's Global Project on Anti-tuberculosis Drug Resistance Surveillance and the Implications of Our Theoretical Results for Tuberculosis Control

Resistance of *M.tuberculosis* to antimycobacterial agents was reported in the 1960's soon after the introduction of effective chemotherapy [12,16,25]. Recently the WHO in collaboration with the International Union Against Tuberculosis and Lung Disease (IUATLD) has completed the first phase of a global surveillance project to assess the prevalence of anti-tuberculosis drug resistance [28]. The survey involved 35 countries on five continents; approximately 5,000 tuberculosis cases, from geographic areas that represented 20% of the world's population, were included [28]. Cases were tested for INH, rifampin (RMP), ethambutol (EMB) and streptomycin (SM) resistance. Prevalence of primary resistance (to any drug) varied from 2% (Czech Republic) to 41% (Dominican Republic), with a median prevalence of 10.4% [28]. Prevalence of acquired resistance (to any drug) varied from 5.3% (New Zealand) to 100% (Ivanovo Oblast, Russia), with a median prevalence of 36% [28]. WHO/IUATLD also suggest that their results are an underestimate of the problem, because the countries included in their surveillance survey had better tuberculosis control than average [28]. Their results illustrate that new tuberculosis control strategies may be necessary, particularly strategies that are targeted at preventing the transmission of drug resistance.

Our results imply that to prevent an explosive rise in drug resistance in developing countries, it is essential to not only increase treatment rates, improve case-holding rates and reduce treatment delays, but also to treat drug-resistant cases with effective drug regimens. Our current and previous analyses [4,9] have shown that if resistant strains are very transmissible, they will cause a very high incidence of primary drug resistance, and the emergence of such strains will ensure that certain epidemic control strategies are likely to be counterproductive. Hence, in order to predict the outcome of epidemic control strategies it is important to conduct empirical studies which can quantitatively measure the biology of drug-resistant strains. Laboratory and epidemiological data have indicated that the observed INH-resistant and multidrug-resistant (MDR) strains are of reduced fitness in comparison with drug-sensitive *M.tuberculosis* strains [28]; but further studies need to be conducted in order to assess the relative infectivity, pathogenicity and virulence of drug-resistant strains in comparison to drug-sensitive strains. Our analyses also illustrate that further empirical studies, perhaps based on collecting molecular epidemiological data, need to be conducted to determine the role of exogeneous reinfection and the effect of treatment delays in the transmission of tuberculosis.

In this paper, we have discussed a theoretical framework, based upon mathematical transmission models, for understanding tuberculosis epidemics.

We have shown how this framework can be used for predicting tuberculosis epidemic dynamics and for designing control strategies. The theoretical framework that we have discussed has significant implications for the development of health policy. Our analyses have shown that if efforts are only focused on controlling drug-sensitive tuberculosis and if the drug-resistant strains are fairly transmissible, then the drug-resistant epidemic is likely to continue to increase and tuberculosis control will be unsuccessful. By using mathematical models as health policy tools, we can focus and clarify the debate on how to control tuberculosis. Within our theoretical framework, when designing or improving control strategies there are at least four options to consider: (i) increasing treatment rates; (ii) decreasing treatment failure rates; (iii) improving the treatment efficacy of drug-resistance; and (iv) reducing treatment delays. Which particular combination of options should be chosen to improve a tuberculosis control program in any particular location can be rationally evaluated by using our theoretical framework. Simple transmission models can be extremely useful in designing epidemic control strategies, because such models can capture the essence of the complexity of the transmission dynamics, yet remain analytically tractable. The simple models that we have presented in this paper can now be used as building blocks for developing more complex models that can be used to design more detailed tuberculosis control strategies.

Acknowledgments. We wish to thank Chuck Daley, Paul Farmer, Julie Gerberding, Phil Hopewell, and Peter Small for their insightful comments and criticisms on earlier versions of this work. Enlightening comments from Jake and Dan Freimer were also greatly appreciated. We also would like to acknowledge NIDA/NIH (Grant Nos. R29DA08153 and RO1-09531) and NIAID (KO8AI01441) for financial support.

References

1. American Thoracic Society, Treatment of tuberculosis and tuberculosis infection in adults and children, Amer. J. Respir. Crit. Care Med. **149** (1994), 1359–1374.

2. Anderson, R. M. and R. M. May, Infectious Diseases of Humans: Dynamics and Control. Oxford University Press, Oxford, 1991.

3. Bloom, B. R. and C. J. L. Murray, Tuberculosis: Commentary on a reemergent killer, Science **257** (1992), 1055–1064.

4. Blower, S. M. and J. L. Gerberding, The dynamics of drug resistant tuberculosis: a theoretical framework, Journal of Molecular Medicine (1998). In press.

5. Blower, S. M. and A. R. McLean, Prophylactic vaccines, risk behavior change and the probability of eradicating HIV in San Francisco, Science **265** (1994), 1451–1454.

6. Blower, S. M. and A. R. McLean, AIDS: Modeling epidemic control, Science **267** (1995), 252–253.

7. Blower, S. M., A. R. McLean, T. Porco, M. Sanchez, P. M. Small, P. Hopewell, and A. Moss, The intrinsic transmission dynamics of tuberculosis epidemics, Nature Medicine **1** (1995), 815–821.

8. Blower, S. M., T. C. Porco and G. Darby, Predicting and preventing the emergence of antiviral drug resistance: HSV-2, Nature Medicine (1998). In press.

9. Blower, S. M., P. M. Small and P. Hopewell, Control strategies for tuberculosis epidemics: new models for old problems, Science **273** (1996), 497–500.

10. Brewer, T. F., S. J. Heymann, G. A. Colditz, M. E. Wilson, K. Auerbach, D. Kane and H. V. Fineberg, Evaluation of tuberculosis control policies using computer simulation, JAMA **276** (1996), 1898–1903.

11. Brudney, K. and J. Dobkin, Resurgent tuberculosis in New York City: HIV, homelessness and the decline of tuberculosis control programs, Am. Rev. Respir. Dis. **144** (1991), 745–749.

12. Canetti, G. Present aspects of bacterial resistance in tuberculosis, Am. Rev. Respir. Dis. **92** (1965), 687–703.

13. Castillo-Chavez, C. and Z. Feng, To treat or not to treat: the case of tuberculosis, Journal of Mathematical Biology **35** (1997), 629–659.

14. Davidson, P. T. Treating tuberculosis: What drugs and How Long? Ann. Int. Med. **112** (1990), 393–394.

15. Goble, M., M. D. R. Iseman, L. D. Madsen, et al. New Engl. J. Med. **328** (1993), 527.

16. Hong Kong Government Tuberculosis Service and British Medical Research Council Cooperative Investigation. Drug resistance in patients with pulmonary tuberculosis presenting at chest clinics in Hong Kong, Tubercle. **45** (1964), 77–95.

17. Krus, V. P. and L. A. Krachev, The mathematical theory of epidemics: A study of the evolution of resistance in microorganisms, Adv. Appl. Prob. **3** (1971), 206–208.

18. Lietman T., T. C. Porco and S. M. Blower, Leprosy and tuberculosis: the epidemiological consequences o f cross-immunity, American Journal of Public Health **87**(12) (1997), 1923–1927.

19. MRC Tuberculosis Chemotherapy Trials Commitee. The treatment of pulmonarytuberculosis with isoniazid, Brit. Med. Journal **2** (1952), 735–746.

20. Pinsky P. and R. Shonkwiler, A gonorrhea model treating sensitive and resistant strains in a multigroup population, Mathematical Biosciences **98** (1990), 103–126.

21. Porco, T. C. and S. M. Blower Quantifying the intrinsic transmission dynamics of tuberculosis epidemics, Theoretical Population Biology (1998). In press.

22. Sanchez, M. A. and S. M. Blower, Uncertainty and sensitivity analysis of the basic reproduction number: Tuberculosis as an example, Amer. J. Epidemiol. **145**(12) (1997), 1127–1138.

23. Schmidt, L. H., A. A. Grover, R. Hoffmann, J. Rehm and R. Sullivan, The emergence of isoniazid-sensitive bacilli in monkeys inoculated with isoniazid-resistant strains, Trans 17th Conference on Chemotherapy of Tuberculosis, VA-Armed Forces (1958), 264.

24. Sutherland, I. and E. Svandon, Endogeneous reactivation and exogenous reinfection; their relative importance with regard to the development of non-primary tuberculosis, Bull. Int. Un. Tuberc. **46** (1971), 75–114.

25. US PHS Cooperative Investigation. Prevalence of drug resistance in previously untreated patients, Am. Rev. Respir. Dis. **89** (1964) 327.

26. Waaler, H. T., A. Geser and S. Andersen, The use of mathematical models in the study of the epidemiology of tuberculosis, AJPH **52** (1962), 1002–1013.

27. WHO Global Report on Tuberculosis, Geneva, 1996.

28. WHO / IUATLD Global Project on Anti-tuberculosis Drug Resistance Surveillance, Anti-tuberculosis Drug Resistance in the World. Geneva, 1997.

Sally Blower
Department of Microbiology & Immunology
University of California San Francisco
513 Parnassus, HSE Room 420
San Francisco, CA 94143
sally@itsa.ucsf.edu

Travis Porco
San Francisco Department of Public Health
Community Health Epidemiology Section
25 Van Ness Avenue, Suite 710
San Francisco, CA, 94102-6033
travis_porco@dph.sf.ca.us

Tom Lietman
F.I. Proctor Foundation
University of California San Francisco
95 Kirkham Av.
Box 0944
San Francisco, CA, 94143-0944
tml@itsa.ucsf.edu

Skew Brownian Motion: A Model for Diffusion with Interfaces?

R. S. Cantrell and C. Cosner

Abstract. Skew Brownian motion is a diffusion process on the real line with a distinguished point. A particle diffusing under skew Brownian motion behaves as if it were experiencing ordinary Brownian motion except at the distinguished point, but at the distinguished point it moves to the left with a probability P or to the right with probability $1 - P$, with P not equal to $1/2$. As such, skew Brownian motion may be a reasonable model for diffusion with interfaces. An application is given to an ecological model with two types of habitat. However, if skew Brownian motion is formulated in terms of diffusion equations, assuming conservation of mass leads to predictions that in some cases a nonzero number of individuals must be at the distinguished point; i.e. that the probability distribution for the position of a particle may include a delta function at the distinguished point. In the ecological context there is some empirical work suggesting that individuals might in fact sometimes congregate on interfaces. It is unclear whether this behavior is problematic in other modeling contexts. The process of skew Brownian motion should be studied further to assess its usefulness in modeling diffusion in the presence of interfaces.

§1. Introduction

Diffusion processes based on the concept of Brownian motion are widely used to describe biological and chemical phenomena in which different species disperse at random and interact. A variation on standard Brownian motion, known as skew Brownian motion, allows for random dispersal but with an interface at which there is a preferred direction of motion. It is the purpose of this article to give a brief description of skew Brownian motion with some references and a description of how we used it to model a problem in population dynamics related to refuge design.

The idea of skew Brownian motion was introduced as an exercise in a book by Ito and McKean [3, §4.2, problem 1]. The properties of the process were explored to some extent in (Walsh [6], Harrison and Shepp [2]). Essentially, skew Brownian motion describes the position of an object moving on the real line via an unbiased random walk, *except* when it reaches the point $x = 0$,

Mathematical Models in Medical and Health Sciences
Mary Ann Horn, Gieri Simonett, and Glenn Webb (eds.), pp. 73–78.

where it moves one direction with probability α or the other with probability $1-\alpha$, $\alpha \neq 1/2$. This last property suggests that skew Brownian motion might be a reasonable starting point for the construction of models for dispersal in the presence of interfaces. In fact, Walsh [6] suggests that it might be used to model "a particle diffusing through a semi-permeable membrane under osmotic pressure". However, if the dispersal process is not allowed to increase or decrease the total amount of dispersing material (or number of dispersing individuals) it turns out to be necessary to allow particles (individuals) to actually remain on or in the interface itself, at least temporarily. This point is not mentioned in any of the references on skew Brownian motion, so we perform the derivation in the next section, along with giving a description and formulation of skew Brownian motion. In the third section we discuss a model based on skew Brownian motion which was developed in (Cantrell and Cosner [1]) to describe population dynamics and dispersal in an environment consisting of different types of habitat when the individuals in the population prefer one habitat type over the other. The main point of that discussion is to provide an illustration of how skew Brownian motion can be used in a model. In the last section we draw a few conclusions about the use of skew Brownian motion in modeling and suggest some directions for further research.

§2. Description and Anomalies of Skew Brownian Motion

Ordinary Brownian motion can be described as the limit of a random walk where at each time step Δt the corresponding spatial step is either Δx or $-\Delta x$, each with probability $1/2$, where the limit is taken so that Δx and Δt approach zero with $(\Delta x)^2/\Delta t = \delta^2$ for some fixed δ. Skew Brownian motion can be constructed in a completely analogous way, except that there is a distinguished point (say $x = 0$) for which the probability of moving to the right is α and the probability of moving to the left is $1 - \alpha$, with $\alpha \neq 1$ in general. (Harrison and Shepp [2].) Both ordinary and skew Brownian motions are diffusion processes which can be associated with semigroups of operators $\{T_t : t \geq 0\}$ via the Chapman-Kolmogorov equations for their transition functions (see [5]). The infinitesimal generator of the semigroup is computed as

$$Af = \lim_{t \downarrow 0} \frac{T_t f - f}{t}$$

and the associated diffusion equation is

$$\frac{du}{dt} = Au. \tag{1}$$

In the case of ordinary Brownian motion the generator is $A = (\delta^2/2)d^2/dx^2$ with domain effectively being $C^2(\mathbb{R})$ ([5, p.18]) so that the diffusion equation (1) can be realized as

$$\frac{\partial u}{\partial t} = \frac{\delta^2}{2} \frac{\partial^2 u}{\partial x^2} \quad \text{for } (x,t) \in \mathbb{R} \times (0, \infty). \tag{2}$$

(The transition function itself can be viewed as the fundamental solution of (2).) It is common practice in mathematical modeling to begin with equation (2) as a description of transport or dispersal via diffusion and then to add additional "reaction" terms to describe chemical reactions, population dynamics, etc., and usually this causes no problems. However, some care must be taken in using that approach for skew Brownian motion if we want a transport mechanism which does not change the total amount of mass, population, or whatever quantity is being described by the model. The corresponding semigroup generator for skew Brownian motion was computed by Walsh [6].

$$Af = \frac{\delta^2}{2} \frac{d^2 f}{dx^2},$$

$$\mathrm{dom} A = \{f \in C^2(\mathbb{R}\backslash\{0\}) : \alpha f'(0+)=(1-\alpha)f'(0-), f''(0+)=f''(0-)\}. \tag{3}$$

The realization of (1) as a differential equation becomes

$$\frac{\partial u}{\partial t} = \frac{\delta^2}{2} \frac{\partial^2 u}{\partial x^2}, \quad (x,t) \in (\mathbb{R}\backslash\{0\}) \times (0,\infty),$$

$$\frac{\alpha \partial u}{\partial x}(0+,t) = (1-\alpha)\frac{\partial u}{\partial x}(0-,t),$$

$$\frac{\partial^2 u}{\partial x^2}(0+,t) = \frac{\partial^2 u}{\partial x^2}(0-,t). \tag{4}$$

If (4) is interpreted in terms of fluxes via Fick's law, the flux $(\delta^2/2)\partial u/\partial x$ will be discontinuous at $x = 0$ if $\alpha \neq 1/2$ and $\partial u/\partial x \neq 0$ at $x = 0+$ or $x = 0-$. This suggests that one should expect material to build up on the interface at $x = 0$, which suggests that there might be a nonzero probability that a diffusing particle will be precisely at the single point $x = 0$, which would be inconsistent with the probability measure for the location of the particle being absolutely continuous with respect to Lebsegue measure. To explore these ideas more carefully we restrict (4) to the interval $[-1,1]$ and impose reflecting (i.e. no flux) boundary conditions at $x = \pm1$. The resulting equation is

$$\frac{\partial u}{\partial t} = \frac{\delta^2}{2} \frac{\partial^2 u}{\partial x^2} \quad \text{on } [(-1,0) \cup (0,1)] \times (0,\infty),$$

$$\frac{\partial u}{\partial x}(\pm1,t) = 0, \quad \alpha\frac{\partial u}{\partial x}(0+,t) = (1-\alpha)\frac{\partial u}{\partial x}(0-,t), \tag{5}$$

$$\frac{\partial^2 u}{\partial x^2}(0+,t) = \frac{\partial^2 u}{\partial x^2}(0-,t).$$

If we think of $u(x,t)$ as a function and integrate (5) over the inverval $[-1,1]$ with respect to x, we obtain

$$\frac{d}{dt}\int_{-1}^{1} u(x,t)dx = \frac{\delta^2}{2}\int_{-1}^{0} \frac{\partial^2 u}{\partial x^2}(x,t)dx + \frac{\delta^2}{2}\int_{0}^{1} \frac{\partial^2 u}{\partial x^2}(x,t)dx$$

$$= \frac{\delta^2}{2}\left[\frac{\partial u}{\partial x}(0-,t) - \frac{\partial u}{\partial x}(0+,t)\right] \tag{6}$$

$$= \frac{\delta^2}{2}\left(\frac{2\alpha-1}{1-\alpha}\right)\frac{\partial u}{\partial x}(0+,t).$$

To obtain a model where the total mass is conserved we would need to augment the continuous distribution u determined by (5) with a point mass or Dirac delta at $x = 0$ multiplied by a time dependent coefficient $p(t)$ satisfying

$$\frac{dp}{dt} = -\frac{\delta^2}{2} \left(\frac{2\alpha - 1}{1 - \alpha} \right) \frac{\partial u}{\partial x}(0+, t). \tag{7}$$

Since $u(x, t)$ can be determined from (5) (e.g. via the sort of methods used in [1]), equation (7) together with initial data for u and for the total mass at $t = 0$ will determine $p(t)$. The density will then be $u(x, t) + p(t)\delta(x)$, with $p(t) \neq 0$ in general.

§3. An Application

In [1] the goal was to model a situation where a population inhabits a region consisting of two different types of habitat, diffuses freely within each habitat type, but has a preferred direction (i.e. preferred choice of habitat) at the interface between habitat types. We used skew Brownian motion as the paradigm for describing movement at an interface with a preferred direction. The specific scenario we examined was that of a refuge consisting of favorable habitat surrounded by a buffer zone of somewhat unfavorable habitat, with the exterior of the buffer zone assumed to be immediately lethal to the population. The model assumed a local population growth rate r inside the refuge and a death rate $-s$ in the buffer zone. The refuge was taken to be the interval $(0, 2L)$ and the buffer zone to be $(-\ell, 0) \cup (2L, 2L + \ell)$. The model for the population density $u(x, t)$ was then given as

$$\begin{aligned}
\frac{\partial u}{\partial t} &= D_2 \frac{\partial^2 u}{\partial x^2} + ru \quad \text{in } (0, 2L) \times (0, \infty), \\
\frac{\partial u}{\partial t} &= D_1 \frac{\partial^2 u}{\partial x^2} - su \quad \text{in } [(-\ell, 0) \cup (2L, 2L + \ell)] \times (0, \infty),
\end{aligned} \tag{8}$$

$$\begin{aligned}
\alpha D_1 \frac{\partial u}{\partial x}(0+, t) &= (1 - \alpha) D_2 \frac{\partial u}{\partial x}(0-, t), \\
\alpha D_1 \frac{\partial u}{\partial x}(2L-, t) &= (1 - \alpha) D_2 \frac{\partial u}{\partial x}(2L+, t),
\end{aligned} \tag{9}$$

$$\begin{aligned}
D_2 \frac{\partial^2 u}{\partial x^2} + ru \mid_{x=0+} &= D_1 \frac{\partial^2 u}{\partial x^2} - su \mid_{x=0-}, \\
D_2 \frac{\partial^2 u}{\partial x^2} + ru \mid_{x=2L-} &= D_1 \frac{\partial^2 u}{\partial x^2} - su \mid_{x=2L+},
\end{aligned} \tag{10}$$

$$u(-\ell, t) = u(2L + \ell, t) = 0. \tag{11}$$

The equations (8) correspond to standard diffusion and growth or decline within each subregion. The interface condition (9) is based on the condition for skew Brownian motion, modified to account for the different diffusion rates in the two regions, with α again representing the probability that an individual on the interface will move into the refuge. If $\alpha = 1/2$ the condition is equivalent to matching fluxes across the interface. For $\alpha > 1/2$ there is a preference for moving into the refuge. The equation (10) arises from the requirement that the domain of the generator A of the diffusion processes should be restricted to functions $f(x)$ on $(-\ell, 2L + \ell)$ such that $(Af)(x)$ is continuous. (This requirement is imposed so that individuals never get permanently stuck at any location and so there are no impenetrable barriers to dispersal; see [3, p.83–100].) Finally, the boundary condition (11) simply means that individuals reaching the boundary die immediately so the density there is zero.

The model (8)-(11) can be analyzed via separation of variables. In [1] the main goal was to determine the dependence of the average population growth rate on the parameters r, s, ℓ, L, and α. The average population growth rate is determined as the principal eigenvalue of the operator A for which (8)-(11) give the realization of $du/dt = Au$. The corresponding eigenvalue problem for A is given by the following, which arise from (8), (10), and (11):

$$D_2 \frac{\partial^2 \phi}{dx^2} + r\phi = \sigma\phi \quad \text{in} \ (0, 2L),$$
$$D_1 \frac{\partial^2 \phi}{\partial x^2} - s\phi = \sigma\phi \quad \text{in} \ (-\ell, 0) \cup (2L, 2L + \ell), \tag{12}$$

$$\alpha D_1 \frac{\partial \phi}{\partial x} \mid_{x=0+} = (1 - \alpha) D_2 \frac{\partial \phi}{\partial x} \mid_{x=0-},$$
$$\alpha D_1 \frac{\partial \phi}{\partial x} \mid_{x=2L-} = (1 - \alpha) D_2 \frac{\partial \phi}{\partial x} \mid_{x=2L+}, \tag{13}$$

$$\phi(-\ell) = \phi(2L + \ell) = 0. \tag{14}$$

In view of (12), equation (10) becomes the requirement that $\phi(x)$ must be continuous at $x = 0, 2L$. It is possible to solve (12)-(14) by constructing the eigenfunction ϕ in terms of trigonometric and (possibly) hyperbolic functions and then using the matching conditions at $x = 0$ and $x = 2L$ to determine σ via a transcendental equation. The conclusions of [1] were then obtained by studying the dependence of σ on the parameters r, s, α, ℓ, L. A typical sort of conclusion is that the average growth rate is most sensitive to an increase of the size ℓ of the buffer zone when both the buffer zone and the refuge are small, but the sensitivity to the size of ℓ decreases rapidly as ℓ gets larger ([1, section 4]). Many other results on parameter dependence are also obtained. The key point for the current discussion, however, is simply that a model based on skew Brownian motion proved to be tractable and yielded reasonable and useful conclusions in an applied context.

As is shown by the analysis in [1] it is not always necessary for the mathematical analysis to account for the possibility that there may be a nonzero number of individuals actually *on* the interfaces at any given time. However, this is a point that should be considered when evaluating the model from an applied viewpoint. There is some empirical evidence that when confronted by a barrier dispersing individuals of some species may stop or move along the barrier rather than crossing it or reversing direction [4]. For such species a

prediction that some individuals may remain at the interface for some time
is at least plausible. However, such an assumption might not be plausible in
other contexts, so the modelling approach should be used with some care.

§4. Conclusions

The concept of skew Brownian motion seems to have some potential applications in biological modelling because it can lead to reasonably tractable models
which allow for a preferred direction of movement at an interface. However,
skew Brownian motion does not appear to have been widely studied from the
mathematical viewpoint, so if it is used in a model some care must be taken
in the analysis and interpretation of the model. The observation that skew
Brownian motion seems to require the introduction of a point mass at the
origin to avoid a gain or loss of particles via dispersal (i.e. without reaction
dynamics) may be problematic in some applications, although not in others.
In any case this point requires further study. Another issue which deserves
some attention is that of formulating skew Brownian motion in more than one
space dimension. Some other possible directions for further research are described in [1]. We hope that the present discussion will interest some readers
enough that they will examine skew Brownian motion themselves and draw
their own conclusions.

Acknowledgments. This research has been partially supported by NSF
Grant DMS 96-25741

References

1. Cantrell, R. S. and C. Cosner, Diffusion models for population dynamics
   incorporating individual behavior at boundaries: applications to refuge
   design, preprint.

2. Harrison, J. M. and L. A. Shepp, On skew Brownian motion, The Annals
   of Probability **9** (1981), 309–313.

3. Ito, K. and H. P. McKean Jr., *Diffusion processes and their sample paths*,
   Springer-Verlag, New York, 1965.

4. Kaiser, H., Small spatial scale heterogeneity influences predation success
   in an unexpected way: model experiments on the functional response of
   predatory mites (Acarina), Oecologia (Berlin) **56** (1983), 249–256.

5. Taira, K., *Diffusion processes and partial differential equations*, Harcourt
   Brace Jovanovich, New York, 1988.

6. Walsh, J. B., A diffusion with discontinuous local time, Asterisque **52-53**
   (1978), 37–45.

Spatio-Temporal Dynamics of the Immune System Response to Cancer

M. A. J. Chaplain, V. A. Kuznetsov,
Z. H. James and L. A. Stepanova

Abstract. In this paper, a mathematical model describing the one-dimensional growth of a solid tumour (for example, a malignant melanoma of the skin) in the presence of an immune system response, is presented. In particular, attention is focussed upon the interaction of tumour cells with so-called tumour-infiltrating cytotoxic lymphocytes (TICLs), in a small, multicellular tumour, without central necrosis and at some stage prior to angiogenesis. At this stage the immune cells and the tumour cells are in a state of dynamic equilibrium (cancer dormancy). The resulting system of three nonlinear partial differential equations is analysed and numerical simulations are presented. The numerical simulations demonstrate the existence of cell distributions that are quasi-stationary in time but unstable and heterogeneous in space. The resulting rich spatio-temporal dynamic behaviour of the system is compared with actual experimental evidence.

§1. Introduction

A neoplasm (tumour) may be defined as an abnormal mass of tissue whose growth exceeds that of normal tissue, is un-coordinated with that of the normal tissue, and persists in the same excessive manner after cessation of the stimuli which evoked the change [24]. A cancer, or malignant tumour, is a tumour that invades surrounding tissues, traverses at least one basement membrane zone, grows in the mesenchyme at the primary site and has the ability to grow in a distant mesenchyme, forming secondary cancers or metastases. Tumours which originate spontaneously in humans or animals usually grow slowly. Many months, years, or even dozens of years, are required for their clinical manifestation [36, 39, 41] and the precise nature of this phenomenon remains unclear. One of the reasons for the slow growth of tumours and, in some cases, for their regression, may be the reaction of the immune system to the nascent tumour cells. Many authors point out, that intensive lymphoid, granulocyte and monocyte infiltration in a tumour, especially pronounced at

Mathematical Models in Medical and Health Sciences
Mary Ann Horn, Gieri Simonett, and Glenn Webb (eds.), pp. 79–97.

the early stages, correlates with a favourable prognosis [3, 20, 21]. However, the possible involvement of the immune system in the control of growth and development, including metastases in humans, is still a matter of some debate. Indeed, some researchers do not confirm the prognostic role of lymphoid infiltration in a tumour. Moreover, data have been reported which suggests a stimulating effect of certain cells of the immune system on the growth of tumours [28, 29]. These apparent contradictions may be associated with, and partly explained by the fact that carcinogenesis is a multi-stage process and that right from its inception there exists a complex tissue architecture within the tumour. Indeed, a tumour is a highly intricate, heterogeneous structure consisting of various cells which secrete a considerable quantity of biologically active compounds into the local environment [11].

The early stage of primary tumour formation often occurs in the absence of a vascular network. According to [9, 33], this stage may last up to several years. The tumour nodule grows to an approximate size of 1–3 mm in diameter, containing close to $(1-3) \times 10^6$ cells and then growth slows down and/or ceases. This limitation of growth is attributed by researchers to the competition between tumour cells for metabolites, the competition between tumour cells and cells of the immune system for metabolites and/or a direct cytostatic/cytotoxic effect produced by the tumour cells on each other. In addition, the early (avascular) stage and the subsequent stages of tumour growth are characterized by a chronic inflammatory infiltration of neutrophils, eosinophils, basophils, monocytes/macrophages, T-lymphocytes, B-lymphocytes and natural killer (NK) cells [21, 37, 42]. These cells penetrate the interior of the tumour and accumulate in it due to attractants secreted from the tumour tissue and the high locomotive ability of activated immune cells [32]. During the avascular stage, tumour development can be effectively eliminated by tumour-infiltrating cytotoxic lymphocytes (TICLs) [18]. The TICLs may be cytotoxic lymphocytes (CTLs), NK cells and/or lymphokine activated killer (LAK) cells [7, 10, 20, 42]. The cytostatic/cytotoxic activity of granulocytes and monocytes/macrophages located in the tumour is determined less frequently [7, 10, 38]. In some cases, relatively small tumours are in cell-cycle arrest or there is a balance between cell proliferation and cell death. This steady-state of fully malignant, but regulated under growth control, could continue many months or years [40]. In many (but not at all) cases such a latent form of a small numbers of malignant tumours is mediated by cellular immunity [40]. Clinically, such latent forms of tumours have been referred to as "cancer dormancy".

An important factor, which may influence the outcome of the interactions between tumour cells and TICLs in a solid tumour, is the distribution of the TICLs. A thick shell of lymphoid infiltration is often revealed around the tumour [3, 4] and even near the central hypoxic zone [19]. This would define an internal structure, whereby the regions of cell proliferation and cell death alternate, with the TICLs located near the groups of dying tumour cells [25]. In spite of some progress into the investigation of TICLs and their mechanisms of interaction with tumour cells, our understanding of the spatio-temporal dynamics of TICLs in small tumours and in micrometastases *in vivo* is still rather limited. It is perhaps not surprising therefore, that this complicated picture has not yet received an adequate explanation. Certainly, other components of the immune system (e.g., cytokines) are involved in modulating the local cellular immune response dynamics. Many cytokines are produced during cell-cell interactions, which can be focussed to perform their function over short ranges in space and over short intervals of time. Interestingly, strong local immune reactions are induced by the release of interleukin-1 (IL-1), IL-2, IL-3, IL-4, IL-5, IL-6, IL-7, IL-8, IL-10, IL-12, IL-13, IL-15, G-CSF, GM-CSF, INF-α, TNF-α, INF-γ etc. Each of these cytokines recruits and activates some distinct cell population, which could be tumour-infiltrating cells, or the tumour cells themselves [10, 31, 35]. Besides immune reactions, other processes (e.g., cell proliferation, development, locomotion and apoptosis) are governed in a feedback fashion by their own intensity. The experimental analysis of such *in vivo* functions requires gene transfer technology and adoptive cell transfer studies, among others. Such studies are, however, hampered by the availability of *in vitro* cloned TICLs and by the frustrating experience that these *in vitro* propagated killer cells perform relatively badly *in vivo*, due to, for example, the down-regulation of their homing receptors and up-regulation of many of the cytokines amongst other things.

It is difficult to control experimentally all of the interacting elements in a tumour. Furthermore, complex biological systems, such as the immune system and a cancer *in vivo*, do not always behave or act as predicted by experimental investigations *in vitro* [29]. Thus mathematical modelling and computer simulations can be helpful in understanding some important features in these elaborate systems [1, 2].

Recently, Owen and Sherratt [26] have also developed a model with the possibility of spatio-temporal irregularities within a growing tumour using a model of tumour cell and macrophage interactions. In this paper, a mathematical model describing the spatio-temporal dynamics of "dormant" tumour, under the control of the immune response of TICLs, is presented. The complex dynamics of the interactions between immune cells and tumour cells, in a small dormant tumour, without central necrosis and at some stage prior to angiogenesis are discussed. Analytical and numerical analysis of the model to be presented here demonstrate that the complex behaviour of the system depends upon certain parameters, in particular, on the "diffusion" (random motility) rate of tumour cells and immune cells (lymphocytes).

§2. The Mathematical Model

Let us consider a simplified process of a small, growing, avascular tumour which produces signals (e.g. secretes chemicals) which attract a population of lymphocytes. These signals are recognised by TILs and and the tumour is directly attacked by TICLs [13, 14, 17]. The humoral immune response, the interactions between cells of the immune system and dynamics of cytokines in the tumour will be accounted for indirectly, because data related to these processes is often contradictory and many important mechanisms of cytokine dynamics in tumours are unknown.

Local interactions between TICLs and tumour cells *in vivo* may be described by the following simplified kinetic scheme:

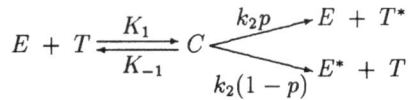

$$E + T \underset{K_{-1}}{\overset{K_1}{\rightleftharpoons}} C \underset{k_2(1-p)}{\overset{k_2p}{\longrightarrow}} \begin{matrix} E + T^* \\ E^* + T \end{matrix}$$

where E, T, C, E^* and T^* are the local concentrations of TICLs, tumour cells, TICL-tumour cell complexes, inactivated TICLs and 'lethally hit' or 'programmed-for-lysis' tumour cells, respectively. The parameters k_1, k_{-1} and k_2 are non-negative kinetic constants: k_1 and k_{-1} describe the rate of binding of TICL to tumour cells and detachment of TICL from tumour cells *without* damaging cells; k_2 is the rate of detachment of TICL from tumour cells, resulting in irreversibly programming tumour cells for lysis with probability p or inactivating TICLs with probability $(1 - p)$. Substantiation of the above scheme (for CTLs) has already been discussed at greater length in [15]. Using the law of mass action, the above kinetic scheme can be "translated" into a system of ordinary differential equations cf. [15].

For the sake of simplicity we will consider the case of a one-dimensional tumour growth, (i.e., we shall assume that the cells lie on a straight line). This corresponds to the situation of the most malignant development of a primary neoplasm: that is, to invasive growth, when a cancer (e.g., malignant melanoma) grows not on the surface of the skin, but vertically downwards, growing directly into the tissue below. Invasive growth is extremely insidious and dangerous, giving rise to metastases or secondary tumours [5, 6].

The influence of other tissue cells on TICLs and tumour cells will be taken into account by specifying precise values for the model parameters, together with appropriate initial and boundary conditions.

For a simplified description of the spatio-temporal growth of a solid tumour in the very early stages of its development, we will use a simple reaction-diffusion equation of the form

$$\frac{\partial T}{\partial t} = \frac{\partial}{\partial x}\left[D\frac{\partial T}{\partial x}\right] + F(T), \tag{1}$$

where $T(x,t)$ is the population density of tumour cells at the point x in space and at time t, D is the diffusion coefficient of the tumour cells (a measure of the random motility of the tumour cells) and $F(T)$ is the nonlinear function which takes into account mutual competition between tumour cells and/or a limit on the maximum density of cells per unit area due to their finite sizes cf. [8, 30]. In particular, the growth dynamics of solid tumours may be described adequately by the logistic equation [15, 22, 23],

$$F(T) = a(1 - bT)T. \tag{2}$$

We suppose that when the front of invading tumour cells moves into the tissue to a certain depth, they encounter TICLs which are migrating towards them. The dynamics of the interaction between TICLs and tumour cells may be presented in the following form:

$$\frac{\partial E}{\partial t} = \frac{\partial}{\partial x}\left[D_1\frac{\partial E}{\partial x}\right] + F_1(E,T,C), \tag{3}$$

$$\frac{\partial T}{\partial t} = \frac{\partial}{\partial x}\left[D_2\frac{\partial T}{\partial x}\right] + F_2(E,T,C), \tag{4}$$

$$\frac{\partial C}{\partial t} = F_3(E,T,C), \tag{5}$$

$$\frac{\partial E^*}{\partial t} = F_4(E^*,C), \tag{6}$$

$$\frac{\partial T^*}{\partial t} = F_5(T^*,C), \tag{7}$$

where E, T, C, E^*, and T^* are the population densities of: unbound TICLs, unbound tumour cells, TICL-tumour cell complexes, inactivated TICLs and 'lethally hit' tumour cells, respectively; $D_i(i = 1, 2)$ are the cell diffusion (random motility) coefficients.

We assume that inactivated and 'lethally hit' cells are quickly eliminated from the tissue (for example, by macrophages) and do not substantially influence the immune processes being analysed. A slightly more complicated model might consider the re-introduction of these inactivated TICLs at some later stage. Also, we shall confine ourselves to consider the situation in which the cell diffusion (random motility) coefficients are independent of the spatio-temporal disposition of the cells (i.e., they are constant).

As suggested in the ordinary differential equation model [15] of the CTL response to the growth of an immunogenic tumour, the functions of local changes in the population density $F_i(i = 1 \ldots 5)$ are defined as follows:

$$F_1(E,T,C) = sh(x - l) + \frac{fET}{g+T} - d_1E - k_1ET + (k_{-1} + k_2p)C, \tag{8}$$

$$F_2(E,T,C) = a(1 - bT)T - k_1ET + (k_{-1} + k_2(1 - p))C, \tag{9}$$

$$F_3(E,T,C) = k_1ET - (k_{-1} + k_2)C, \tag{10}$$

$$F_4(E^*,C) = k_2(1 - p)C - d_2E^*, \tag{11}$$

$$F_5(T^*,C) = k_2pC - d_3T^*. \tag{12}$$

In addition to terms arising from the kinetic scheme decribed previously (by application of the law of mass action), we have included terms to account for (1) the "normal" immune response to the tumour cells, with s the 'normal', non-enhanced by the presence of tumour cells, rate of flow of mature TICLs into the tumour; (2) death or loss of the various cells, where d_1, d_2 and d_3 are positive constants representing the rates of elimination of E, E^* and T^*, respectively, resulting from spontaneous death and/or migration from the region of tissue being considered; (3) a logistic growth rate for the tumour cells. The maximal growth rate of the tumour cells population is a, which incorporates both cell multiplication (mitosis) and death. Owing, for example, to competition for resources, mutual inhibition of growth and limited tissue space, the maximum density of the tumour cells is defined, and is represented by the parameter b^{-1}; and (4) a term representing the observed accumulation of TICLs in response to the tumour - in the region of tumour cell localization, the maximum rate of accumulation of the TICL population, due to the presence of the tumour, is f. Both TICL multiplication due to stimulation by the tumour cells, and enhanced TICL migration induced by TICL-tumour cell interactions, after which there is the production of many attractor factors for lymphocytes (e.g., IL-1, IL-2, IL-8, INF-γ, etc.) may contribute to this process [12, 27]. It is important to note that a maximum rate of stimulated accumulation of TICLs is consistent with limitations in the rate of transport of TICLs to the tumour. These rate limitations could occur in the circulation, in the rate of exit from the circulation or in the rate of movement through the tissue to the tumour. The density of tumour cells, at which the maximum rate of accumulation of TICLs diminishes by a factor of two, is g. Finally, we have assumed that the tumour does not metastasize and that there is no migration of TICL-tumour cell complexes.

It is easy to see that equations (6) and (7) are only coupled to the full system through the complexes C, i.e., T^* and E^* have no effect on each other or the variables T and E. Thus, for the remainder of this paper, it is sufficient to analyse equations (3), (4) and (5) which essentially dictate the behaviour of the complete system.

An area of tissue for the above system is determined by the one-dimensional spatial domain $[0, x_0]$, where x_0 is the length of the region being considered. We assume that there are two distinct regions in this interval - one region entirely occupied by tumour cells, the other entirely occupied by the immune cells. We propose that an initial interval of tumour localization is $[0, l]$, where $l = 0.2x_0$ and the function $h(x - l)$ is defined as follows:

$$h(x - l) = 0 \quad \text{if} \quad x - l \le 0, \qquad h(x - l) = 1 \quad \text{if} \quad x - l > 0.$$

Although in our model there is only a normal rate of flow of mature TICLs in the part of the region $[l, x_0]$, this assumption is not crucial. We have performed an analysis of the model where the rate of flow of TICLs (s) is present throughout the entire spatial domain $[0, x_0]$ with little or no difference in the final results.

Boundary and Initial Conditions

Zero-flux boundary conditions (BC) of the form

$$\frac{\partial E}{\partial x}(0, t) = 0, \qquad \frac{\partial E}{\partial x}(x_0, t) = 0,$$
$$\frac{\partial T}{\partial x}(0, t) = 0, \qquad \frac{\partial T}{\partial x}(x_0, t) = 0, \tag{13}$$

$$\frac{\partial C}{\partial x}(0,t) = 0, \qquad \frac{\partial C}{\partial x}(x_0,t) = 0.$$

are imposed, with initial conditions (IC) given by:

$$
E(x,0) = \begin{cases} 0 & \text{if } 0 \le x \le l, \\ E_0(1 - \exp{(-1000(x-l)^2)}) & \text{if } l < x \le x_0, \end{cases}
$$
$$
T(x,0) = \begin{cases} T_0(1 - \exp{(-1000(x-l)^2)}) & \text{if } 0 \le x \le l, \\ 0 & \text{if } l < x \le x_0, \end{cases} \qquad (14)
$$
$$
C(x,0) = \begin{cases} 0 & \text{if } x \notin [l-\epsilon, l+\epsilon], \\ C_0 \exp{(-1000(x-l)^2)} & \text{if } x \in [l-\epsilon, l+\epsilon]. \end{cases}
$$

where

$$E_0 = \frac{s}{d_1}, \qquad T_0 = \frac{1}{b}, \qquad C_0 = \min(E_0, T_0), \qquad 0 < \epsilon \ll 1.$$

These conditions correspond to the case of a tumour that appears below the outer surface of a tissue (e.g., in the basal cell layer of the epidermis) and propagates into deeper levels of the tissue, i.e., invades the dermis (vertical tumour growth). This account could describe a nodular melanoma which has no clinically or histologically evident radial growth phase. Presumably though, a short radial growth phase does exist but dermal invasion occurs so rapidly that a preinvasive stage is not apparent [24].

Thus, if the system is subjected to the zero-flux boundary conditions above, tumour cells and TICLs will be unable to penetrate both the outer boundary at $x = 0$ (i.e., cells cannot move through the upper layer of the skin) and the inner boundary at $x = x_0$. The latter situation may be interpreted as the existence of a strong, physical barrier which is totally impenetrable to all cell types. However, tumour cells are still able to assemble at the inner barrier and complexes are able to form at both boundaries.

Figure 1 depicts qualitatively the ICs described in equation (14) (after the non-dimensionalization of the next section), which shows a front of tumour cells encountering a front of TICLs, resulting in the formation of TICL-tumour cell complexes. In the absence of a tumour, the homogeneous steady-state density of the TICLs is s/d_1 and this is the value we take for the initial density of TICLs at the boundary $x = x_0$. Similarly, in the absence of an immune response, the homogeneous steady-state density of the tumour cells is $1/b$ and this is what we take as the initial density of tumour cells at the boundary $x = 0$. Thus, when the fronts of the two cell populations meet, the maximum density of TICL-tumour cell complexes will be $\min(E_0, T_0)$.

The exact solution of the above system cannot be obtained analytically. For an analysis of the model by numerical methods and in order to compare it with experimental observations, it is necessary to determine realistic values for the parameters.

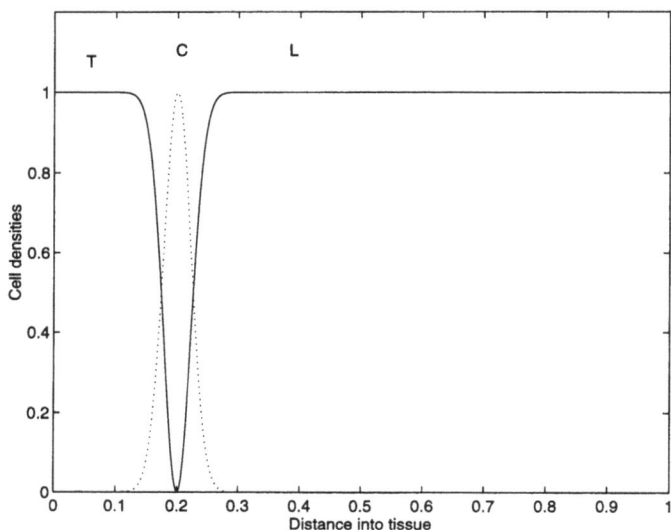

Fig. 1. Initial conditions used for the tumour cells (T), complexes (C) and tumour in infiltrating cytotoxic lymphocytes (L).

§3. Estimation of Parameters

An adequate description of the growth of a BCL_1 lymphoma in the spleen of recipient mice, chimeric with respect to the Major Histocompatability Complex (MHC), was provided by the ordinary differential equation model of [15], using estimated parameters obtained in [16]. Using these estimates the transition of the lymphoma into a clinically undetected, 'dormant' state, represented by a stable focus was demonstrated. The parameters were determined to have the following values:

$$a = 0.18 \text{ day}^{-1}, \qquad\qquad b = 2.0 \times 10^{-9} \text{ cells}^{-1},$$
$$k_1 = 1.3 \times 10^{-7} \text{ day}^{-1} \text{ cells}^{-1}, \qquad k_{-1} = 24.0 \text{ day}^{-1},$$
$$k_2 = 7.2 \text{ day}^{-1}, \qquad\qquad p = 0.9997,$$
$$d_1 = 0.0412 \text{ day}^{-1}, \qquad\qquad f = 0.1245 \text{ day}^{-1},$$
$$g = 2.02 \times 10^7 \text{ cells}, \qquad\qquad s = 1.36 \times 10^4 \text{ day}^{-1} \text{ cells}.$$

Finally, we need to calculate the diffusion (random motility) coefficients of the TICLs and tumour cells. A tumour may be infiltrated by TICLs as a result of passive migration or active transport. In the first case, the diffusion (random motility) coefficient can be evaluated employing Einstein's formula:

$$D_1 = \frac{kT}{6\pi R_1 \eta},$$

where k is Boltzmann's constant, T is the temperature in degrees Kelvin, R_1 is the average radius of a TICL and η is the viscosity coefficient of the medium. At $T = 310k$ (37°C), $R_1 = 4\mu m$ and $\eta = \eta_{\text{water}}$, $D_1 = 7.0 \times 10^{-5}$ cm^2 day^{-1}. This value is close to the diffusion coefficient of CTLs *in vitro*; obtained by T.L. Rothstein et al., 1978 [34], studying sequential killing of immobilised allogenic tumour cells by CTLs.

Diffusion of tumour cells in tissue is conditioned largely by the replication of the cells and the growth of the tumour. The diffusion coefficient may be estimated from the following equation [30]:

$$D_2 = R_2^2 a,$$

where R_2 is the average radius of a tumour cell and a is the rate of duplication of the tumour cell population. Assuming $R_2 = 4\mu m$ and $a = 0.2$ day^{-1}, $D_2 = 1.3 \times 10^{-6}$cm^{2}day^{-1}.

We know that TICLS are capable of infiltrating solid or lymphoma-like tumours rather rapidly [14, 20, 32, 37] and it is apparent, that if the movement of the TICLs and/or tumour cells is an active process induced by chemoattractants, the value of the diffusion coefficients of these cells may be appreciably greater and perhaps even reach approximately 10^{-2} cm^2 day^{-1} [12, 14]. Thus, the intervals of variation of the diffusion coefficients may be large, obviously depending upon the physical and biochemical properties of the surrounding tissue matrix and concentration of various chemoattractants.

Before proceeding with the numerical analysis, we use the standard practice of non-dimensionalization which enables the important dimensionless parameters that govern the behaviour of the system to be identified.

§4. Non-Dimensionalization

We non-dimensionalise equations (3), (4) and (5), the boundary conditions and initial conditions. An order-of-magnitude density scale is selected for the E, T and C cell densities, of E_0, T_0 and C_0, respectively; as suggested by the initial conditions. Time is scaled relative to the diffusion rate of the TICLs; i.e., $t_0 = x_0^2 D_1^{-1}$ and the space variable is scaled relative to the length of the region under consideration. Then, on making the following substitutions:

$$\bar{E} = \frac{E}{E_0}, \qquad \bar{T} = \frac{T}{T_0}, \qquad \bar{C} = \frac{C}{C_0},$$
$$\bar{x} = \frac{x}{x_0}, \qquad \bar{t} = \frac{t}{t_0}, \qquad \sigma = \frac{st_0}{E_0} = d_1 t_0,$$
$$\rho = f t_0, \qquad \mu = \frac{k_1 t_0 T_0 E_0}{C_0} = k_1 t_0 T_0, \qquad \eta = \frac{g}{T_0},$$
$$\epsilon = \frac{t_0 C_0(k_{-1}+k_2 p)}{E_0}, \qquad \omega = \frac{D_2 t_0}{x_0^2}, \qquad \alpha = a t_0,$$
$$\phi = k_1 t_0 E_0, \qquad \lambda = \frac{t_0 \bar{C}_0(k_{-1}+k_2(1-p))}{T_0}, \qquad \chi = t_0(k_{-1}+k_2).$$

and omitting the accents, equations (3), (4) and (5) may be re-written as:

$$\frac{\partial E}{\partial t} = \frac{\partial^2 E}{\partial x^2} + \sigma h(x-l) + \frac{\rho ET}{\eta + T} - \sigma E - \mu ET + \epsilon C, \qquad (15)$$

$$\frac{\partial T}{\partial t} = \omega \frac{\partial^2 T}{\partial x^2} + \alpha(1 - \beta T)T - \phi ET + \lambda C, \tag{16}$$

$$\frac{\partial C}{\partial t} = \mu ET - \chi C, \tag{17}$$

After non-dimensionalization, the boundary conditions become:

$$\frac{\partial E}{\partial x}(0,t) = 0, \quad \frac{\partial E}{\partial x}(1,t) = 0,$$

$$\frac{\partial T}{\partial x}(0,t) = 0, \quad \frac{\partial T}{\partial x}(1,t) = 0, \tag{18}$$

$$\frac{\partial C}{\partial x}(0,t) = 0, \quad \frac{\partial C}{\partial x}(1,t) = 0.$$

with our initial conditions taking the following form:

$$E(x,0) = \begin{cases} 0 & \text{if } 0 \le x \le l \\ (1 - \exp(-1000(x - l)^2)) & \text{if } l < x \le 1 \end{cases}$$

$$T(x,0) = \begin{cases} (1 - \exp(-1000(x - l)^2)) & \text{if } 0 \le x \le 1 \\ 0 & \text{if } l < x \le 1 \end{cases} \tag{19}$$

$$C(x,0) = \begin{cases} 0 & \text{if } x \notin [l - \epsilon, l + \epsilon] \\ \exp(-1000(x - l)^2) & \text{if } x \in [l - \epsilon, l + \epsilon] \end{cases}$$

Values for the ten non-dimensional parameters are obtained from the estimated dimensional parameters in section 4. Both diffusion coefficients were taken to be 10^{-6} cm^2 day^{-1}, since these are close to the estimates obtained in the previous section. By employing a numerical method, we obtain solutions for the above non-dimensionalized system, in the following section.

§5. Numerical Simulation Results

In the numerical simulations which follow, it was convenient to normalise the spatial variable in such a manner that $x_0 = 1$cm, giving $l = 0.2$cm. The non-dimensionalized model was solved numerically using two different methods: (i) A NAG routine D03PGF (This routine integrates parabolic partial differential equations via the method of lines and Gear's method) and (ii) the method of uniform networks based on an absolutely stable implicit difference scheme. Both methods produced results which were the same to within an accuracy of 6 decimal places. Additionally, for every case examined, we plotted the temporal dynamics of each cell population. This was achieved by estimating the total number of each type of cell (lymphocytes, tumour cells, complexes) within the tissue at each time-step using a numerical quadrature scheme based on Simpson's Rule.

With $D_1 = D_2 = 10^{-6}$ cm^2 day^{-1}, the system exhibits rich spatio-temporal dynamics and a rather complicated behaviour as shown in Figures 2, 3, 4 and 5.

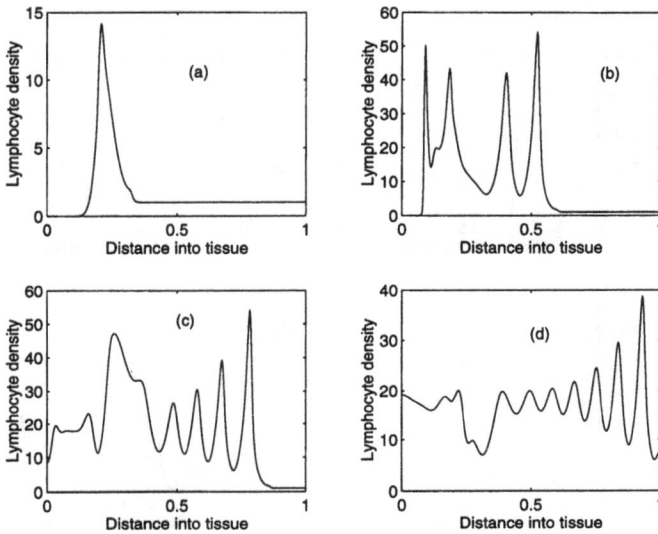

Fig. 2. Spatial distribution of TICL density within the tissue at times corresponding to 100, 400, 700 and 1000 days, respectively.

Figure 2(a-d) shows the spatial distribution of TICL density within the tissue at times corresponding to 100, 400, 700 and 1000 days respectively. The figures show a heterogeneous spatial distribution of TICL density throughout the tissue. Figure 3(a-d) shows the corresponding spatial distribution of tumour cell density within the tissue at times corresponding to 100, 400, 700 and 1000 days. The figures show a train of solitary-like waves invading the tissue and subsequently creating a spatially heterogeneous distribution of tumour cell density throughout.

The dynamic of this spatial heterogeneity appears to persist as the long time behaviour of the system in Figure 4(a-d) shows. The times here correspond to 3000, 5000, 7000 and 10000 days respectively. Figure 5(a-d) shows the corresponding spatial distribution of tumour cell-lymphocyte complexes within the tissue at times corresponding to 100, 400, 700 and 1000 days respectively.

In addition to observing the above spatio-temporal distributions of each cell type within the tissue, the temporal dynamics of the overall populations of each cell type (i.e., total cell number) was examined. This was achieved by calculating the (scaled) total number of each cell type within the whole tissue space using numerical quadrature. Figure 6 shows the variation in the (scaled) number of TICLs within the tissue over time (approximately 80 years, an estimated average lifespan). Initially, the total number of TICLs within the tissue increases and then subsequently oscillates around some stationary level (approximately 18). Long-time numerical calculations indicated that this

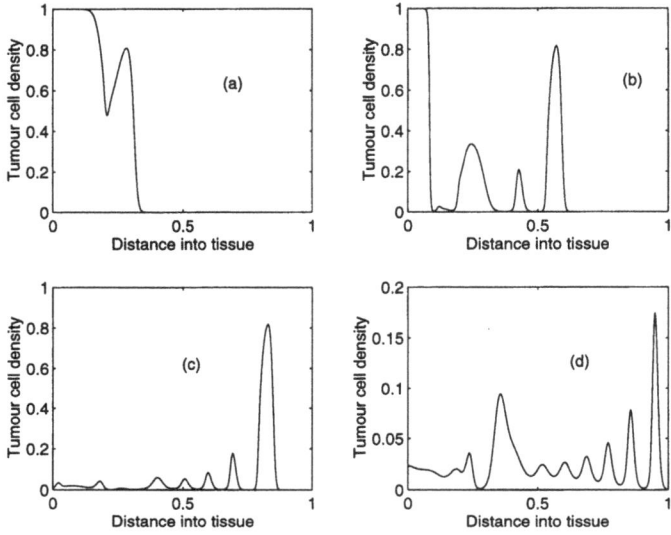

Fig. 3. Spatial distribution of tumour cell density within the tissue at times corresponding to 100, 400, 700 and 1000 days, respectively.

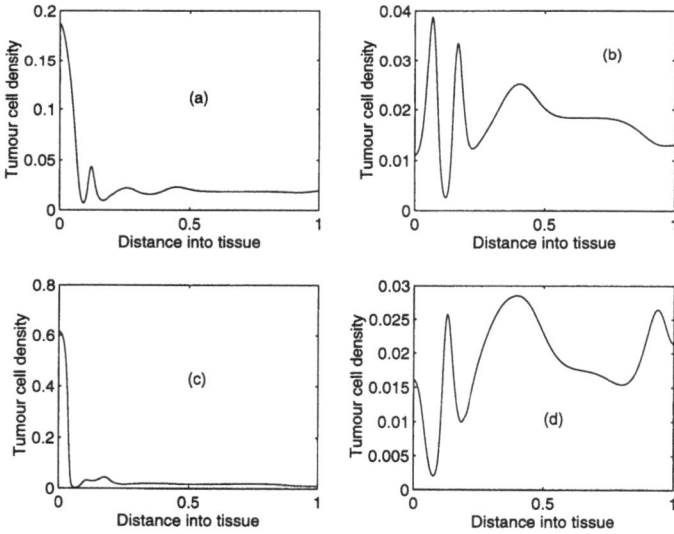

Fig. 4. Spatial distribution of tumour cell density within the tissue at times corresponding to 3000, 5000, 7000 and 10000 days, respectively.

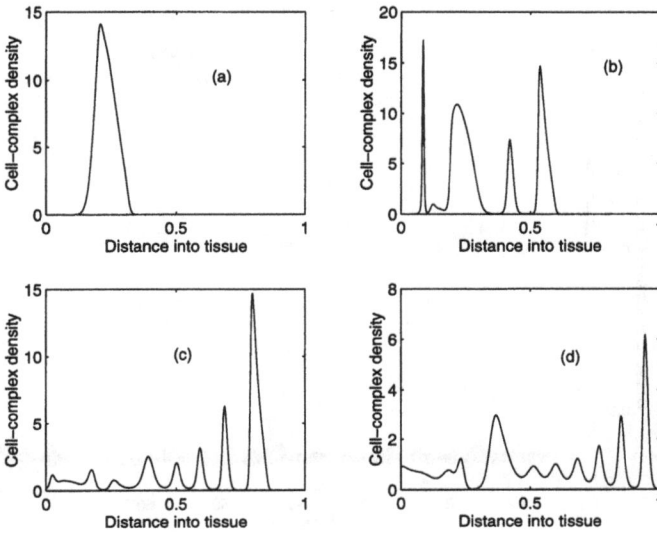

Fig. 5. Spatial distribution of tumour cell-TICL complex density within the tissue at times corresponding to 100, 400, 700 and 1000 days, respectively.

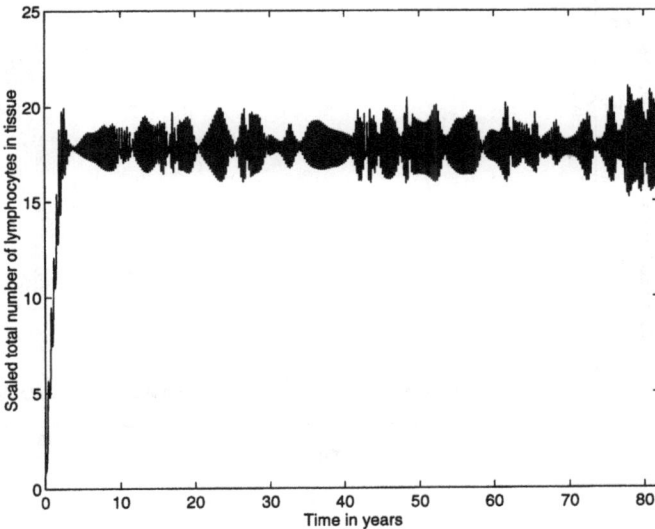

Fig. 6. Total number of lymphocytes within tissue over a period of 80 years.

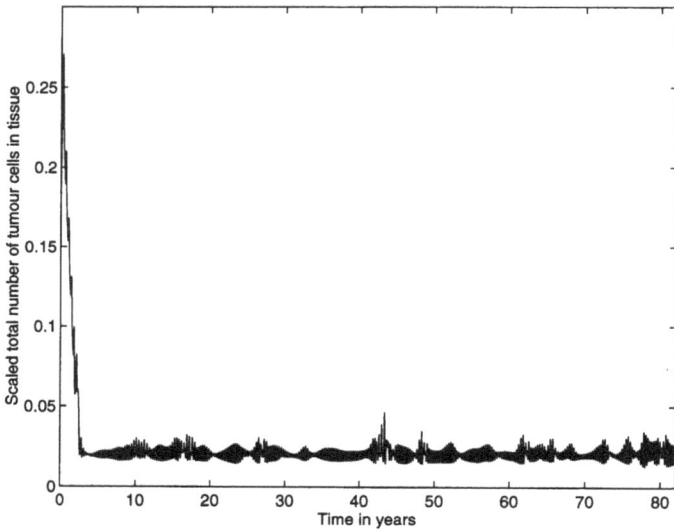

Fig. 7. Total number of tumour cells within tissue over a period of 80 years.

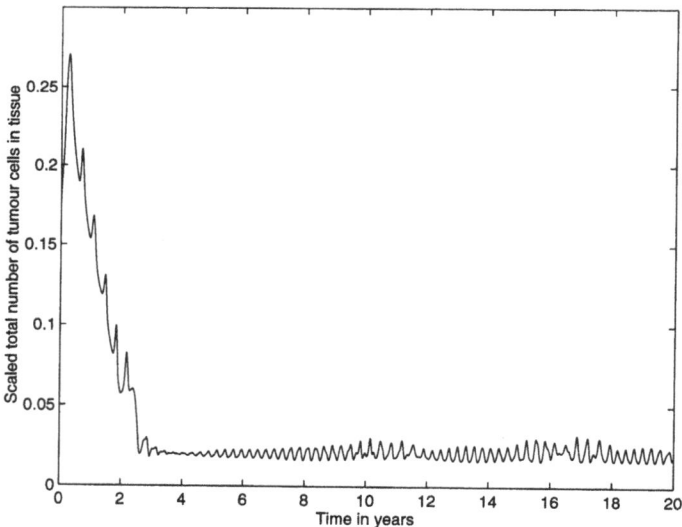

Fig. 8. Total number of tumour cells within tissue over a period of 20 years illustrating the early dynamics. The number of tumour cells initially decreases before settling down to an oscillatory behaviour around a stationary level of approximately 0.02.

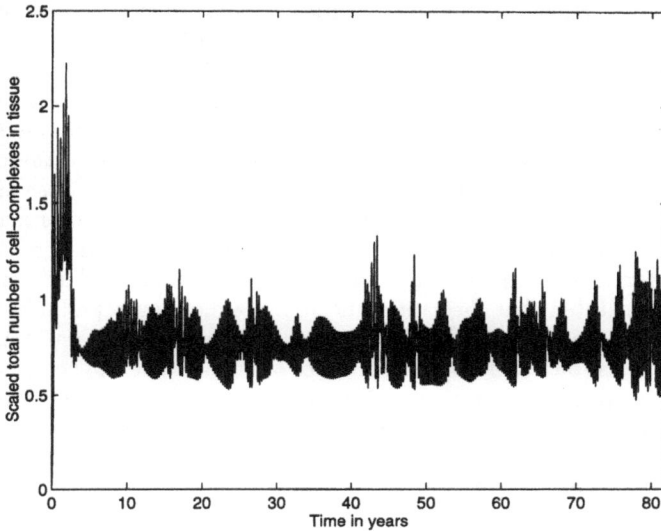

Fig. 9. Total number of tumour cell-TICL complexes within tissue over a period of 80 years.

behaviour will persist for all time.

A similar scenario is observed for the tumour cell population. From Figure 7, we observe that initially, the tumour cell population decreases in number before subsequently oscillating around some stationary value (approximately 0.02) for all time. Figure 8 provides a more detailed view of the early oscillations. Figure 9 gives the corresponding temporal dynamics of the complexes.

The above simulations appear to indicate that eventually the tumour cells develop very small-amplitude oscillations about a 'dormant' state, indicating that the TICLs have successfully managed to keep the tumour under control. The numerical simulations demonstrate the existence of cell distributions that are quasi-stationary in time but unstable and heterogeneous in space.

§6. Conclusion

The numerical predictions of the model make it possible to comprehend the mechanisms involved in the appearance of spatio-temporal heterogeneities detected in solid tumours infiltrated by cytotoxic lymphocytes. These are described in numerous immunomorphological investigations [3, 25]. However, in the material discussed above, only some general problems associated with the mathematical theory, of the interaction of TICLs with TCs have been examined. Other issues to be further investigated include stability, the specific character of the dynamic behaviour of the system (both spatial and temporal), and the role of parameters, especially those of diffusion, on the cells in the tissue. The investigation and solution of these 'formal' problems are not only of theoretical importance, but of practical importance as well.

We hope, that the effects caused by the nonlinearity of the system, which still must be found in the analysis of mathematical models, will make it possible for researchers and clinicians to have a better idea of the complicated and sometimes counter-intuitive outcome of processes occurring in tumours. We note that this model could easily be extended to consider the case of radially symmetric, spherical, tumour growth, which corresponds to the situation of a small tumour, growing from within a tissue prior to vascularization. Additionally, the familiar concept of a central necrotic core could also be incorporated. It has been stated that the rate of macrophage and neutrophil accumulation in a spheroid depends on the density of tumour cells and is determined by a law analogous to that of Michaelis-Menten kinetics, while the accumulation of immune lymphocytes in a tumour is determined by the three-cell cooperation of lymphocytes, macrophages and tumour cells [16]. This data could provide further adaptations to our model, incorporating new cell types and increasing the realism of the system.

References

1. Adam, J. A., The dynamics of growth-factor-modified immune response to cancer growth: One dimensional models, Math. Comp. Modell. **17** (1993), 83–106.

2. Adam, J. A. and N. Bellomo (eds.), *A Survey of Models for Tumor-Immune System Dynamics*, Birkhauser, Boston, 1996.

3. Berezhnaya, N. M., L. V. Yakimovich, R. A. Semenova-Kobzar, V. D. Lyulkin and A. Yu. Papivets. The effect of interleukin-2 on proliferation of explants of malignant soft-tissue tumours in diffusion chambers, Experimental Oncology **8** (1986), 39–42.

4. Brocker, E. B., G. Zwaldo, B. Holzmann, E. Macher and C. Sorg, Inflammatory cell infiltrates in human melanoma at different stages of tumour progression, Int. J. Cancer **41** (1988), 562–567.

5. Clark, W. H., Tumour progression and the nature of cancer, Brit. J. Cancer **64** (1991), 631–644.

6. Clark, W. H., D. E. Elder and M. Vanhorn, The biologic forms of malignant melanoma, Human Pathology **17** (1986), 443–450.

7. Deweger, R. A., B. Wilbrink, R. M. P. Moberts, D. Mans, R. Oskam and W. den Otten, Immune reactivity in SL2 lymphoma-bearing mice compared with SL2-immunized mice, Cancer Immun. Immunotherapy **24** (1987), 1191–1192.

8. Durand, R. E. and R. M. Sutherland, Growth and cellular characteristics of multicell spheroids, Recent Results in Cancer Research **95** (1984), 24–49.

9. Folkman, J., How is blood-vessel growth regulated in normal and neo-plastic tissue, Proc. Amer. Assoc. Cancer Res. **26** (1985), 384–385.

10. Forni, G., G. Parmiani, A. Guarini and R. Foa, Gene Transfer in tumour therapy, Annals Oncol. **5** (1994), 789–794.

11. Franks, L. M. and N. Teich (eds.), *Introduction to the Cellular and Molecular Biology of Cancer*, Oxford University Press, New York, 1986.

12. Friedl, P., P. B. Noble and K. S. Zanker, T-Lymphocyte Locomotion in a 3-Dimensional Collagen Matrix – Expression and Function of Cell-Adhesion Molecules, J. Immunol. **154** (1995), 4973–4985.

13. Ioannides, C. G. and T. L. Whiteside, T-cell recognition of human tumours – Implications for molecular immunotherapy of cancer, Clin. Immunol. Immunopath. **66** (1993), 91–106.

14. Jaaskelainen, J., A. Maenpaa, M. Patarroyo, C. G. Gahmberg, K. Somersalo, J. Tarkkanen, M. Kallio and T. Timonen, Migration of recombinant Il-2-activated T-cells and natural killer cells in the intercellular space of human H-2 glioma spheroids in vitro – A study on adhesion molecules involved, J. Immunol. **149** (1992), 260–268.

15. Kuznetsov, V. A., I. A. Makalkin, M. A. Taylor and A. S. Perelson, Nonlinear dynamics of immunogenic tumours: Parameter estimation and global bifurcation analysis, Bull. Math. Biol. **56** (1994), 295–321.

16. Kuznetsov, V. A., V. P. Zhivoglyadov and L. A. Stepanova, Kinetic approach and estimation of the parameters of cellular interaction between the immune system and a tumour, Arch. Immunol. Therap. Exper. **41** (1993), 21–32.

17. Kawakami, Y., M. I. Nishimura, N. P. Restifo, S. L. Topalian, B. H. O'Neil, J. Shilyansky, J. R. Yannelli and S. A. Rosenberg, T-cell recognition of human-melanoma antigens, J. Immunotherapy, **14** (1993), 88–93.

18. Loeffler, D. and S. Ratner, In vivo localization of lymphocytes labeled with low concentrations of HOECHST-33342, J. Immunol. Meth. **119** (1989), 95–101.

19. Loeffler, D., G. Heppner and E. Lord, Influence of hypoxia on T-lymphocytes in solid tumours, Proc. Amer. Assoc. Cancer Res. **29** (1988), 378.

20. Lord, E. M. and G. Burkhardt, Assessment of in situ host immunity to syngeneic tumours utilizing the multicellular spheroid model, Cell. Immunol. **85** (1984), 340–350.

21. Lord, E. M. and G. Nardella, The multicellular tumour spheroid model. 2. Characterization of the preliminary allograft response in unsensitized mice. Transplantation **29** (1980), 119–124.

22. Marušić, M., Ž. Bajzer, S. Vuk-Pavlović and J. P. Freyer, Analysis of the growth of multicellular tumour spheroids by mathematical models, Cell Prolif. **27** (1994), 73–94.

23. Marušić, M., Ž. Bajzer, S. Vuk-Pavlović and J. P. Freyer, Tumour growth *in vivo* and as multicellular spheroids compared by mathematical models, Bull. Math. Biol. **56** (1994), 617–631.

24. MacSween, R. N. M. and K. Whaley (eds.) *Muir's Textbook of Pathology*, 13th edition, Edward Arnold, London, 1992.

25. Nesvetov, A. M. and A. S. Zhdanov, Relationship of the morphology of the immune response and the histological structure of tumours in stomach cancer patients, Voprosy Onkologii **27** (1981), 25–31.

26. Owen, M. R. and J. A. Sherratt, Pattern formation and spatio-temporal irregularity in a model for macrophage-tumour interactions, J. Theor. Biol. **189** (1997), 63–80.

27. Pleass, R. and R. Camp, Cytokines induce lymphocyte migration in vitro by direct, receptor-specific mechanisms, Euro. J. Immunol. **24** (1994), 273–276.

28. R. T. Prehn, The dose-response curve in tumour-immunity, Inter. J. Immunopharmacol. **5** (1983), 255–257.

29. R. T. Prehn, Stimulatory effects of immune reactions upon the growths of untransplanted tumours, Cancer Res. **54** (1994), 908–914.

30. Prigogine, I. and R. Lefever, Stability problems in cancer growth and nucleation, Comp. Biochem. Physiol. **67** (1980), 389–393.

31. Puri, R. K. and J. P. Siegel, Interleukin-4 and cancer therapy, Cancer Invest. **11** (1993), 473–486.

32. Ratner, S. and G. H. Heppner, Mechanisms of lymphocyte traffic in neoplasia, Anticancer Res. **6** (1986), 475–482.

33. Retsky, M. W., R. H. Wardwell, D. E. Swartzendruber and D. L. Headley, Prospective computerized simulation of breast-cancer – Comparison of computer-predictions with 9 sets of biological and clinical data, Cancer Res. **47** (1987), 4982–4987.

34. Rothstein, T. L., M. G. Mage, J. Mond and L. L. McHugh, Guinea pig antiserum to mouse cytotoxic T-lymphocytes and their precursors, J. Immunol. **120** (1978), 209–215.

35. Schwartzentruber, D. J., S. L.Topalian, M. Mancini and S. A. Rosenberg, Specific release of granulocyte-macrophage colony-stimulating factor, tumour necrosis factor-α and IFN-γ by human tumour-infiltrating lymphocytes after autologous tumour stimulation, J. Immunol. **146** (1991), 3674–3681.

36. Siu, H., E. S. Vitetta, R. D. May and J. W. Uhr, Tumour dormancy. Regression of BCL tumour and induction of a dormant tumour state in mice chimeric at the major histocompatibility complex, J. Immunol. **137** (1986), 1376–1382.

37. Sordat, B., H. R. MacDonald and R. K. Lees, The multicellular spheroid as a model tumour allograft. 3. Morphological and kinetic analysis of

spheroid infiltration and destruction, Transplantation **29** (1980), 103–112.

38. Suzuki, Y., C. M. Liu, L. P. Chen, D. Bennathan and E. F. Wheelock, Immune regulation of the L5178Y murine tumour dormant state. 2. Interferon-gamma requires tumour necrosis factor to restrain tumour cell growth in peritoneal cell cultures from tumour dormant mice, J. Immunol. **139** (1987), 3146–3152.

39. Uhr, J. W., T. Tucker, R. D. May, H. Siu and E. S. Vitetta, Cancer dormancy: Studies of the murine BCL lymphoma, Cancer Res. (Suppl.), **51** (1991), 5045s–5053s.

40. Uhr, J. W., R. H. Scheurmann, N. E. Street and E. S. Vitetta, Cancer dormancy: Opportunities for new therapeutic approaches, Nature Med. **3** (1997), 505–509.

41. Wheelock, E. F., K. J. Weinhold and J. Levich, The tumour dormant state, Adv. Cancer Res. **34** (1981), 107–140.

42. Wilson, K. M. and E. M. Lord, Specific (EMT6) and non-specific (WEHI-164) cytolytic activity by host cells infiltrating tumour spheroids, Brit. J. Cancer **55** (1987), 141–146.

M. A. J. Chaplain
Department of Mathematics
University of Dundee
Dundee DD1 4HN
United Kingdom
chaplain@mcs.dundee.ac.uk

V. A. Kuznetsov
Laboratory of Experimental and Computational Biology
Division of Basic Sciences
National Cancer Institute, FCRDC
Frederic, MD 21702-1201

Z. H. James
Department of Mathematical Sciences
University of Bath
Claverton Down
Bath BA2 7AY
United Kingdom

L. A. Stepanova
Laboratory of Mathematical Immunobiophysics
Institute of Biochemical Physics
Russian Academy of Sciences
Moscow, 117977
Russia

An Age and Maturity Structured Model of Cell Population Dynamics

Janet Dyson, Rosanna Villella-Bressan and Glenn Webb

§1. Introduction

We consider a model of cell population dynamics in which individuals are distinguished by age and maturity. The model is applicable to a proliferating cell population in which population growth results from both division and immigration. The density $u(t, a, x)$ of the population with respect to age a and maturity x at time t satisfies the equations

$$u_t(t, a, x) + u_a(t, a, x) + x u_x(t, a, x)$$
$$= \eta(a, x) u(t, a, x), \quad t > 0, \, a > 0, \, 0 \leq x \leq 1$$
$$u(t, 0, x) = \int_0^\infty b(a, x) u(t, a, x) \, da, \quad t > 0, \, 0 \leq x \leq 1 \qquad (AMP)$$
$$u(0, a, x) = \phi(a, x), \quad a > 0, \, 0 \leq x \leq 1.$$

The term $\eta(a, x)$ represents loss of population due to such processes as mortality, emigration and the disappearance of dividing cells, as well as a gain of population due to immigration from external sources. The gain of population due to the division process is represented in the boundary term as an input of cells of age 0, as modulated by the division modulus $b(a, x)$.

For an *in vivo* population of normal cells a cell line consisting of successive generations of dividing cells terminates after a finite number of divisions. This finiteness of cell line is known as the Hayflick limit. Although tumor cell populations may contain immortal cell lines, normal cell populations may require an immigration of more primitive cell types to maintain population renewal. A convenient way to model the immigration of more primitive cells is to introduce a structure variable corresponding to cell maturity. Population is thus gained at any maturity value x by both the arrival of immigrants of age $a > 0$ with maturity x and the entry of newly divided daughter cells of age $a = 0$ with maturity x. In this sense maturity represents level of morphological development rather than progress in the cell cycle (which is represented by

Mathematical Models in Medical and Health Sciences
Mary Ann Horn, Gieri Simonett, and Glenn Webb (eds.), pp. 99–116.
Copyright © 1998 by Vanderbilt University Press, Nashville, TN.
ISBN 0-8265-1310-7.

cell age). The equations in (AMP) account for these gain and loss processes, as well as the aging of cells in a 1-1 correspondence with time ($da/dt = 1$) and an exponential rate of maturation of cells in time ($dx/dt = x$).

The premise of the age-maturity structured model of cell population dynamics is that maturation is a continuous process and may take place at any point in the cell cycle. It is asserted in [12] that the assumption of a continuous maturation-proliferation hypothesis is required for consistency with data for blood cell production systems. The model (AMP) provides a means to understand qualitative distinctions between normal and abnormal blood cell production systems. The solutions of (AMP) are asymptotically stable (normal) if the initial values are positive at the minimum maturity value $x = 0$, and chaotic (aplastic anemic) if the initial values are 0 at the minimum maturity value $x = 0$. The interpretation of this qualitative behavior is that the system will recover from an initial shock only if there is a sufficient supply of the most primitive precursor cells.

Using the method of characteristics we transform this problem into an integral equation. We solve this equation and show that the solutions yield a semigroup of linear operators in the space $Y = C([0,1], L^1(0,\infty))$. We then study instability, hypercyclicity and chaotic behavior of the semigroup of the solutions. The model (AMP) is linear in the population density $u(t,a,x)$ and thus describes a proliferating cell population only over a limited time interval before nonlinear regulation takes place. In future work the authors will extend this model to nonlinear cases which are, in particular, applicable to models of normal and abnormal blood production systems [2, 5, 6, 10, 13, 15, 16].

§2. Existence and Uniqueness of the Solution

Consider the equation

$$u_t(t,a,x) + u_a(t,a,x) + xu_x(t,a,x) = \eta(a,x)u(t,a,x), \tag{1}$$

$t > 0$, $a > 0$, $0 \le x \le 1$, and the initial condition

$$u(0,a,x) = \phi(a,x), \quad a > 0, 0 \le x \le 1 \tag{2}$$

where $\phi \in Y = C([0,1], L^1(0,\infty))$. The norm of ϕ is

$$\|\phi\| = \sup_{x \in [0,1]} \int_0^\infty |\phi(a,x)| \, da = \sup_{x \in [0,1]} |\phi(\cdot,x)|_{L^1},$$

where $|\cdot|_{L^1}$ is the norm in $L^1(0,\infty)$.

It can be shown, using the method of characteristics, that a classical solution of (1), (2) satisfies the integral equation

$$u(t,a,x) = \exp \int_0^t \eta(r + a - t, xe^{r-t}) \, dr \, \phi(a - t, xe^{-t}) \quad \text{if } t < a,$$

$$= \exp \int_{t-a}^t \eta(r + a - t, xe^{r-t}) \, dr \, u(t - a, 0, xe^{-a}) \quad \text{if } t > a. \tag{3}$$

We also impose the boundary condition

$$u(t, 0, x) = \int_0^\infty b(a, x) u(t, a, x) \, da \tag{4}$$

and we set

$$B(t, x) = u(t, 0, x). \tag{5}$$

Then $B(t, x)$ satisfies the integral equation

$$\begin{aligned}
B(t, x) &= \Phi(t, x) + \int_0^t b(a, x) \exp \int_{t-a}^t \eta(r + a - t, xe^{r-t}) \, dr \\
&\qquad\qquad\qquad\qquad \times B(t - a, xe^{-a}) \, da \\
&= \Phi(t, x) + \int_0^t b(t - s, x) \exp \int_s^t \eta(r - s, xe^{r-t}) \, dr \\
&\qquad\qquad\qquad\qquad \times B(s, xe^{-(t-s)}) \, ds
\end{aligned} \tag{6}$$

where

$$\Phi(t, x) = \int_t^\infty b(a, x) \exp \int_0^t \eta(r + a - t, xe^{r-t}) \, dr \, \phi(a - t, xe^{-t}) \, da. \tag{7}$$

If we set

$$k(\sigma, x) = b(\sigma, x) \exp \int_0^\sigma \eta(r, xe^{r-\sigma}) \, dr,$$

equation (6) becomes

$$B(t, x) = \Phi(t, x) + \int_0^t k(t - s, x) B(s, xe^{-(t-s)}) \, ds. \tag{8}$$

We now have

Theorem 1. *Suppose that $b(a, x)$ and $\eta(a, x)$ are continuous in $[0, \infty) \times [0, 1]$ and satisfy*

$$0 \le b(a, x) \le b, \quad \eta(a, x) \le \eta,$$

where b and η are constant. Then equation (8) has a unique solution such that $|B(t, x)|$ is bounded for each t. Also

$$|B(t, x)| \le b \, e^{(\eta + b)t} \|\phi\|. \tag{9}$$

Thus the integral problem (3), (4) has a unique solution $u^\phi(t, a, x)$ such that $u^\phi(t, \cdot, x) \in L^1$ and $|u^\phi(t, \cdot, x)|_{L^1}$ is bounded for each t, and

$$\int_0^\infty |u^\phi(t, a, x)| \, da \le e^{(\eta + b)t} \|\phi\|. \tag{10}$$

Proof: Define $B_n(t, x)$ inductively by

$$B_0(t, x) = \Phi(t, x)$$
$$B_n(t, x) = \Phi(t, x) + \int_0^t k(t - s, x) B_{n-1}(s, x e^{-(t-s)}) \, ds. \tag{11}$$

The hypotheses on $b(a, x)$ and $\eta(a, x)$ imply that

$$|\Phi(t, x)| \leq b e^{\eta t} \|\phi\| \text{ and } 0 \leq k(\sigma, x) \leq b e^{\eta \sigma},$$

so, by induction, we see that

$$|B_n(t, x) - B_{n-1}(t, x)| \leq \frac{t^n}{n!} b^{n+1} e^{\eta t} \|\phi\|. \tag{12}$$

So $B_n(t, x)$ is uniformly convergent for (t, x) on compact subsets of $[0, \infty) \times [0, 1]$ to a solution of the integral equation (8); and this solution satisfies (9) because

$$|B(t, x)| \leq \sum_{n=0}^{\infty} \frac{b^{n+1} t^n}{n!} e^{\eta t} \|\phi\| = b e^{(\eta + b) t} \|\phi\|. \tag{13}$$

We prove now uniqueness. Suppose $\phi = 0$.

Then if $B(t, x)$ satisfies the integral equation we have

$$|B(t, x)| \leq \int_0^t b e^{\eta(t-s)} |B(s, x e^{-(t-s)})| \, ds. \tag{14}$$

Set $|B(t, \cdot)|_\infty = \sup_{[0,1]} |B(t, x)|$ and take the sup over x, to get

$$|B(t, \cdot)|_\infty \leq \int_0^t b e^{\eta(t-s)} |B(s, \cdot)|_\infty \, ds.$$

Then, by Gronwall's inequality, $|B(t, \cdot)|_\infty = 0$, and so $B(t, x) = 0$, as required. Also from (3)

$$\int_0^t |u^\phi(t, a, x)| \, da \leq \int_0^t e^{\eta a} |B(t - a, x e^{-a})| \, da \leq \int_0^t e^{\eta a} b e^{(\eta + b)(t-a)} \|\phi\| \, da$$
$$\leq e^{\eta t} b \|\phi\| \int_0^t e^{b(t-a)} \, da = e^{\eta t} \|\phi\| (e^{bt} - 1)$$

and

$$\int_t^\infty |u^\phi(t, a, x)| \, da \leq e^{\eta t} \int_t^\infty |\phi(a - t, x e^{-t})| \, da \leq e^{\eta t} \|\phi\|.$$

and (10) follows immediately. $\square$

It is easy to prove inductively that

$$B_m(t,x) = \Phi(t,x)+$$

$$\sum_{n=1}^{m} \int_0^t \{\int_s^t \int_s^{s_{n-1}} \cdots \int_s^{s_2} k(t-s_{n-1},x)\, k(s_{n-1}-s_{n-2}, x\, e^{-(t-s_{n-1})}) \quad (15)$$

$$\ldots k(s_1 - s, x\, e^{-(t-s_1)})\, ds_1 \ldots ds_{n-1}\} \Phi(s, xe^{-(t-s)})\, ds,$$

and so $B(t,x)$ is given explicitly by

$$B(t,x) = \Phi(t,x)+ \qquad\qquad\qquad\qquad (16)$$

$$\sum_{n=1}^{\infty} \int_0^t \{\int_s^t \int_s^{s_{n-1}} \cdots \int_s^{s_2} b(t-s_{n-1},x)\, b(s_{n-1}-s_{n-2}, x\, e^{-(t-s_{n-1})})$$

$$\ldots b(s_1 - s, x\, e^{-(t-s_1)})\, \exp\Big(\int_{s_{n-1}}^t \eta(r-s_{n-1}, xe^{r-t})\, dr+$$

$$\int_{s_{n-2}}^{s_{n-1}} \eta(r-s_{n-2}, xe^{r-t})\, dr + \cdots + \int_s^{s_1} \eta(r-s, xe^{r-t})\, dr\Big)$$

$$ds_1 \ldots ds_{n-1}\} \Phi(s, xe^{-(t-s)})\, ds.$$

Hence

$$u^\phi(t,a,x) = \exp \int_0^t \eta(r+a-t, x\, e^{r-t})\, dr\; \phi(a-t, xe^{-t}) \quad \text{if } t < a, \qquad (17)$$

$$= \exp \int_{t-a}^t \eta(r+a-t, x\, e^{r-t})\, dr\{\Phi(t-a, x\, e^{-a})+$$

$$\sum_{n=1}^{\infty} \int_0^{t-a} \{\int_s^{t-a} \int_s^{s_{n-1}} \cdots \int_s^{s_2} b(t-a-s_{n-1}, x\, e^{-a})$$

$$b(s_{n-1}-s_{n-2}, x\, e^{-(t-s_{n-1})}) \ldots b(s_1 - s, x\, e^{-(t-s_1)})$$

$$\exp\Big(\int_{s_{n-1}}^{t-a} \eta(r-s_{n-1}, xe^{r-t})\, dr+$$

$$+ \int_{s_{n-2}}^{s_{n-1}} \eta(r-s_{n-2}, xe^{r-t})\, dr + \cdots + \int_s^{s_1} \eta(r-s, xe^{r-t})\, dr\Big)\, ds_1 \ldots ds_{n-1}\}$$

$$\Phi(s, xe^{-(t-s)})\, ds\} \quad \text{if } t > a.$$

From now on we say that the function u^ϕ given by (17) is the solution of (AMP) with initial data ϕ.

§3. The Semigroup of the Solutions

We now associate to the solutions of the problem (AMP) a strongly continuous semigroup of linear operators in the space $Y = C([0,1], L^1(0,\infty))$ and study properties of this semigroup.

Let $\phi \in Y$ and define

$$(T(t)\phi)(a, x) = u^\phi(t, a, x). \tag{18}$$

Hence

$$T(t)\phi(a, x) = \exp \int_0^t \eta(r + a - t, xe^{r-t})\, dr\, \phi(a - t, xe^{-t}) \text{ if } t < a$$

$$= \exp \int_{t-a}^t \eta(r + a - t, xe^{r-t})\, dr\, B(t - a, xe^{-a}) \text{ if } t > a. \tag{19}$$

Denote by Y_0 the space $\{\phi \in Y,\ \phi(a, 0) = 0\}$. We have the following result:

Theorem 2. *If $b(a, x)$ and $\eta(a, x)$ are uniformly continuous and satisfy*

$$0 \le b(a, x) \le b, \quad \eta(a, x) \le \eta,$$

where b and η are constant, then $T(t)$ is a strongly continuous semigroup of type $\omega = \eta + b$ on Y, that is for each $t \ge 0$, $T(t)$ is a linear bounded operator in Y and

i) $T(0) = I$,

ii) $T(t)T(\tau) = T(t + \tau)$,

iii) $t \to T(t)\phi$ *is continuous for all $\phi \in Y$.*

iv) $\|T(t)\phi\| \le e^{\omega t}\|\phi\|$, *where $\omega = \eta + b$.*

Also

v) $T(t)$ *maps Y_0 into Y_0,*

vi) $\phi \ge 0$ *implies $T(t)\phi \ge 0$,*

vii) *if there is a $\delta > 0$ such that $\phi(a, x) = 0$ for $x \in [0, \delta]$, then $T(t)\phi(a, x) = 0$ for $t > -\log \delta$ and all $x \in [0, 1]$.*

We sketch the proof via a number of propositions, assuming the conditions of the Theorem throughout.

We first note that

Proposition 3. *If $\phi \in Y$ then $T(t)\phi \in Y$.*

Proof: The result is proved by first showing that both $\Phi(t, x)$ and $B(t, x)$ are continuous in x for fixed t, and bounded on bounded subsets of $[0, \infty) \times [0, 1]$. It can then be shown that $u^\phi \in Y$ using a standard uniform continuity argument. $\square$

It is then easy to see that if $\phi \in Y_0$ then also $T(t)\phi \in Y_0$ and that if $\phi \ge 0$ then also $T(t)\phi \ge 0$.

A uniqueness argument shows that $T(t)T(\tau) = T(t + \tau)$, and a compactness argument then shows that $T(t)$ is strongly continuous. We also have

Proposition 4. *If $\phi(a, x) = 0$ for $x \in [0, \delta]$, $\delta > 0$, then $u^\phi(t, a, x) = 0$ for $t > -\log \delta$ and all $x \in [0, 1]$ and all a.*

Proof: Note that if $t > -\log \delta$ then $xe^{-t} < \delta$ and so $\phi(s, xe^{-t}) = 0$ for all x. Thus, using (7) $\Phi(s, xe^{-(t-s)}) = 0$ for all s, x and the result follows from (17). $\square$

The proof of Theorem 2 is then complete.

§4. Some Remarks on Linear Chaotic Semigroups in Y_0

Let $W(t)$ be a strongly continuous semigroup of linear operators in a Banach space Z with norm $\|\cdot\|$.

A condition which has been always associated with chaos is sensitive dependence on initial conditions.

The semigroup $W(t)$ has *sensitive dependence on initial conditions* if there is a $\beta > 0$ such that for any $x \in Z$ and $\epsilon > 0$ there is y and $\tilde{t}$ such that $\|y - x\| < \epsilon$ and $\|W(\tilde{t})y - W(\tilde{t})x\| \geq \beta$.

We say that $x \in Z$ is *stable* if given $\epsilon > 0$ there exists $d > 0$ such that if $\|z - x\| < d$ then $\|W(t)z - W(t)x\| < \epsilon$ for all $t \geq 0$. We say that x is *unstable* if it is not stable.

It is easy to see that as $W(t)$ is a linear semigroup then $W(t)$ has sensitive dependence on initial conditions if and only if at least one point of Z is unstable (in which case all points are unstable and any β in the definition would do).

Following Devaney, [4], and Webb, [17], we give the following definition.

The semigroup $W(t)$ is *chaotic* if
   i) $W(t)$ is *topologically transitive*, that is, given two open sets in Z, U and V, there exist $x \in U$ and $t \geq 0$ such that $x \in U$ and $W(t)x \in V$.

   ii) The set of *periodic points*, that is the set of $x \in Z$ such that $W(t)x = x$ for some $t > 0$, is dense in Z.

 iii) $W(t)$ *has sensitive dependence on initial conditions*.

Condition (iii) was proved to be a consequence of the first two in [1].

In fact as $W(t)$ is linear, (iii) is a consequence of (i).

Proposition 5. *If the semigroup $W(t)$ is topologically transitive then it has sensitive dependence on initial conditions.*

Proof: Let $\beta > 0$ and $V_\beta = \{x \in Y, \|x\| > \beta\}$ and, given $\epsilon > 0$, set $U_\epsilon = \{x \in Y, \|x\| < \epsilon\}$. There exists $\phi \in U_\epsilon$ and $\tilde{t} \geq 0$ such that $T(\tilde{t})\phi \in V_\beta$. So 0 is unstable and the result follows. $\square$

The semigroup $W(t)$ is *hypercyclic* if there is a $x \in Z$ such that the set

$$\{W(t)x, \, t \geq 0\}$$

is dense in Z.

Examples of linear hypercyclic semigroups can be found in [2, 3, 7, 8, 9, 10, 11, 14, 16, 17].

It has been proved in [3] that

Proposition 6. *The semigroup $W(t)$ is hypercyclic if and only if is topologically transitive.*

The following proposition, also in [3], gives sufficient conditions for hypercyclicity.

Proposition 7. *Consider the sets*

$$Z_1 = \{x \in Z, \lim_{t \to \infty} W(t)x = 0\}$$

and

$$Z_2 = \{x \in Z, \text{ for all } \epsilon > 0 \text{ there exist}$$
$$y \in Z \text{ and } t \geq 0 \text{ with } \|y\| < \epsilon \text{ and } \|W(t)y - x\| < \epsilon\}.$$

If Z_1 and Z_2 are dense in Z then $W(t)$ is hypercyclic.

We suppose now that $T(t)$ is a semigroup in $Y_0 = \{\phi \in Y, \phi(a,0) = 0\}$ and consider the following condition

(H) If $\phi(a,x) = 0$ for $x \in [0,\delta]$, where $0 < \delta \leq 1$ then there exists τ_δ such that $T(t)\phi = 0$ for $t > \tau_\delta$.

Proposition 8. *Suppose that $T(t)$ is a strongly continuous semigroup in Y_0 which satisfies condition (H).*

Suppose that there exists $\phi_0 \in Y_0$ such that $T(t)\phi_0$ does not tend to 0 as t tends to ∞. Then 0 is unstable.

Proof: There exist $\epsilon > 0$ and $t_n \to \infty$ such that

$$\|T(t_n)\phi_0\| > \epsilon \text{ for all } n.$$

Suppose that 0 is stable. So there exists $d > 0$ such that

$$\text{if } \|\phi\| < d \text{ then } \|T(t)\phi\| < \epsilon \text{ for all } t \geq 0.$$

Choose $\delta_1 > 0$ and $\phi_1 \in Y_0$ such that $\phi_1(a,x) = \phi_0(a,x)$ for $x \in [0,\delta_1]$ and $\|\phi_1\| < d$, so that

$$\|T(t)\phi_1\| \leq \epsilon \text{ for all } t \geq 0,$$

and there exist τ_1 such that

$$T(t)\phi_1 = T(t)\phi_0 \text{ if } t > \tau_1.$$

So if $t > \tau_1$, then $\|T(t)\phi_0\| < \epsilon$, in contradiction with (20). $\square$

This proposition can be compared with Proposition 10 of [6].

We say that $w \in Y$ is *eventually periodic* if there exists $\tau \geq 0$ such that $T(\tau)w$ is a periodic point.

We have the following result

Proposition 9. *Suppose that $T(t)$ is a strongly continuous semigroup in Y_0 which satisfies condition (H).*

Then, if $T(t)$ has at least one periodic point, the set of eventually periodic points is dense in Y_0. In fact if u is a periodic point, the set of w such that $T(\tau)w = u$ is dense for some $\tau \geq 0$.

Proof: Suppose that u is a periodic point and that $T(\bar{t})u = u$, $\bar{t} > 0$. Let $v \in Y_0$ and $\epsilon > 0$. Let $\delta > 0$ be such that if $0 \leq x \leq \delta$ then $|u(\cdot,x)|_{L^1} < \frac{\epsilon}{2}$ and $|v(\cdot,x)|_{L^1} < \frac{\epsilon}{2}$. We can choose $w \in Y_0$ such that $w(\cdot,x) = u(\cdot,x)$ if $x \in [0,\delta]$ and $\|w - v\| \leq \epsilon$.

But if $t > \tau_\delta$, $T(t)w = T(t)u$. Choose $\bar{n} \in \mathbb{N}$ such that $\bar{n}\bar{t} > \tau_\delta$. Then $T(\bar{n}\bar{t})w = T(\bar{n}\bar{t})u = u$. $\square$

Corollary 10. *Suppose that $T(t)$ is a strongly continuous semigroup in Y_0 which satisfies condition (H).*

If $T(t)$ has one periodic point then 0 is unstable.

Proof: Let u be periodic and $\|u\| = \beta$. Let $\epsilon > 0$, then there are w and τ such that $\|w\| < \epsilon$ and $T(\tau)w = u$ and so $\|T(\tau)w\| \geq \beta$. $\square$

In fact this corollary is also a consequence of Proposition 8. It is easy now to prove

Proposition 11. *Suppose that $T(t)$ is a strongly continuous semigroup in Y_0 which satisfies condition (H).*

Suppose that the set of periodic points of $T(t)$ is dense in Y_0. Then $T(t)$ is also topologically transitive; hence chaotic.

Proof: We prove that $T(t)$ is topologically transitive. Let U and V open sets of Y_0. Let $u \in V$ be periodic. Then by Proposition 9 there exist $w \in U$ and τ such that $T(\tau)w = u$. $\square$

§5. Instability of $T(t)$ in Y_0

Now let $T(t)$ be the semigroup generated by the solutions of (AMP) in Y_0.

We have proved in Theorem 2 that $T(t)$ satisfies condition (H). It is then easy to prove the following instability result.

Theorem 12. *Suppose that $b(a, x)$ and $\eta(a, x)$ are uniformly continuous in $[0, \infty) \times [0, 1]$ and that there exist constants b, η_1 and η_2 such that*

$$0 \leq b(a, x) \leq b, \quad 0 < \eta_1 \leq \eta(a, x) \leq \eta_2.$$

Then there exists $\phi_0 \in Y_0$ such that the solution of (AMP), $u^{\phi_0}(t, a, x)$, does not tend to 0 as t tends to ∞.

Hence every $\phi \in Y_0$ is unstable.

Proof: Take $\phi_0(a, x) = e^{-pa}x^q$ where $p > 0$ and $0 < q < \eta_1$. So $u^{\phi_0}(t, a, x) \geq 0$. If $t < a$, from (3)

$$u^{\phi_0}(t, a, x) \geq e^{\eta_1 t}\phi(a - t, x e^{-t}) = e^{(\eta_1 - q)t}x^q e^{-p(a-t)},$$

so

$$\int_0^\infty u^{\phi_0}(t, a, x)\, da \geq \int_t^\infty e^{(\eta_1 - q)t}x^q e^{-p(a-t)}\, da = \frac{x^q e^{(\eta_1 - q)t}}{p}.$$

So $\|u^{\phi_0}(t, \cdot, \cdot)\| \geq \frac{e^{(\eta_1 - q)t}}{p} \to \infty$ as $t \to \infty$. The result follows from Proposition 8. $\square$

§6. Hypercyclicity of $T(t)$ in X_0

Let $T(t)$ be the semigroup generated by the solutions , u^ϕ, of (AMP) in Y. Given $\phi \in Y$, we define

$$v^\phi(t,x) = \int_0^\infty u^\phi(t,a,x)\,da = \int_0^\infty (T(t)\phi)(a,x)\,da,$$

so $v^\phi(t,x)$ gives the density of the population of cells of all age which at time t have maturity x.

If we set

$$(S(t)\phi)(x) = v^\phi(t,x), \qquad t \geq 0,$$

$S(t)$ maps Y into $X = C[0,1]$, is linear and is such that, for all $\phi \in Y$,

i) $S(0)\phi = \int_0^\infty \phi(a,x)\,da$,

ii) $S(t+s)\phi = S(t)T(s)\phi = S(s)T(t)\phi$,

iii) $t \to S(t)\phi$ is continuous and

$$|S(t)\phi|_\infty \leq e^{\omega t}\|\phi\|.$$

Also, if we set $X_0 = \{f \in X,\ f(0) = 0\}$,

iv) S(t) maps Y_0 into X_0.

v) $\phi \geq 0$ implies $S(t)\phi \geq 0$,

vi) if there is a $\delta > 0$ such that $\phi(a,x) = 0$ for $x \in [0,\delta]$ then $S(t)\phi = 0$ for $t > -\log\delta$.

Suppose that $T(t)$ is hypercyclic in Y_0 and let $\phi \in Y_0$ be such that the set $\{T(t)\phi,\ t \geq 0\}$ is dense in Y_0. Then the set $\{S(t)\phi,\ t \geq 0\}$ is dense in X_0. In fact, let $\psi \in X_0$. Then there is $\tilde{t}$ such that $\|T(\tilde{t})\phi(a,x) - e^{-a}\psi(x)\| \leq \epsilon$ and so for all $x \in [0,1]$, $\int_0^\infty |T(\tilde{t})\phi(a,x) - e^{-a}\psi(x)|\,da \leq \epsilon$ and so, as $\int_0^\infty e^{-a}\,da = 1$, $|\int_0^\infty T(\tilde{t})\phi(a,x)\,da - \psi(x)| \leq \epsilon$.

We are led to the following definition.

Definition 6.1. *We say that $T(t)$ is hypercyclic in X_0 if $S(t)$ is hypercyclic, that is if there exists $\phi \in Y_0$ such that the set*

$$\{S(t)\phi,\ t \geq 0\}$$

is dense in X_0.

Note that $\{S(t)\phi,\ t \geq 0\} = \{v^\phi(t,x),\ t \geq 0\}$.

We prove the following hypercyclicity result.

Theorem 13. *Suppose that $b(a,x) = b(a)$ and $\eta(a,x) = \mu(x) + \nu(a) \geq \eta_1 > 0$ and are uniformly continuous in $[0,1] \times [0,\infty)$. Then $T(t)$ is hypercyclic in X_0.*

The proof will use the following proposition which is the analogue of Proposition 7 for the present situation.

Proposition 14. *Consider the sets*

$$Y_{00} = \{\phi \in Y_0 : \lim_{t \to \infty} \int_0^\infty u^\phi(t, a, x)\, da = 0\}$$

and

$X_{0,\infty} = \{z \in X_0 :$ *for all* $\epsilon > 0$ *there exist*

$$\phi \in Y_0 \text{ and } t \geq 0 \text{ with } \|\phi\| < \epsilon \text{ and } |\int_0^\infty u^\phi(t, a, x)\, da - z|_\infty < \epsilon\}.$$

If Y_{00} and $X_{0,\infty}$ are dense in Y_0 and X_0 respectively then the semigroup $T(t)$ is hypercyclic in X_0.

The proof is a natural adaptation of that of Proposition 7 given in [3]; see also [7].

So the theorem follows from the next two propositions.

Proposition 15. *Y_{00} is dense in Y_0.*

Proof: If for $\delta > 0$, $\phi(a, x) = 0$ for all $x \in [0, \delta]$, then $u^\phi(t, a, x) = 0$ for $t > -\log \delta$. But these functions are dense in Y_0. □

Proposition 16. *Suppose that $b(a, x) = b(a)$ and $\eta(a, x) = \mu(x) + \nu(a) \geq \eta_1 > 0$ and are uniformly continuous in $[0, 1] \times [0, \infty)$. Then $X_{0,\infty} = X_0$.*

Proof: Take

$$\phi_n(a, x) = e^{-pa}x^{q_n}\exp(-\int_0^{t_0}\mu(xe^r)\,dr), \qquad \text{if } 0 \leq x \leq e^{-t_0},$$

$$= \phi_n(a, e^{-t_0}) \qquad \text{if } e^{-t_0} \leq x \leq 1,$$

where $p > 0$ and $0 < q_n < \eta_1$ and t_0 will be fixed later. Suppress the n for the present.

Then if $a > t_0$,

$$u^\phi(t_0, a, x) = \exp\int_0^{t_0}(\mu(xe^{r-t_0}) + \nu(r + a - t_0))\,dr$$

$$e^{-p(a-t_0)}x^q\,e^{-qt_0}\exp(-\int_0^{t_0}\mu(xe^{r-t_0})\,dr)$$

$$= x^q\,g_q(t_0, a),$$

where $g_q(t_0, a) = e^{-qt_0}\exp\int_0^{t_0}\nu(r + a - t_0)\,dr\,e^{-p(a-t_0)}$.

If $a < t_0$

$$u^\phi(t_0, a, x) = x^q\, e^{-qt} \exp(\int_0^{t_0} \mu(xe^r)\,dr) \exp(\int_{t_0-a}^{t_0} \nu(r+a-t)\,dr)$$

$$\{\int_0^\infty b(s+t-a) \exp \int_0^{t_0-a} \nu(r+s)\,dr\, e^{-ps}\,ds \exp(-\int_0^{t_0} \mu(xe^r)\,dr)+$$

$$+\sum_{n=1}^\infty \int_0^{t_0-a} (\int_s^{t_0-a} \cdots \int_s^{s_2} b(t_0-a-s_{n-1})\ldots b(s_1-s)$$

$$\exp(\int_{s_{n-1}}^{t_0-a} \nu(r-s_{n-1})\,dr + \cdots + \int_s^{s_1} \nu(r-s)\,dr)ds_1\ldots ds_{n-1})$$

$$\int_0^\infty b(\alpha+s)\exp\int_0^s \nu(r+\alpha)\,dr\, e^{-p\alpha}\,d\alpha\,ds \exp(-\int_0^{t_0}\mu(xe^r)\,dr)\}$$

$$= x^q f_q(t,a), \ \text{say}$$

where $f_q(t,a) \geq 0$.
Hence, if we set

$$h_q(t_0) = \int_0^{t_0} f_q(t_0,a)\,da + \int_{t_0}^\infty g_q(t_0,a)\,da,$$

then $h_q(t_0) \geq \int_{t_0}^\infty g_q(t_0,a)\,da$, and so

$$\exp(\int_0^{t_0}\mu(xe^r)\,dr)\, h_q(t_0) \geq \frac{1}{p} e^{(\eta_1-q)t_0}. \tag{21}$$

Now choose q_n such that $\mathrm{span}(x^{q_n})$ is dense in X_0 and $0 < q_n < \eta_1$.
So given $z \in X_0$, there exist α_n, $n \in F$, $F \subset \mathbb{N}$ finite, such that

$$|z(x) - \sum \alpha_n x^{q_n}|_\infty < \epsilon.$$

Take

$$\phi(a,x) = \frac{\sum \alpha_n x^{q_n} e^{-pa} \exp(-\int_0^{t_0}\mu(xe^r)\,dr)}{h_{q_n}(t_0)} \quad \text{if } 0 \leq x \leq e^{-t_0},$$

$$= \phi(a, e^{-t_0}) \quad \text{if } e^{-t_0} \leq x \leq 1.$$

We have

$$|\phi(\cdot,x)|_{L^1} \leq \sum \frac{|\alpha_n|}{p\, h_{q_n}(t_0)\exp(\int_0^{t_0}\mu(xe^r)\,dr)} \quad \text{for } 0 \leq x \leq e^{-t_0},$$

and so by (21),

$$\|\phi\| = \sup_{x\in[0,e^{-t_0}]} |\phi(\cdot,x)|_{L^1} \leq \sum |\alpha_n| e^{-(\eta_1-q_n)t_0}.$$

Choose t_0 such that $\sum |\alpha_n| e^{-(\eta_1 - q_n)t_0} < \epsilon$. Then

$$\int_0^\infty u^\phi(t_0, a, x)\, da = \sum \frac{\alpha_n}{h_{q_n}(t_0)} \int_0^\infty u^{\phi_n}(t_0, a, x)\, da$$
$$= \sum \frac{\alpha_n\, x^{q_n}}{h_{q_n}(t_0)} h_{q_n}(t_0) = \sum \alpha_n\, x^{q_n},$$

and the result is proved. $\square$

Note. If η is constant and if there is a $p > 0$ such that $\int_0^\infty b(a)e^{-pa}\, da = 1$ then Proposition 16 can be proved very easily. In fact with this p take $\phi_n = e^{-pa} x^{q_n}$ as before. Then $u^{\phi_n}(t, a, x) = e^{(\eta - q_n + p)t} e^{-pa} x^{q_n}$ because this satisfies (AMP).

Now take $\phi = p e^{-pa} \sum \alpha_n x^{q_n} e^{-(\eta - q_n + p)t_0}$ and choose t_0 large enough such that $\|\phi\| < \epsilon$. Then

$$\int_0^\infty u^\phi(t_0, a, x)\, da = \sum \alpha_n x^{q_n} e^{(\eta - q_n + p)t_0} e^{-(\eta - q_n + p)t_0},$$

and again the result follows.

§7. Chaotic Behaviour of $T(t)$ in X_0

We now look at the existence of periodic points of $T(t)$ and at its chaotic behaviour in X_0.

Note that if $\phi \in Y$ is periodic so that $T(\bar{t})\phi = T(0)\phi$ for some $\bar{t} > 0$, then also $S(\bar{t})\phi = S(0)\phi$, and so $v^\phi(t + \bar{t}, x) = v^\phi(t, x)$.

Denote by Π the set of periodic points of $T(t)$ and suppose that Π is dense in Y_0. Then the set $\{S(0)\phi, \phi \in \Pi\}$ is dense in X_0. In fact, given $\psi \in X_0$ there is $\phi \in \Pi$ such that $\|\phi(a, x) - e^{-a}\psi(x)\| \le \epsilon$ and so for all $x \in [0, 1]$, $|\int_0^\infty \phi(a, x)\, da - \psi(x)| \le \epsilon$.

We are led to the following definition.

Definition 7.1. *We say that $T(t)$ is chaotic in X_0 if $S(t)$ is hypercyclic and the set*

$$P = \{\, S(0)\phi,\ \phi \in Y_0 \text{ is a periodic point of } T(t)\}$$

is dense in X_0.

Note that $S(0)\phi = v^\phi(0, x) = \int_0^\infty \phi(a, x)\, da$.

We have the analogous result to Proposition 11.

Proposition 17. *Suppose that the set P is dense in X_0. Then $S(t)$ is hypercyclic, hence $T(t)$ is chaotic in X_0.*

Proof: We prove that $X_{0,\infty} = X_0$. Given $z \in X_0$ and $\epsilon > 0$, there exists $\phi \in P$ such that

$$\left| \int_0^\infty \phi(a, x)\, da - z \right| < \epsilon.$$

But the set of $w \in Y_0$ such that $T(\tilde{t})w = \phi$ is dense in Y_0, so there exist $w \in Y_0$ $\tilde{t}$ such that $\|w\| < \epsilon$ and $T(\tilde{t})w = \phi$. And so $S(\tilde{t})w = \int_0^\infty \phi(a,x)\,da$ and

$$|S(\tilde{t})w - z|_\infty < \epsilon;$$

so $z \in X_{0,\infty}$ and $X_{0,\infty} = X_0$. $\square$

We now give sufficient conditions such that P is dense in X_0. We can find periodic points of $T(t)$ by separating the variables. The following proposition is easily proved.

Propsition 18. *Suppose that $b(a,x) = b(a) \geq 0$ and $\eta(a,x) = \mu(x) + \nu(a)$ are uniformly continuous and bounded.*

Suppose also that we can choose $r > 0$ such that

$$e^{-ra} \exp \int_0^a \nu(\alpha)\,d\alpha \in L^1(0,\infty),$$

$$\int_0^\infty b(a)e^{-ra} \exp \int_0^a \nu(\alpha)\,d\alpha\,da = 1$$

and

$$x^r \exp(-\int_x^1 \frac{\mu(s)}{s}\,ds) \to 0 \text{ as } x \to 0,$$

then for any $k \in \mathbb{R}$

$$e^{-ikt}e^{-ra} \exp(\int_0^a \nu(\alpha)d\alpha)x^r \exp(-\int_x^1 \frac{\mu(s)}{s}\,ds)\,x^{ik}$$

is a periodic solution of (AMP). So in particular

$$e^{-ra} \exp(\int_0^a \nu(\alpha)d\alpha)x^r \exp(-\int_x^1 \frac{\mu(s)}{s}\,ds)\,x^{ik}$$

are periodic points of $T(t)$.

It follows that

$$e^{-ra} \exp(\int_0^a \nu(\alpha)d\alpha)x^r \exp(-\int_x^1 \frac{\mu(s)}{s}\,ds) \sum_{n \in F} \alpha_n e^{i\beta n \log x} e^{-i\beta nt}$$

where F is any finite subset of $\mathbb{Z}$ and $\alpha_n \in \mathbb{C}$, $\beta \in \mathbb{R}$ is also a periodic solution of (AMP), so

$$e^{-ra} \exp(\int_0^a \nu(\alpha)d\alpha)x^r \exp(-\int_x^1 \frac{\mu(s)}{s}\,ds) \sum_{n \in F} \alpha_n e^{i\beta n \log x}$$

is a periodic point of $T(t)$. We denote by V the set of such points and prove that

$$W = \{\int_0^\infty \phi(a,x)\,da,\ \phi \in V\}$$

is dense in X_0. Note that if $\phi \in V$ then

$$\int_0^\infty \phi(a,x)\,da = x^r \exp(-\int_x^1 \frac{\mu(s)}{s}\,ds)\,A \sum_{n \in F} \alpha_n e^{i\beta n \log x}$$

where $A = \int_0^\infty e^{-ra} \exp(\int_0^a \nu(\alpha)d\alpha)\,da$.

Thus it is sufficient to prove the following density result.

Proposition 19. *Suppose that $f \in C_0[0,1]$ is such that $f(x) > 0$ for $x \in (0,1]$. Then given $z \in C_0[0,1]$ and $\epsilon > 0$ there exist $\alpha_n \in \mathbb{C}$, $\beta \in \mathbb{R}$ and F a finite subset of $\mathbb{Z}$ such that*

$$|z(x) - f(x) \sum_{n \in F} \alpha_n e^{i\beta n \log x}| < \epsilon. \tag{22}$$

Proof: We may consider only those z such that

$$z(x) = 0 \text{ for } x \in [0, \bar{\delta}] \text{ where } 0 < \bar{\delta} < 1,$$

since such z are dense in $C_0[0,1]$.

Let $M = \sup_{[0,1]} |f(x)|$,

$$K = \sup_{(0,1]} |\frac{z(x)}{f(x)}| \tag{23}$$

and choose δ, $0 < \delta \le \bar{\delta}$, such that $K|f(x)| < \epsilon/2$ for $x \in [0, \delta]$.

Consider first $x \in [\delta, 1]$. We make the transformation $x = e^{-s}$, so that $s \in [0, -\log \delta]$, and define

$$w(s) = \frac{z(e^{-s})}{f(e^{-s})}, \qquad 0 \le s \le -\log \delta,$$

so, by 23, $|w(s)| \le K$ for $s \in [0, -\log \delta]$. We extend w to $[0, -2\log \delta]$ in such way that $w(-2\log \delta) = w(0)$ and $|w(s)| \le K$.

Now there exist α_n such that

$$|w(s) - \sum \alpha_n \exp \frac{2\pi i n s}{-2\log \delta}| \le \frac{\epsilon}{2M}, \qquad s \in [0, -2\log \delta]. \tag{24}$$

Thus

$$|\frac{z(e^{-s})}{f(e^{-s})} - \sum \alpha_n \exp \frac{\pi i n s}{-\log \delta}| \le \frac{\epsilon}{2M}, \qquad s \in [0, -2\log \delta],$$

so

$$|z(x) - f(x) \sum \alpha_n \exp \frac{\pi i n \log x}{\log \delta}| \le \frac{\epsilon}{2M}|f(x)| \le \frac{\epsilon}{2}.$$

Now look at $x \in (0, \delta]$. From (24)

$$|\sum \alpha_n \exp \frac{\pi i n \log x}{\log \delta}| \le \frac{\epsilon}{2M} + K \text{ for all } x > 0.$$

Also $z(x) = 0$. So

$$|z(x) - f(x) \sum \alpha_n \exp \frac{\pi i n \log x}{\log \delta}| =$$

$$= |f(x) \sum \alpha_n \exp \frac{\pi i n \log x}{\log \delta}| \le |f(x)|(\frac{\epsilon}{2M} + K) \le \epsilon.$$

Thus (22) holds with $\beta = \frac{\pi}{\log \delta}$. $\square$

Thus taking $f(x) = x^r \exp(-\int_x^1 \frac{\mu(s)}{s} ds)$ we have, using Proposition 17,

Theorem 20. *Suppose $b(a, x) = b(a) \geq 0$ and $\eta(a, x) = \mu(x) + \nu(a)$ are uniformly continuous and bounded above. Suppose also that we can choose r such that*

$$e^{-ra} \exp \int_0^a \nu(\alpha)\, d\alpha \in L^1(0, \infty),$$

$$\int_0^\infty b(a) e^{-ra} \exp \int_0^a \nu(\alpha)\, d\alpha\, da = 1$$

and

$$x^r \exp\left(-\int_x^1 \frac{\mu(s)}{s}\, ds\right) \to 0 \text{ as } x \to 0.$$

Then $T(t)$ is chaotic in X_0.

A very simple case in which such r exists is when

$$\eta(a, x) = \eta > 0 \quad \text{and} \quad \int_0^\infty b(a)\, da > 1.$$

In this case there exists $\gamma > 0$ such that

$$\int_0^\infty b(a)\, e^{-\gamma a}\, da = 1,$$

and we can choose $r = \gamma + \eta$.

In fact then for all $k \in \mathbb{R}$ the functions

$$e^{-\gamma a} x^{\gamma + \eta} x^{-ik}$$

belong to Y_0 and are periodic points of $T(t)$ as

$$e^{ikt} e^{-\gamma a} x^{\gamma + \eta} x^{-ik}, \quad k \in \mathbb{R}$$

are classical solutions of (AMP).

More generally, if

$$\eta(a, x) = \eta, \quad \int_0^\infty b(a) e^{-\gamma a}\, da = 1 \text{ where } \gamma > 0, \text{ and } \gamma + \eta > 0,$$

then again we can choose $r = \gamma + \eta$.

References

1. Banks, J., J. Brooks, G. Cairns, G. Davis and P. Stacey, On Devaney's definition of chaos, Amer. Math. Monthly **99** (1992), 332–335.

2. Brunowsky, P. and J. Komornik, Ergodicity and exactness of the shift on $C[0, \infty)$ and the semiflow of a first-order partial differential equation, J. Math. Anal. Appl. **104** (1984), 235–245.

3. Desch W. and W. Shappacher and G. Webb, Hypercyclic and chaotic semigroups of linear operators, preprint.

4. Devaney, R., *A First Course in Dynamical Systems: Theory and Experiment*, Addison-Wesley, , 1992.

5. Dyson, J., R. Villella Bressan and G. Webb, A singular transport equation modelling a proliferating maturity structured problem cell population, Canad. Appl. Math. Quar. **1** (1996), 65–95.

6. Dyson J., R. Villella Bressan and G. Webb, A semilinear transport equation with delays, submitted.

7. Dyson J., R. Villella Bressan and G. Webb, Hypercyclicity of solutions of a transport equation with delays, Nonlinear Analysis T.M.A. **29** (1997), 1343–1351.

8. Emamirad H., Hpercyclicité du semi-groupe de transport et le théorème de représentation de Lax et Phillips, C.R. Acad.Sci. Paris, Série 1 **325** (1997), 157–162.

9. Godefroy G. and J. H. Shapiro, Operators with dense, invariant, cyclic vector manifolds, J. Funct. Anal. **98** (1991), 229–269.

10. Lasota A., Stable and chaotic solutions of a first order partial differential equation, Nonlinear Anal. **5** (1981), 1181–1193.

11. Mac Cluer C. R., Chaos in linear distributed systems, Trans. ASME **114** (1992), 322–324.

12. Mackey M. and P. Dormer, Continuous maturation of proliferating erythroid precursors, Cell Tissue Kinet.**15** (1982), 381–392.

13. Mackey M. and R. Rudnicki, Global stability in a delayed partial differential equation describing cellular replication, J. Math. Biol. **33** (1994), 89–109.

14. Protopoescu V. and Y.Y. Azmy, Topological chaos for a class of linear models, Math. Mod. and Meth. in Appl. Scien. **2** (1992), 70–90.

15. Rey A. and M. Mackey, Multistability and boundary layer development in a transport equation with delayed arguments, Canad. Appl. Math. Quar. **1** (1993), 61–81.

16. Rudnicki R., Strong ergodic properties of a first order partial differential equation, J. Math. Anal. Appl. **133** (1988), 941–956.

17. G. Webb, Lectures on chaotic dynamical systems, Lectures given at the University of Padova, May 1996.

Janet Dyson
Mansfield College
University of Oxford
Oxford, England
janet.dyson@mansfield.oxford.ac.uk

Rosanna Villella-Bressan
Dipartimento di Matematica Pura ed Applicata
Universita' di Padova
Padova, Italy
rosannav@math.unipd.it

Glenn Webb
Department of Mathematics
Vanderbilt University
Nashville, TN 37240
webbgf00@ctrvax.vanderbilt.edu

A New Mathematical Model
of Schistosomiasis

Zhilan Feng and Fabio Augusto Milner

Abstract. We propose a new deterministic model for schistosomiasis, based on a system of ordinary differential equations. The numbers of human (definitive) hosts, uninfected and infected snail (intermediate) hosts, and cercaria are used as the main dependent variables. We show that model is well posed and study its asymptotic behavior. The model allows for the existence of two nontrivial steady states. When both exist, we show the local asymptotic stability of the smaller one.

§1. Introduction

In modeling our environment one of the most difficult choices we have to make is the amount of detail we are willing to put into the model. This is usually limited by the detail we are capable of modeling due to our limited ability to gather information. This choice requires a delicate balance between the need for enough detail to resolve important characteristics of the dynamics of the interactions and our ability to obtain data in sufficient detail to use the model.

After some pioneer work on host-parasite systems during the first half on this century [12,22], deterministic modeling of the propagation of infectious diseases was the object of many papers following the work of Kermack and McKendrick [21] with the introduction of S–I–R models, see, for example [29]. More recently, the age structure of the population was also considered [30]. This allows one to model natality and mortality processes which may be age and/or density dependent, as well as the vertical transmission of and the immunity to the disease [9]. All of these studies were concerned with microparasitic diseases, i.e., those transmitted by viruses or bacteria.

The first deterministic models for host-macroparasite systems [10,11], derived less than 25 years ago, were quite simple and soon proved to be unsatisfactory [25]. Then some authors developed other deterministic models [6,17,19], as well as stochastic ones [7,23].

One of the central issues to address in the modeling is the integration of the processes influencing the distribution of parasites in the host population

Mathematical Models in Medical and Health Sciences
Mary Ann Horn, Gieri Simonett, and Glenn Webb (eds.), pp. 117–128.
Copyright © 1998 by Vanderbilt University Press, Nashville, TN.
ISBN 0-8265-1310-7.

[5]. Parasite recruitment cannot be described in a completely random manner as was previously thought [15]. Very recently age-structured and hybrid models were introduced [13,18,19,28]. The study of threshold phenomena is very important for its useful applications in epidemiology and has been the object of several studies [9]. However, for host-parasite systems it has barely started [20].

We shall consider *Schistosoma mansoni*, a human blood fluke which causes schistosomiasis. Campaigns against *S. mansoni* focus upon treatment of infected human patients with Praziquantal. Schistosomiasis is one of the most prevalent diseases in the world, with approximately 200 million people worldwide carrying the parasites in 74 nations. Typical symptoms are fever, rash, bronchitis, hepatosplenomegaly, diarrhea, cirrhosis, portal hypertension. Fortunately, it is not too lethal, but it still causes approximately 750,000 deaths per year. The life cycle of the parasite includes several stages: eggs, miracidia, cercaria, and worm (adult).

Several mathematical and medical studies have addressed specifically the dynamics of schistosomiasis and other parasites in human populations [24,31], using systems similar to the one we are interested in.

The theoretical implications associated with parasite regulation of host population size and stability, have increased in importance in the research of the last twenty years [2,3,6,8,15,26]. In particular, mathematical models describing the dynamics of host-parasite interactions that exhibit regulatory phenomenon have been proposed and studied, e.g. in [1,4,6,7,16,17,27]. It is demonstrated that parasites may regulate the growth of its host's population provided they exhibit an overdispersed pattern of distribution within the host population. Models in [6] are for host-parasite interactions when the parasites have direct life cycles which involve only a single host population and one stage of the parasites. In [27] a free-living stage of parasites was considered in the model. Multiple stages of parasites and two hosts are considered in [14]. The definitive host, however, is assumed to have a constant population size and hence the role of the parasites on population regulation is ignored. It is also assumed in [14] that a constant proportion of intermediate host population is infected at all time.

In our model we try to describe the known biology of schistosome life-cycles more accurately without making the models unmanageably complicated.

§2. A New Model and Its Well-Posedness

We consider a new model that involves various stages in the life cycle of schistosome parasites, variable population sizes of human hosts and intermediate snail hosts with different assumptions on the host growth rates.

Our model is based on several assumptions, including the following:

(H1) Human host population grows exponentially in the absence of parasites;

(H2) Snail population grows logistically in the absence of parasites;

(H3) Infected snails do not reproduce;

(H4) Distribution of parasites among human hosts is overdispersed,

(H5) Birth rates of hosts are greater than their death rates, $b_j - \mu_j > 0$,
   $j = h, s$.

These are very realistic hypotheses. The difference in the average life span of humans and hosts is between one and two orders of magnitude. Consequently, during the time a only few generations of humans come and go, great many generations of snail will have passed and their populations would be at an equilibrium. For such disease free populations, a logistic model is frequently a very good approximation. On the other hand, shistosomiasis is a disease prevalent mostly in countries with a high birth rate, for which the growth is still exponential. Concerning the infertility of the snails, it has been observed in the laboratory and in the field that cercaria cause the castration of their snail hosts, forcing them to stop reproducing. The negative binomial distribution of parasites among hosts has been shown to be a very good fit of available data in several studies. Finally, demographic data consistently shows birth rates to exceed death rates for both types of hosts.

Let H, P, S, I, M, C denote the numbers of human hosts, adult parasites, uninfected snails and infected snails, free-living miracidia, free-living cercaria, respectively. Introduce the following (positive) demographic and epidemiological parameters.

b_h = birth rate of humans

μ_h = natural death rate of human hosts

α = parasite-induced death rate of human hosts, per parasite

β = production rate of cercaria per infected snail

λ = attachment rate of cercaria to human hosts

k = "clumping parameter" of the binomial

μ_p = death rate of parasites

r = treatment-induced death rate of parasites

b_s = birth rate of snails

μ_s = natural death rate of (uninfected) snails

L = carrying capacity of environment for snails

ρ = contact rate (per snail) of uninfected snails with miracidia

S_0 = constant for the "saturation fraction"

d_s = parasite-induced death rate of snails

b_p = mean number of eggs (miracidia) laid per parasite

ζ = "efficacy" of cercaria in infecting humans ($0 \le \zeta \le 1$)

H_0 = constant for the "saturation fraction"

We then describe the dynamics of the schistosome–snail–human interactions through the following system of equations:

$$\begin{cases} \dfrac{d}{dt}H = (b_h - \mu_h)H - \alpha P, \\[2mm] \dfrac{d}{dt}P = C\lambda - \alpha\left(\dfrac{k+1}{k}\right)\dfrac{P^2}{H} - (\mu_h + \mu_p + \alpha + r)P, \\[2mm] \dfrac{d}{dt}S = (b_s - \mu_s)\left(1 - \dfrac{S+I}{L}\right)S - \rho M \dfrac{S}{S_0 + S}, \\[2mm] \dfrac{d}{dt}I = \rho M \dfrac{S}{S_0 + S} - (\mu_s + d_s)I, \\[2mm] M = b_p P, \qquad C = \beta I, \qquad \lambda = \zeta \dfrac{H}{H_0 + H}. \end{cases} \qquad (1)$$

The system can be obtained 'a la Anderson and May, [6], by writing an infinite dimensional system of ODEs, one for each class of hosts having exactly i parasites ($i \geq 0$) and assuming that parasites are distributed among humans according to a negative binomial distribution with clumping parameter k.

The first equation says that, in the absence of parasitism, the size of the human population grows exponentially while parasitism takes a toll proportional to the number present. The first assumption is reasonable since most countries with a high prevalence of schistosomiasis have very high birth rates. The attachment rate of cercaria is taken here to be constant, although it should probably be a function of the length of infection of the snail. However, the introduction of age of infection will force the change of the ODE modeling the dynamics of infected snails to a PDE, making the system mathematically more complicated. This will be done elsewhere.

Concerning the well-posedness of system (1), we just note that from the theory of systems of ordinary differential equations we immediately have local existence and uniqueness of solutions for any non-negative initial values. Moreover, as long as they exist, solutions stay non-negative. Even though at first glance the system might seem singular at $H = 0$, if we define the mean parasite load of humans, $X = P/H$, we obtain for it the following nonsingular equation to replace the second one in (1):

$$\frac{d}{dt}X = \frac{\zeta\beta I}{H_0 + H} - (b_h + \mu_p + \alpha + r)X - \frac{\alpha}{k}X^2.$$

Using then very standard techniques, one can derive a priori the exponential boundedness of solutions, from where the unique existence of a global solution follows.

§3. Equilibria and a modified reproductive number $\mathcal{R}_0$

It is evident from (1) that the system always admits the disease-free (trivial) steady state

$$E = (H, P, S, I) = (\infty, 0, L, 0).$$

This should be understood in the sense that, in the absence of parasitism, the dynamics of humans and snails is entirely decoupled and, consequently, the former grow exponentially to ∞ while the latter stabilize at the carrying capacity L.

Let us turn to the existence of nontrivial equilibria $E^* = (H^*, P^*, S^*, I^*)$, i.e., constant solutions of (1) for which $P^* > 0$.

For convenience, we shall introduce now the following notation.

$$\delta = \mu_h + \mu_p + \alpha + r, \tag{2}$$

$$\gamma = \frac{\rho b_p (b_h - \mu_h)}{(\mu_s + d_s)\alpha}, \tag{3}$$

$$\eta = \frac{\beta}{\delta \frac{b_h - \mu_h}{\alpha} + \alpha(1 + \frac{1}{k})(\frac{b_h - \mu_h}{\alpha})^2}. \tag{4}$$

It follows easily from (1) and (2) that, at equilibrium, we have

$$P = \frac{(b_h - \mu_h)}{\alpha} H, \tag{5}$$

$$\beta \lambda I = P \left[\alpha \frac{(k+1)}{k} \frac{P}{H} + \delta \right]. \tag{6}$$

Now (5) gives

$$\frac{P}{H} = \frac{(b_h - \mu_h)}{\alpha},$$

which used with (4)–(6) leads to the relation

$$\beta \lambda I = \frac{H \beta}{\eta},$$

whereby, using (1),

$$I = \frac{H}{\lambda \eta} = \frac{H_0 + H}{\zeta \eta}. \tag{7}$$

Also, at equilibrium, (1) yields the relation

$$\rho b_p P \frac{S}{S_0 + S} = (\mu_s + d_s)I, \tag{8}$$

which, combined with (3), (5), and (7), immediately leads to

$$\frac{H}{H_0 + H} \frac{S}{S_0 + S} = \frac{1}{\gamma \zeta \eta} = \frac{1}{\mathcal{R}_0}. \tag{9}$$

Here $\mathcal{R}_0$ is a modified reproductive number, given by

$$\mathcal{R}_0 = \zeta \eta \gamma = \frac{\zeta \beta \rho b_p}{(\mu_s + d_s)(\delta + (1 + \frac{1}{k})(b_h - \mu_h))}.$$

We see from (9) that $\mathcal{R}_0 \geq 1$ and the equality can only hold if both H_0 and S_0 vanish, which contradicts our assumptions. Hence, $\mathcal{R}_0 > 1$.

Next note that, at equilibrium, (1) also yields the relation

$$(b_s - \mu_s)\left(1 - \frac{S+I}{L}\right)S = (\mu_s + d_s)I, \tag{10}$$

which shows that

$$S - \frac{S^2}{L} - \frac{IS}{L} = \frac{\mu_s + d_s}{b_s - \mu_s}I.$$

Equivalently,

$$S(L - S) = I\left(\frac{\mu_s + d_s}{b_s - \mu_s}L + S\right),$$

that is,

$$I = \frac{S(L - S)}{S + \frac{\mu_s + d_s}{b_s - \mu_s}L}. \tag{11}$$

We now see from (5), (8) and (11) that, once S^* has been found, the equilibria (H^*, P^*, I^*) of the system are given by

$$H^* = \frac{\alpha}{(b_h - \mu_h)}P^*, \tag{12}$$

$$P^* = \frac{(\mu_s + d_s)(S_0 + S^*)I^*}{\rho b_p S}, \tag{13}$$

$$I^* = \frac{S^*(L - S^*)}{S^* + \frac{\mu_s + d_s}{b_s - \mu_s}L}. \tag{14}$$

Finally, the combination of (10) with (12)–(14) leads, after long but straightforward calculations, to the following quadratic equation for S^*.

$$a_0 S^2 + a_1 S + a_2 = 0, \tag{15}$$

where

$$\begin{cases} a_0 = \mathcal{R}_0 - 1, \\ a_1 = H_0\gamma - S_0 - L(\mathcal{R}_0 - 1), \\ a_2 = L\left(S_0 + H_0\gamma\frac{\mu_s + d_s}{b_s - \mu_s}\right). \end{cases} \tag{16}$$

Since it is always $a_0 > 0$ and $a_2 > 0$, one can easily prove the following theorem about non-trivial equilibria.

Theorem 1.
 i) If $a_1 \geq 0$, then (1) admits no positive equilibrium;
 ii) If $a_1 < 0$, and $a_1^2 = 4a_0a_2$, then (1) admits exactly one positive equilibrium;
iii) If $a_1 < 0$, and $a_1^2 > 4a_0a_2$, then (1) admits two positive equilibria.

Proof: In view of (12)–(14) we only need to see that in cases ii) and iii) the solutions S^* of (15) are smaller than L. And this follows from a straightforward calculation using (16). $\square$

§4. Stability of Non-Trivial Equilibria

Consider the case when there are two distinct positive equilibria, denoted by E_* and E^*, corresponding to the two roots of (15) S_* and S^* with $S_* < S^*$. We shall now study the eigenvalues of the Jacobian at E^*. In order to simplify the notation, we introduce the following positive quantities:

$$r_h = b_h - \mu_h, \qquad r_s = b_s - \mu_s, \qquad \nu_s = \mu_s + d_s,$$

$$q = \delta + 2(1 + 1/k)\, r_h, \qquad q_1 = q - (1 + 1/k)\, r_h = \delta + (1 + 1/k)\, v r_h.$$

Then the Jacobian at E^* is

$$J(E^*) = \begin{pmatrix} r_h & -\alpha & 0 & 0 \\ j_{21} & -q & 0 & \beta\lambda\frac{H^*}{H_0+H^*} \\ 0 & -\rho b_p\frac{S^*}{S_0+S^*} & j_{33} & -r_s\frac{S^*}{L} \\ 0 & \rho b_p\frac{S^*}{S_0+S^*} & \rho b_p\frac{S_0\,P^*}{(S_0+S^*)^2} & -\nu_s \end{pmatrix}, \qquad (17)$$

where

$$\begin{cases} j_{21} = \dfrac{\beta\lambda I^* H_0}{(H_0 + H^*)^2} + (1 + \dfrac{1}{k})\dfrac{r_h^2}{\alpha} = \dfrac{r_h q_1}{\alpha}\dfrac{H_0}{H_0 + H^*} + (1 + \dfrac{1}{k})\dfrac{r_h^2}{\alpha}, \\[3mm] j_{33} = r_s(1 - \dfrac{S^* + I^*}{L} - \dfrac{S^*}{L}) - \dfrac{\rho b_p P^* S_0}{(S_0 + S^*)^2} = -r_s\dfrac{S^*}{L} + \dfrac{\rho b_p P^* S^*}{(S_0 + S^*)^2}. \end{cases} \qquad (18)$$

In order to simplify the analysis, we notice the following facts. All the rates (number/year) and probability-like parameters (β and ρ) are in the order of $O(10^{-2}) - O(1)$, and the constants H_0 and S_0 may be in the order of $O(1) - O(10)$. However the carrying capacity L (for snails) can be very large (for example, in the order of $O(10^4) - O(10^5)$) so that $\frac{1}{L}$ is much smaller than other parameters involved in the model. Let $\epsilon = \frac{1}{L}$. Then

$$S^* = \frac{1}{\epsilon} - \frac{2(\gamma + \delta)H_0}{\mathcal{R}_0 - 1} + O(\epsilon),$$

$$H^* = \frac{H_0}{\mathcal{R}_0 - 1} + O(\epsilon),$$

where γ, δ are given by (3) and (2), respectively. We now list some obvious consequences of these relations for future use.

$$\begin{cases} \dfrac{H^*}{H_0 + H^*} = \dfrac{1}{\mathcal{R}_0} + O(\epsilon), \\[3mm] \dfrac{H_0}{H_0 + H^*} = 1 - \dfrac{1}{\mathcal{R}_0} + O(\epsilon), \\[3mm] \dfrac{S^*}{S_0 + S^*} = 1 - \epsilon S_0 + O(\epsilon^2). \end{cases} \qquad (19)$$

Note that it follows from (18) that

$$\dot{j}_{21} = \frac{r_h q_1}{\alpha}(1 - \frac{1}{\mathcal{R}_0}) + (1 + \frac{1}{k})\frac{r_h^2}{\alpha} + O(\epsilon),$$

$$\dot{j}_{33} = -r_s + O(\epsilon),$$

(20)

and it is also clear that

$$\frac{\rho b_p S_0 P_*}{(S_0 + S^*)^2} = O(\epsilon^2).$$

(21)

Then we have from (17) and (19)–(21),

$$|wI - J(E^*)| = \left[(w - r_h)\left((w + q)(w + \nu_s) - \frac{\rho b_p \beta H^* S^*}{(S_0 + S^*)(H_0 + H^*)}\right)\right.$$
$$\left. + \dot{j}_{21}\alpha(\nu_s + w)\right](w - \dot{j}_{33}) + O(\epsilon^2)$$
$$= (w^3 + c_1 w^2 + c_2 w + c_3)(w - \dot{j}_{33}) + O(\epsilon^2),$$

where, using (9),

$$c_1 = \nu_s - r_h + q,$$

$$c_2 = \nu_s q - r_h \nu_s - q r_h + \dot{j}_{21}\alpha - \frac{\rho b_p \beta}{\mathcal{R}_0}$$
$$= \nu_s q - r_h \nu_s - q r_h + \dot{j}_{21}\alpha - \nu_s q_1 + O(\epsilon)$$
$$= \nu_s q - r_h \nu_s - q_1(\nu_s + r_h \frac{1}{\mathcal{R}_0}) + O(\epsilon),$$

(22)

$$c_3 = -r_h \nu_s q + \dot{j}_{21}\alpha \nu_s + r_h \frac{\rho b_p \beta}{\mathcal{R}_0}$$
$$= r_h \nu_s q_1(1 - \frac{1}{\mathcal{R}_0}) + O(\epsilon).$$

Here we have also used the fact that

$$\dot{j}_{21}\alpha = r_h(q - \frac{1}{\mathcal{R}_0}q_1) + O(\epsilon).$$

Since, (20), $\dot{j}_{33} = -r_s + O(\epsilon)$, we see that $\dot{j}_{33} < 0$ when ϵ is small. Thus we only need to study the three roots of the equation

$$w^3 + c_1 w^2 + c_2 w + c_3 = 0,$$

(23)

where c_i $(i = 1, 2, 3)$ are given in (22). We shall study the characteristic equation without the terms $O(\epsilon)$. Then, using the Implicit Function Theorem, it follows that the same conclusion holds for the original equation.

Lemma 2. *All the roots of (23) have negative real parts if the following inequality holds*

$$\frac{kq}{\nu_s} < 1. \tag{24}$$

Proof: By the Routh-Hurwitz criterion, all the roots of (23) have negative real parts if $c_1 > 0, c_3 > 0$ and $c_1 c_2 - c_3 > 0$. So, we shall see that these relations hold if (24) does.

First note that $\mathcal{R}_0 > 1$ gives $c_3 > 0$, and it is also clear that

$$c_1 = \nu_s - r_h + q = \nu_s + \delta + (1 + \frac{2}{k})r_h > 0.$$

Next we remark that

$$c_1 c_2 - c_3 = (\nu_s - r_h + q)(q\nu_s - r_h\nu_s - q_1\nu_s - q_1 r_h\frac{1}{\mathcal{R}_0}) + \nu_s r_h q_1(\frac{1}{\mathcal{R}_0} - 1)$$

$$= r_h\left(r_h\nu_s + r_h q_1\frac{1}{\mathcal{R}_0} + \frac{\nu_s}{k}(\nu_s + q - kq) - qq_1\frac{1}{\mathcal{R}_0}\right). \tag{25}$$

But (24) implies that

$$\frac{\nu_s}{k}(\nu_s + q - kq) > \frac{\nu_s}{k}q \geq q^2, \tag{26}$$

and, since $\mathcal{R}_0 > 1$ and $q_1 < q$,

$$qq_1\frac{1}{\mathcal{R}_0} < qq_1 < q^2. \tag{27}$$

It follows now from (25)–(27) that $c_1 c_2 - c_3 > 0$, which concludes the proof. $\square$

Remark 3. *The inequality (24) is satisfied for most parameter values in a realistic range.*

As a consequence of the lemma, we have the following stability result.

Theorem 4. *If (24) holds, and a_0, a_1, a_2 are as in part iii) of Theorem 1, then the equilibrium E^* is locally asymptotically stable.*

The results from many numerical simulations seems to indicate that E_* is unstable, but we do not have a rigorous proof for this fact.

§5. Conclusions

We presented a new model for schistosomiasis, consisting of four ODEs, one each for the number of human hosts, uninfected snails, infected snails, and parasites. The model is based on several quite realistic assumptions, such as the logistic growth of snails in the absence of parasites, the exponential growth of humans in the same situation, the infertility of infected snails, and the overdispersion of the parasite distribution in humans.

We have shown that the model is well posed, and that it may have zero, one, or two positive equilibria. For this last case, we showed that the one corresponding to the lower number of parasites is stable. The one corresponding to the larger number of parasites seems to be unstable, based on numerical simulations. In numerical simulations it was also observed that periodic solutions are possible.

The model clearly exhibits the regulatory effect of parasites in humans, since it changes from exponentially increasing solutions to steady states or periodic solutions, by varying some of the parameters.

Future work should include sensitivity analysis to the changes in the various parameters of the model, the study of the instability of the other positive equilibrium, and also the effect of including age of infection for snails.

References

1. Anderson, R. M., Mathematical models of host-helminth parasite interactions, in *Ecological Stability*, M. B. Usher and M. H. Williamson (eds.), Chapman and Hall, London, 1974, 43–69.

2. Anderson, R. M., The regulation of host population growth by parasitic species, Parasitology **76** (1978), 119– 157.

3. Anderson, R. M., The influence of parasitic infection on the dynamics of host population growth, in *Population Dynamics*, R. M. Anderson, B. D. Turner and L. R. Taylor (eds.), Blackwell Scientific Publishers, Oxford, 1979, 245–281.

4. Anderson, R. M., Depression of host population abundance by direct life cycle macroparasites, J. Theor. Biol **82** (1980), 283–311.

5. Anderson, R. M. and D. M. Gordon, Processes influencing the distribution of parasite numbers within host populations with special emphasis on parasite-induced host mortalities, Parasitology **85** (1982), 373–398.

6. Anderson, R. M. and R. M. May, Regulation and stability of host-parasite population interactions. I. Regulatory processes, J. Animal Ecology **47** (1978), 219–247.

7. Barbour, A. D. and M. Kafetzaki, A host-parasite model yielding heterogeneous parasite loads, J. Math. Biol. **31** (1993), 157–176.

8. Bradley, D. J., Stability in host-parasite systems, in *Ecological Stability*, M. B. Usher and M. H. Williamson (eds.), Chapman and Hall, London, 1974, 71–97.

9. Busenberg, S. N., K. Cooke and M. Iannelli, Endemic thresholds and stability in a class of age structured populations, SIAM J. Appl. Math **48** (1985), 1379–1395.

10. Crofton, H. D., A quantitative approach to parasitism, Parasitology **62** (1971), 179–193.

11. Crofton, H. D., A model of host-parasite relationships, Parasitology **63** (1971), 343–364.

12. Debach, P. and H. S. Smith, Are populations oscillations inherent in the host-parasite relation? Ecology **22** (1941), 363–369.

13. Dietz, K., Overall population patterns in the transmission cycle of infectious disease agents, in *Population Biology of Infectious Diseases*, R. M. Anderson and R. M. May (eds.), Springer Verlag, Berlin, 1982, 87–102.

14. Dobson, A. P., The population Biology of parasite-induced changes in host behavior, The Quarterly Review of Biology **63** (1988), 139–165.

15. Eisen, S., An alternative model based on random distributions for density-dependent regulation in host-parasite systems, The American Midland Naturalist **109(2)** (1983), 230–239.

16. Hadeler, K. P., An integral equation for helminthic infections: stability of the non-infected population, in *Trends in Theoretical and Practical Nonlinear Differential Equations*, V. Lakshmikantham (ed.), Lecture Notes in Pure and Applied Mathematics, vol. 90, Marcel Dekker, 1984, 231–240.

17. Hadeler, K. P. and K. Dietz, An integral equation for helminthic infections: global existence of solutions, in *Recent Trends in Mathematics*, Conf. Proc. Reinhardsbrunn, Teubner-Verlag, Leipzig, 1982.

18. Hadeler, K. P. and K. Dietz, Nonlinear hyperbolic partial differential equations for the dynamics of parasite populations, Comp. Math. Applic. **9** (1983), 415–430.

19. Hadeler, K. P. and K. Dietz, Population dynamics of killing parasites which reproduce in the host, J. Math. Biol. **21** (1984), 45–55.

20. Heesterbeek, J. A. P. and M. G. Roberts, Threshold quantities for helminth infections, J. Math. Biol. **33** (1995), 415–434.

21. Kermack, W. O. and A. G. McKendrick, Contributions to the mathematical theory of epidemics, Proc. Royal Soc., Series A **115** (1927), 700–721.

22. Kostitzin, *Symbiose, Parasitisme, et Évolution*, Hermann, Paris, 1934.

23. Leyton, M. K., Stochastic models in populations of helminthic parasites in the definitive host. II. Sexual mating functions, Math. Biosc. **3** (1968), 413–419.

24. MacDonald, G., The dynamics of helminth infections with spatial reference to schistosomes, Trans. Royal Soc. Trop. Med. Hyg. **59** (1965), 489–506.

25. May, R. M., Dynamical aspects of host-parasite associations: Crofton's model revisited, Parasitology **75** (1977), 259–276.

26. May, R. M. and R. M. Anderson, Regulation and stability of host-parasite population interactions. II. Destabilizing processes, J. Animal Ecology **47** (1978), 249–267.

27. May, R. M. and R. M. Anderson, Population biology of infectious diseases II, Nature **280** (1979), 455–461.

28. Nasell, I., *Hybrid Models of Tropical Infections*, Lecture Notes in Biomathematics, vol. 59, 1985.

29. Waltman, P., *Deterministic Threshold Models in the Theory of Epidemics*, Lecture Notes in Biomathematics, vol. 1, Springer Verlag, Berlin, 1974.

30. Webb, G. F., *Theory of Nonlinear Age-Dependent Population Dynamics*, Marcel Dekker Inc., New York, 1985.

31. Wu, Z., K. Bu, L. Yuan, G. Yang, J. Zhu and Q. Liu, Factors contributing to reinfection with schistosomiasis japonica after treatment in the lake region of China, Acta Tropica **52 (2)** (1993), 83–88.

Zhilan Feng
Department of Mathematics
Purdue University
West Lafayette, IN 47907-1395
zfeng@math.purdue.edu

Fabio Augusto Milner
Department of Mathematics
Purdue University
West Lafayette, IN 47907-1395
milner@math.purdue.edu
http://www.math.purdue.edu/ milner

Positive Profit in a Predator-Prey Situation

K. Renee Fister and Suzanne Lenhart

Abstract. An optimal control of a parabolic predator-prey system, in which the interaction terms are Lotka-Volterra type is considered. Both species are harvested for economic profit: hence, the controls are the proportion of the populations to harvest. Specific conditions are analyzed so that maximum profit is realized.

§1. Introduction

We consider optimal control of harvesting in a predator-prey parabolic system with Neumann boundary conditions. Solutions of the system represent population densities of the prey and the predator species. In addition, the system has Lotka-Volterra type growth terms with local interaction terms representing the predator-prey situation. Moreover, the controls are a proportion of the species populations to be harvested.

Given our controls f_1, f_2, the corresponding prey and predator state variables, $u = u(f_1, f_2)$ and $v = v(f_1, f_2)$ satisfy the state system

$$
\begin{aligned}
L_1 u &= u(a_1 - d_1 u) - c_1 uv - f_1 u & &\text{in } Q = \Omega \times (0, T), \\
L_2 v &= v(a_2 - d_2 v) + c_2 uv - f_2 v & & \\
u(x, 0) &= u_0(x), \quad v(x, 0) = v_0(x) & &\text{for } x \in \Omega, \\
\frac{\partial u}{\partial \nu} &= 0, \quad \frac{\partial v}{\partial \nu} = 0 & &\text{on } \partial\Omega \times (0, T),
\end{aligned}
\tag{1}
$$

where we use the notation

$$
L_1 u \equiv u_t - \sum_{i,j=1}^{n} (a_{ij}^1 u_{x_j})_{x_i} + \sum_{i=1}^{n} b_i^1 u_{x_i},
$$

$$
L_2 v \equiv v_t - \sum_{i,j=1}^{n} (a_{ij}^2 v_{x_j})_{x_i} + \sum_{i=1}^{n} b_i^2 v_{x_i}.
$$

In addition, $\nu_i = \sum_{j=1}^{n} a_{ij} n_j$ is the ith component of the conormal vector.

Mathematical Models in Medical and Health Sciences
Mary Ann Horn, Gieri Simonett, and Glenn Webb (eds.), pp. 129–137.
Copyright © 1998 by Vanderbilt University Press, Nashville, TN.
ISBN 0-8265-1310-7.

The functions f_1 and f_2 are controls that represent harvesting a proportion of the population. The coefficients a_1, a_2, d_1, d_2 are the standard Lotka-Volterra (logistic) growth terms, with a_1, a_2 denoting growth and d_1, d_2 signifying crowding. The c_1, c_2 coefficients represent interaction effects. The $-c_1 uv$ term is a decay term for the prey population; whereas, the $c_2 uv$ term is a growth term for the predator population.

To discuss our controls appropriately, we define the class of admissible controls,

$$A = A(\Gamma_1, \Gamma_2) \equiv \{(f_1, f_2)|0 \leq f_i \leq \Gamma_i \text{ a.e. } \Omega \times (0,T), \ i = 1,2\}.$$

Our objective is to illustrate the positivity of the following payoff functional

$$J(f_1 \ f_2) = \int_Q \{K_1 u f_1 + K_2 v f_2 - M_1 f_1^2 - M_2 f_2^2\} dx dt$$

over this admissible control class, where $K_1 u f_1$, $K_2 v f_2$ represent the revenue of harvesting and $M_1 f_1^2$, $M_2 f_2^2$ denote the cost of the controls. In addition, K_i, M_i are positive for $i = 1, 2$. We recognize that this functional combines the controls and their effects on the populations. Prior to determining the conditions for positive profit, we need a characterization of an optimal control pair. Hence, we maximize the functional over the admissible class of controls to characterize f_1^*, f_2^* such that

$$J(f_1^*, \ f_2^*) = \max_{(f_1, \ f_2) \in A} J(f_1, \ f_2).$$

In this paper, we utilize a control model to represent the dynamics in a diffusive Lotka-Volterra equation. Because of the dispersive nature of the predator and prey species, the population dynamics of these species is dependent on space and time. This dependence is evident by the use of a parabolic diffusive Lotka-Volterra PDE. However, we assume that a given species does not diffuse across the boundary, due to possibly unsuitable environmental conditions outside of our region. The functions $u_0(x)$ and $v_0(x)$ give the initial density distributions of the prey and predator species inside our spatial area.

When thinking of harvesting in a predator-prey system, one can think of the simple (fish) example with capelin as the prey and cod as the predator (Akenhead et al. [1]). See Mesterton-Gibbons [8] for an optimal control problem with combined harvesting in a predator-prey system in the ordinary differential equations case. Our paper treats the predator-prey situation with spatial diffusion, yielding a PDE system. Waltman [12] and Murray [9] provide insight into competitive and predator prey models. In addition, Cañada, Gámez, and Montero [2] analyze the profitability of harvesting species modelled by a diffusive Lotka-Volterra elliptic system. They prove that the payoff functional is positive under certain conditions. Specifically, the payoff functional is positive if the principal eigenvalue of the negative intrinsic growth rate of the species is negative.

Existence of solutions of the system (1) via a monotone iteration scheme and existence of an optimal control via a maximizing sequence argument have already been established [4]. In addition, an optimal control has also been characterized in terms of the optimality system, which is the state system coupled with the adjoint system. We determined the optimality system by differentiating the payoff functional with respect to the control and by evaluating the result at an optimal control. Moreover, uniqueness of solutions to the optimality system has been established on a small time interval. Furthermore, we have a precise characterization of the unique optimal control.

In this paper, we determine certain restrictions on the bounds of the optimal control pair in order for positive profit to be realized. The positivity of the objective functional is important for the feature of "profit", and this technique can be applied to other parabolic systems modeling populations.

§2. Characterization of Optimal Control

The following assumptions are made throughout this paper:

(a) Ω is a smooth bounded domain in $\mathbb{R}^n$;

(b) $u_0(x)$, $v_0(x) \in L^\infty(\Omega)$;

(c) $0 < u_0(x) < B$, $0 < v_0(x) < B$ for some $B \in \mathbb{R}$;

(d) a_i, c_i, d_i, $f_i \in L^\infty(Q)$, $i = 1, 2$;

(e) $a_{ij}^k \in C^2(\overline{Q})$, $a_{ij}^k = a_{ji}^k$, $b_i^k \in C^1(\overline{Q})$ for $k = 1, 2$;

(f) $\vec{b} \cdot \vec{n} \geq 0$, $\vec{b} = (b_i)$ $i = 1, \ldots, n$, where $\vec{n}$ is the outward unit normal on $\partial\Omega \times (0, T)$;

(g) $\sum_{i,j=1}^n a_{ij}^k \xi_i \xi_j \geq \theta \sum_{i=1}^n \xi_i^2$, $k = 1, 2$, where $\theta > 0$.

The ellipticity condition, (g), guarantees that the conormal direction ν is outward. The underlying state space for system (1) is

$$V = L^2((0, T); H^1(\Omega)).$$

Using repeated indices summation convention, we define the bilinear form:

$$a^k(t, u, \phi) = \int_\Omega a_{ij}^k u_{x_j} \phi_{x_i} + \int_\Omega b_i^k u_{x_i} \phi$$

for $u, \phi \in V$ and $k = 1, 2$. We are interested in weak solutions, $u, v \in V$, in the following sense:

$$\int_0^T \langle u_t, \phi \rangle + \int_0^T a^1(t, u, \phi) = -\int_Q c_1 uv\phi - \int_Q d_1 u^2 \phi + \int_Q (a_1 - f_1) u\phi,$$

$$\int_0^T \langle v_t, \psi \rangle + \int_0^T a^2(t, v, \psi) = \int_Q c_2 uv\psi - \int_Q d_2 v^2 \psi + \int_Q (a_2 - f_2) v\psi,$$

for all $\phi, \psi \in V$ where the $\langle \, , \, \rangle$ inner product is the duality between $(H^1(\Omega))^*$ and $H^1(\Omega)$. In addition, existence of a unique solution to the state system as proclaimed in the next theorem is proved via an iteration scheme and *a priori* estimates.

Theorem 2.1. *([4, Theorem 2.1]) Given $(f_1, f_2) \in A$, there exists a unique solutions (u, v) in $V \times V$ solving system (1).*

A maximizing sequence argument is used to prove the existence of an optimal control.

Theorem 2.2. *([4, Theorem 2.2]) There exists a pair of optimal controls in A that maximizes the functional $J(f_1, f_2)$.*

We examine the optimality system which consists of the state system coupled with the adjoint system. To obtain this optimality system, the payoff functional is differentiated with respect to the controls to obtain necessary conditions for the optimality system. Since the payoff functional contains u and v, u and v are also differentiated with respect to the controls. *A priori* estimates are needed for convergence of these difference quotients to "derivative" functions. These functions solve a linearized version of the state system. To compute an optimal control pair, the adjoint system is introduced with a transversality condition and appropriate boundary conditions. Thus, we state the following theorem from [4] pertaining to the adjoints and to a characterization of our optimal control pair.

Theorem 2.3. *([4, Theorem 3.2]) Given an optimal pair (f_1, f_2) and corresponding solutions u, v, there exists $(p, q) \in V \times V$ satisfying the adjoint system*

$$
\begin{aligned}
L_1^* p &= K_1 f_1 + a_1 p - 2 d_1 u p - c_1 v p - f_1 p + c_2 v q & &\text{in } Q, \\
p(x, T) &= 0 & &\text{for } x \in \Omega, \\
\frac{\partial p}{\partial \nu} + (b^1 \cdot \vec{n}) p &= 0 & &\text{on } \partial\Omega \times (0, T),
\end{aligned}
\tag{2}
$$

$$
\begin{aligned}
L_2^* q &= K_2 f_2 + a_2 q - 2 d_2 v q - c_1 u p - f_2 q + c_2 u q & &\text{in } Q, \\
q(x, T) &= 0 & &\text{for } x \in \Omega, \\
\frac{\partial q}{\partial \nu} + (b^2 \cdot \vec{n}) q &= 0 & &\text{on } \partial\Omega \times (0, T),
\end{aligned}
\tag{3}
$$

and furthermore

$$
f_1 = \min\left(\left(\frac{(K_1 - p)u}{2 M_1} \right)^+, \Gamma_1 \right),
$$

$$
f_2 = \min\left(\left(\frac{(K_2 - q)v}{2 M_2} \right)^+, \Gamma_2 \right).
$$

Remark. Note the transversality conditions on the adjoint variables are at $t = T$. In addition, the notation used in the representation for the optimal control pairs is

$$
s^+ = \begin{cases} s & \text{if } s \geq 0, \\ 0 & \text{if } s < 0. \end{cases}
$$

Moreover, the adjoint operators are as follows

$$L_1^* p = -p_t - \sum_{i,j=1}^{n} (a_{ij}^1 p_{x_i})_{x_j} - \sum_{i=1}^{n} (b_i^1 p)_{x_i},$$

$$L_2^* q = -q_t - \sum_{i,j=1}^{n} (a_{ij}^2 q_{x_i})_{x_j} - \sum_{i=1}^{n} (b_i^2 q)_{x_i}.$$

Using the relationship between our optimal control pair and the associated adjoint variables from this theorem, we now form the following optimality system

$$L_1 u = u(a_1 - d_1 u) - c_1 uv - \min\left(\left(\frac{(K_1 - p)u}{2M_1} \right)^+, \Gamma_1 \right) u \quad \text{in } Q,$$

$$L_2 v = v(a_2 - d_2 v) + c_2 uv - \min\left(\left(\frac{(K_2 - q)v}{2M_2} \right)^+, \Gamma_2 \right) v,$$

$$L_1^* p = K_1 \min\left(\left(\frac{(K_1 - p)u}{2M_1} \right)^+, \Gamma_1 \right) + a_1 p - 2d_1 up - c_1 vp$$

$$\qquad - \min\left(\left(\frac{(K_1 - p)u}{2M_1} \right)^+, \Gamma_1 \right) p + c_2 vq,$$

$$L_2^* q = K_2 \min\left(\left(\frac{(K_2 - q)v}{2M_2} \right)^+, \Gamma_2 \right) + a_2 q - 2d_2 vq - c_1 up$$

$$\qquad - \min\left(\left(\frac{(K_2 - q)v}{2M_2} \right)^+, \Gamma_2 \right) q + c_2 uq,$$

$$u(x,0) = u_0(x), \quad v(x,0) = v_0(x),$$

$$p(x,T) = 0 = q(x,T), \qquad x \in \Omega,$$

$$\frac{\partial u}{\partial \nu} = 0 = \frac{\partial v}{\partial \nu}, \quad \frac{\partial p}{\partial \nu} + (b^1 \cdot \vec{n})p = 0, \quad \frac{\partial q}{\partial \nu} + (b^2 \cdot \vec{n})q = 0, \quad \partial \Omega \times (0,T).$$

(4)

Since an optimal pair (f_1, f_2) exists, u, v exist as solutions to the state system (1), and p, q exist as solutions to (2) and (3). Therefore, a solution to the optimality system exists.

A uniqueness result for the optimality system which characterizes the unique optimal control pair is also given in [4]. In conclusion, we have that the optimal control pair

$$f_1 = \min\left(\left(\frac{(K_1 - p)u}{2M_1} \right)^+, \Gamma_1 \right), \quad f_2 = \min\left(\left(\frac{(K_2 - q)v}{2M_2} \right)^+, \Gamma_2 \right),$$

characterized in terms of (u, v, p, q), is the unique solution of the optimality system.

§3. Positivity of the Payoff Functional

To analyze the positivity of the payoff functional, we determine the positivity of its integrand. However, on the set where $f_1 = 0$ and $f_2 = 0$, the integrand of the payoff functional is zero. Hence, we determine conditions on Γ_1 and Γ_2 so that this cannot occur. Note that $\| \cdot \|$ is the same as $\| \cdot \|_\infty$.

Theorem 3.1. *For Γ_1 and Γ_2 sufficiently small, depending only on the coefficients of the state system, we have* $\max\limits_{(f_1,f_2)\in A} J(f_1, f_2) > 0.$

Proof: Let U and Z be supersolutions for u and v respectively. We determine the upper bounds on U and Z via a parabolic maximum principle [10, Chapter 3]. U and Z satisfy the following

$$
\begin{aligned}
L_1 U &= a_1 U \quad \text{in } Q, \\
U(x,0) &= u_0(x) \quad \text{for } x \in \Omega, \\
\frac{\partial U}{\partial \nu} &= 0 \quad \text{on } \partial\Omega \times (0,T),
\end{aligned}
\tag{5}
$$

$$
\begin{aligned}
L_2 Z &= a_2 Z + c_2 U Z \quad \text{in } Q, \\
Z(x,0) &= v_0(x) \quad \text{for } x \in \Omega, \\
\frac{\partial Z}{\partial \nu} &= 0 \quad \text{on } \partial\Omega \times (0,T).
\end{aligned}
\tag{6}
$$

Let $U = e^{\gamma t} W$ where γ is to be chosen. Then substitution into (5) yields

$$
\begin{aligned}
L_1 W + (\gamma - a_1 W) &= 0 \quad \text{in } Q, \\
W(x,0) &= u_0(x) \quad \text{for } x \in \Omega, \\
\frac{\partial W}{\partial \nu} &= 0 \quad \text{on } \partial\Omega \times (0,T),
\end{aligned}
\tag{7}
$$

where $\gamma > a_1$.

   Via a parabolic maximum principle [10], the maximum of W must occur on the boundary. So $W \leq \|u_0\|$. Moreover,

$$
U \leq \|u_0\| e^{\gamma T}.
$$

Using the bound on U, we find a bound on Z in (6), rewritten as

$$
\begin{aligned}
L_2 Z - (a_2 + c_2 U)Z &= 0 \quad \text{in } Q, \\
Z(x,0) &= v_0(x) \quad \text{for } x \in \Omega, \\
\frac{\partial Z}{\partial \nu} &= 0 \quad \text{on } \partial\Omega \times (0,T).
\end{aligned}
$$

Let $Z = e^{\tilde{\eta} t} Y$ where $\tilde{\eta}$ is to be chosen. Then, using (6), we have

$$
\begin{aligned}
L_2 Y + (\tilde{\eta} - a_2 - c_2 U)Y &= 0 \quad \text{in } Q, \\
Y(x,0) &= v_0(x) \quad \text{for } x \in \Omega, \\
\frac{\partial Y}{\partial \nu} &= 0 \quad \text{on } \partial\Omega \times (0,T).
\end{aligned}
\tag{8}
$$

Since U is uniformly bounded in time by $\|u_0\|e^{\gamma T}$, we may choose $\tilde{\eta}$ such that $\tilde{\eta} > a_2 + c_2\|u_0\|e^{\gamma T}$. Hence, we obtain that $\tilde{\eta} - a_2 - c_2 U > 0$. By a parabolic maximum principle [10], the maximum of Y occurs on the boundary so that

$$Y \leq \|v_0(x)\| \quad \text{or} \quad Z \leq \|v_0(x)\|e^{\tilde{\eta}T}.$$

We have just bounded in L^∞ the solutions u and v of the nonlinear state system, by bounds independent of $K_1, K_2, \Gamma_1, \Gamma_2$. Using the above bounds on u and v, our adjoint system has bounded coefficients and is linear in p and q. Using a standard result [11] for linear parabolic systems, there exists a constant C_1 independent of $K_1, K_2, \Gamma_1, \Gamma_2$, and dependent on the coefficients of the adjoint system such that

$$\|p\| \leq C_1 \left[K_1\Gamma_1 + K_2\Gamma_2\right],$$

and

$$\|q\| \leq C_1 \left[K_1\Gamma_1 + K_2\Gamma_2\right].$$

We can take Γ_1 and Γ_2 sufficiently small to obtain that $p(x,t) < K_1$ and $q(x,t) < K_2$ on Q. Thus we have that the optimal controls f_1^* and f_2^* are positive. To understand why, we have

$$\max_{(f_1,f_2)\in A} J(f_1, f_2) > 0,$$

we illustrate a few cases.

On the set where $f_1 = \frac{(K_1 - p)u}{2M_1}$ and $f_2 = \frac{(K_2 - q)v}{2M_2}$, we estimate the integrand of J,

$$\begin{aligned}
&K_1 u f_1 + K_2 v f_2 - M_1 f_1^2 - M_2 f_2^2 \\
&= \frac{(K_1 - p)u}{2M_1}\left(K_1 u - M_1\left(\frac{(K_1 - p)u}{2M_1}\right)\right) \\
&\quad + \frac{(K_2 - q)v}{2M_2}\left(K_2 v - M_2\left(\frac{(K_2 - q)v}{2M_2}\right)\right) \\
&= \frac{(K_1 - p)u}{2M_1}\frac{u}{2}(K_1 + p) + \frac{(K_2 - q)v}{2M_2}\frac{v}{2}(K_2 + q) > 0.
\end{aligned}$$

The integrand of the payoff functional is positive since $u > 0$, $v > 0$, $p > 0$, $K_1 - p > 0$, $q > 0$, and $K_2 - q > 0$ by a parabolic maximum principle.

On the set where $f_1 = \Gamma_1$ and $f_2 = \frac{(K_2 - q)v}{2M_2}$ the integrand becomes

$$\begin{aligned}
&\Gamma_1(K_1 u - M_1\Gamma_1) + \frac{(K_2 - q)v}{2M_2}\left(K_2 v - M_2\left(\frac{(K_2 - q)v}{2M_2}\right)\right) \\
&> \Gamma_1\left(K_1 u - M_1\left(\frac{(K_1 - p)u}{2M_1}\right)\right) + \frac{(K_2 - q)v}{2M_2}\frac{v}{2}(K_2 + q) > 0
\end{aligned}$$

since $\Gamma_1 \leq \frac{(K_1 - p)u}{2M_1}$ in this case.

We can show analogous cases for $f_1 = \frac{(K_1-p)u}{2M_1}$, $f_2 = \Gamma_2$ and $f_1 = \Gamma_1$, $f_2 = \Gamma_2$.

Since the integrand of the payoff functional is positive for the optimal control pair and we integrate over a set of postive measure, then

$$\max_{(f_1,f_2)\in A} J(f_1, f_2) > 0. \quad \square$$

Under appropriate conditions, we have shown that the payoff functional is positive.

Acknowledgments. We want to thank the referee for his/her considerate study and diligence in the reading of this paper.

References

1. Akenhead, S. A., J. Carscadden, G. R. Lilly and R. Wells, Cod-capelin interactions off northeast Newfoundland and Labrador, in *Multispecies Approaches to Fisheries Management Advice*, M.C. Mercer (ed.), Canadian Special Publications of Fisheries and Aquatic Sciences **59** (1980), 141–148.

2. Cañada, A., J. L. Gámez and J. A. Montero, An optimal control problem for a nonlinear elliptic equation arising from population dynamics, in *Calculus of variations, applications and computations*, Pitman Res. Notes Math. Ser. **326** (1995), 35–40.

3. Evans, L. C., *Weak Convergence Methods for Nonlinear Partial Differential Equations*, in *CBMS Regional Conference Series in Mathematics* **74** American Mathematical Society, Providence, RI, 1990.

4. Fister, K. R., Optimal control of harvesting in a predator-prey parabolic system, Houston Journal of Mathematics **23**(2) (1997), 341–355.

5. Ladyzenskaja, O. A., V. A. Solonnikov and N. N. Ural'ceva, *Linear and Quasi-linear Equations of Parabolic Type*, in *Translations of Mathematical Monographs* **23**, American Mathematical Society, Providence, RI, 1967.

6. Leung, A. W., *Systems of Nonlinear Partial Differential Equations, Applications to Biology and Engineering*, Kluwer Academics Publishers, Dordrecht/Boston, 1989.

7. Lions, J. L., *Optimal Control of Systems Governed by Partial Differential Equations*, Springer-Verlag, New York, 1971.

8. Mesterton-Gibbons, M., On the optimal policy for combining harvesting of predator and prey, Natural Resource Modeling **3** (1988), 63–90.

9. Murray, J. D., *Mathematical Biology*, Springer-Verlag, Berlin, 1980.

10. Protter, M. H. and H. F. Weinberger, *Maximum Principles in Differential Equations*, Prentice-Hall, Englewood Cliffs, 1967.

11. Redlinger, R., Pointwise A Priori Bounds for Strongly Coupled Semilinear Parabolic Systems, Indiana University Mathematics Journal **36**(2) (1998), 441–454.

12. Waltman, P., *Competition Models in Population Biology*, CBMS-NSF Regional Conference Series in Applied Mathematics **45**, Society for Industrial and Applied Mathematics, Philadelphia, 1983.

K. Renee Fister
Dept. of Mathematics and Statistics
Murray State University
Murray, KY 42071
kfister@math.mursuky.edu

Suzanne Lenhart
Dept. of Mathematics
University of Tennessee
Knoxville, TN 37996
lenhart@math.utk.edu

Analysis of a Two Component Reaction Diffusion Model on a Heterogeneous Domain

William E. Fitzgibbon and Jeff Morgan

Abstract. We provide a formal mathematical analysis of a two component reaction diffusion system proposed by Benson, Sherratt and Maini [2]. We comment on the extension of our analysis to more general systems.

§1. Introduction

In this brief note we provide a detailed mathematical analysis of the Schnackenberg reaction diffusion model for morphogenesis. This model was recently studied by Benson, Sharratt and Maini [1] as a model for pattern formation in biological systems. Their work provided a very interesting numerical investigation of the system given by

$$\begin{cases} u_t = u_{xx} + \gamma(A - u + u^2 v), & t > 0,\ 0 < x < 1, \\ v_t = \frac{\partial}{\partial x}[D(x)v_x] + \gamma(B - u^2 v), & t > 0,\ 0 < x < 1,\ x \neq c, \\ u_x = v_x = 0, & t > 0,\ x = 0, 1, \\ v(t, c-) = v(t, c+), & t > 0, \\ d_1 v_x(t, c-) = d_2 v_x(t, c+), & \\ v(0, x) = v_0(x), u(0, x) = u_0(x), & 0 < x < 1, \end{cases} \tag{1}$$

where $A, B, \gamma, d_1, d_2 > 0$, $0 < c < 1$,

$$D(x) = \begin{cases} d_1, & 0 < x < c, \\ d_2, & c < x < 1, \end{cases}$$

and $u_0, v_0 \in C([0,1], [0,\infty))$. We should remark that it is straightforward to prove that (1) has a unique classical, nonnegative solution on a maximal time interval $[0, T_{\max})$. Furthermore, if $T_{\max} < \infty$ then u and/or v blow up in the sup-norm.

The set of equations (1) constitutes a simple reaction diffusion equation. Moreover, if the complication at $x = c$ is removed, then this system is one term

Mathematical Models in Medical and Health Sciences
Mary Ann Horn, Gieri Simonett, and Glenn Webb (eds.), pp. 139–144.
Copyright © 1998 by Vanderbilt University Press, Nashville, TN.
ISBN 0-8265-1310-7.

away from the classic Brusselator model studied throughout the literature (cf.
[1] and the references therein). More generally, if the complication at $x = c$ is
removed, then this system is a special case of a general class of systems which
are nearly balanced (cf. Morgan [9]). Simply note that the inhomogeneous
terms which appear in the partial differential equations for u and v sum to a
quantity which is bounded above by a constant.

§2. Existence of a Global Compact Attractor

Our primary result can be stated as follows:

Theorem 1. *The system (1) has a global compact attractor in $C([0,1])^2$.*

The proof of our result is organized in 5 steps.
1. Prove v is bounded.
2. Prove there exists $M_1 > 0$ such that there exists $T > 0$ such that if $t > T$
   then
   $$\|v(t,\cdot)\|_{\infty,(0,1)} + \|u(t,\cdot)\|_{1,(0,1)} \le M_1.$$
3. Prove that for each $1 < p < \infty$ there exists $M_p > 0$ such that there exists
   $T \ge 0$ such that if $a \ge T$ then
   $$\|u(\cdot,\cdot)\|_{p,(a,a+1)\times(0,1)} \le M_p.$$
4. Prove there exists $M_\infty > 0$ such that there exists $T > 0$ such that if $t \ge T$
   then
   $$\|u(t,\cdot)\|_{\infty,(0,1)} \le M_\infty.$$
5. Apply standard parabolic regularity to obtain a global compact attractor.

Remark 1. The constants M_1, M_p and M_∞ above depend upon A, B and
γ, but are independent of u_0 and v_0.

Remark 2. Actually, the question of global existence for the system (1) is
not straightforward. Although we never treat it directly, it is a consequence
of #3 and #4 above.

Proof of 1: Note that $u \ge w$ where w solves

$$\begin{cases} w_t = w_{xx} + \gamma(A - w), & t > 0,\ 0 < x < 1, \\ w_x = 0, & t > 0,\ x = 0, 1, \\ w = u_0, & t = 0,\ 0 < x < 1. \end{cases}$$

Also, it is straightforward to prove $w \to A$ as $t \to \infty$. Therefore, from the
comparison principle and the equation for v, we have

$$\limsup_{t\to\infty} v(t,x) \le \frac{B}{A^2}.$$

Proof of 2: From above, there exists $\varepsilon > 0$ and $0 < \delta < A$ such that

$$u(t,x) \ge A - (A - \delta)e^{-\gamma(t-\varepsilon)}, \quad \text{for } t \ge \varepsilon.$$

Also,

$$\frac{d}{dt} \int_0^1 (u + 2v) \, dx \le \gamma \, (2B + A) - \int_0^1 (u + \delta^2 v) \, dx, \quad \text{for } t \ge \varepsilon$$

and

$$\frac{d}{dt} \int_0^1 (u + 2v) \, dx \le \gamma \, (2B + A), \quad \text{for } 0 \le t \le \varepsilon.$$

The result follows immediately from these two inequalities and the estimate in #1.

Proof of 3: Suppose $T > 0$ and define a smooth function $G : [0, T] \to [0, 1]$ such that $G(t) = 0$ for all $t \le T/4$ and $G(t) = 1$ for all $t \ge T/2$. Let $a > 0$ and define

$$Q_{a,T} = (a, a + T) \times (0, 1).$$

Finally, set

$$G_a(t) = G(t - a), \quad \text{for } t \ge a.$$

We will apply a duality argument to obtain our result. Similar arguments have been applied in a variety of reaction diffusion settings (cf. [3,5,6,9]). In general, this technique seems to be quite useful. To this end, suppose $1 < p < \infty$ and let $\theta \in L^p (Q_{a,T})$ such that $\|\theta\|_{p, Q_{a,T}} = 1$ and $\theta \ge 0$. Let ϕ be the unique solution to

$$\begin{cases} \phi_t = -\phi_{xx} - \theta & \text{on } Q_{aT}, \\ \phi_x = 0, & t > 0, \, x = 0, 1, \\ \phi = 0, & t = a + T, \, 0 < x < 1. \end{cases}$$

From well know results appearing in Ladyzenskaja et al. [8] we know $\phi \ge 0$ and there exists $C_{p,T} > 0$ (independent of θ) such that

$$\|\phi\|_{p, Q_{a,T}}^{1,2} \le C_{p,T}.$$

(Here $\|\phi\|_{p, Q_{a,T}}^{1,2}$ denotes the Sobolev norm for functions having one time derivative and two spatial derivatives in $L^p (Q_{a,T})$.) The argument duality proceeds as follows. We have

$$\iint_{Q_{a,T}} (u + v) G_a \theta = \iint_{Q_{a,T}} (u + v) \, G_a \, (-\phi_t - \phi_{xx})$$

$$= \iint_{Q_{a,T}} (u_t + v_t) \, G_a \phi + \iint_{Q_{a,T}} (u + v) \, (G_a' \phi - G_a \phi_{xx}).$$

Also, from (1) we have

$$\iint_{Q_{a,T}} (u_t + v_t) \, G_a \phi \le \iint_{Q_{a,T}} [\gamma (A + B) + u_{xx} + (D(x)v_x)_x] \, G_a \phi.$$

If we combine these two inequalities and integration by parts, then we have

$$\iint_{Q_{a,T}} (u+v)\, G_a \theta \le I + II + III + \iint_{Q_{a,T}} (u+v)\, G_a' \phi, \qquad (2)$$

where

$$I = \iint_{Q_{a,T}} \gamma\,(A+B)\, G_a \phi,$$

$$II = (d_2 - d_1) \int_a^{a+T} v(t,c)\phi_x(t,c)dt,$$

$$III = \iint_{Q_{a,T}} (d_1 + d_2 - 1)\phi_{xx} G_a v.$$

However, we can estimate each of I, II and III as follows. We have

$$|I| \le \gamma\,(A+B)\, T^{(p-1)/p} C_{p,T}$$

and

$$|II| \le |d_2 - d_1|\,\|v\|_{\infty,Q_{a,T}}\, T^{(p-1)/p}\, \|\phi_x(\ ,c)\|_{p,(a,a+T)}$$
$$\le |d_2 - d_1|\, K_{p,T}\, \|v\|_{\infty,Q_{a,T}}\,.$$

from Sobolev estimates. Finally,

$$|III| \le |d_1 + d_2 - 1|\,\|v\|_{\infty,Q_{a,T}}\, T^{(p-1)/p} C_{p,T}.$$

Therefore, it follows from these estimates and (2) that

$$\iint_{Q_{a,T}} (u+v)\, G_a \theta \le L_{p,T}\left(1 + \|v\|_{\infty,Q_{a,T}}\right) + \iint_{Q_{a,T}} (u+v)\, G_a' \phi. \qquad (3)$$

We can finish by proceeding in an iterative manner. To this end, define $\phi_1 = \phi$, and iteratively define ϕ_k, for $k > 1$, to be the unique solution to

$$\begin{cases} (\phi_k)_t = -(\phi_k)_{xx} - \phi_{k-1} & \text{on } Q_{a,T}, \\ (\phi_k)_x = 0, & t > 0,\ x = 0,1, \\ (\phi_k) = 0, & t = a+T,\ 0 < x < 1. \end{cases}$$

Then from the estimate on ϕ, we can derive the estimate

$$\|\phi_k\|_{p,Q_{a,T}}^{k,2k} \le (C_{p,T})^{k+1}.$$

Furthermore, from the Sobolev imbedding theorem, there exits a natural number m and a number $N_{p,T}$ so that

$$\|\phi_m\|_{\infty,Q_{a,T}} \le N_{p,T}\, \|\phi_m\|_{p,Q_{a,T}}^{m,2m} \le N_{p,T}\,(C_{p,T})^{m+1}. \qquad (4)$$

Now, let's apply the calculations which lead to (3) once again, with G_a replaced by G'_a and θ replaced by ϕ. These calculations combined with (3) yield

$$\iint_{Q_{a,T}} (u+v)\, G_a \theta \le L_{1,p,T} \left(1 + \|v\|_{\infty,Q_{a,T}}\right) + \iint_{Q_{a,T}} (u+v)\, G''_a \phi_1.$$

If we continue in this manner, then we have

$$\iint_{Q_{a,T}} (u+v)\, G_a \theta \le L_{k,p,T} \left(1 + \|v\|_{\infty,Q_{a,T}}\right) + \iint_{Q_{a,T}} (u+v)\, G_a^{(k+1)} \phi_k.$$

Consequently, if we set $k = m$ and define

$$K_{m,p,T} = L_{m,p,T} \left(1 + \|v\|_{\infty,Q_{a,T}}\right),$$

then we have

$$\iint_{Q_{a,T}} (u+v)\, G_a \theta \le K_{m,p,T} + \iint_{Q_{a,T}} (u+v)\, G_a^{(m+1)} \phi_m$$

$$\le K_{m,p,T} + \|u+v\|_{1,Q_{a,T}} \left\|G_a^{(m+1)}\right\|_{\infty} \|\phi_m\|_{\infty,Q_{a,T}}$$

$$\le K_{m,p,T} + \|u+v\|_{1,Q_{a,T}} \left\|G_a^{(m+1)}\right\|_{\infty} N_{p,T} \left(C_{p,T}\right)^{m+1}$$

from (4). Therefore, duality implies

$$\|u+v\|_{\frac{p}{p-1},Q_{a+T/2,T/2}} \le K_{m,p,T} + \|u+v\|_{1,Q_{a,T}} \left\|G_a^{(m+1)}\right\|_{\infty} N_{p,T} \left(C_{p,T}\right)^{m+1},$$

and the result follows.

Proof of 4: Recall that v is bounded from the estimates above. The boundedness for u follows from classic parabolic regularity applied to the individual equation for u. Simply note that u is uniformly bounded in L^1 and the inhomogeneity can be bounded in $L^p(Q_{T,1})$ independent of T for arbitrarily large p.

Proof of 5: The results above imply the existence of a global bounded attractor. Hence we can use the compactness of the semigroups associated with the individual equations for u and v (cf. Horton [7]) and apply results in Hale [4] to obtain the existence of a global compact attractor for (1). □

§3. Concluding Remarks

The estimates applied above can be carried through in a more general setting, and for a larger class of systems. Indeed, our estimates do not rely on space dimension, and can be applied for the same two component system on a bounded, smooth domain Ω which lies locally on one side of its boundary. In this setting, we assume Ω can be decomposed into subdomains U and W such that $\overline{U} \subset \Omega$, $\overline{U} \cup W = \Omega$ and U is a smooth domain which lies locally on one side of its boundary. Here, the boundary of U plays the role of the point $x = c$, and we refer to this boundary as the interface for the domain. An assumption of continuity and flux continuity is assumed on v across the interface. The details will be contained in one of our forthcoming papers. Related results can be found in [3].

References

1. Auchmuty, J. F. G. and G. Nicolis, Bifurcation analysis of nonlinear reaction-diffusion equations, I. Bull. Math. Biol. **37** (1975), 323–365.

2. Benson, D. L., J. A. Sherratt and P. K. Maini, Diffusion driven instability in an inhomogeneous domain, J. Math. Biology **55** (1993), 365–384.

3. Fitzgibbon, W. E., S. L. Hollis and J. Morgan, Steady state solutions for balanced reaction diffusion systems on heterogeneous domains, Advances in Partial Differential Equations, to appear.

4. Hale, J., *Asymptotic behavior of dissipative systems*, Mathematical Surveys and Monographs **25**, AMS, Providence, 1988.

5. Hollis, S., R. Martin and M. Pierre, Global existence and boundedness in reaction-diffusion systems, SIAM J. Math. Anal. **18** (1987), 744–761.

6. Hollis, S. and J. Morgan, On the blow-up of solutions to some semilinear and quasilinear reaction-diffusion systems, Rocky Mountain J. Math **24**(4) (1994), 1447–1465.

7. Horton, P., An analysis of reaction diffusion systems on heterogeneous domains, Ph.D. Dissertation, Texas A&M University, Spring 1998.

8. Ladyzenskaja, O., N. Solonnokov and N. Ural'ceva, *Linear and Quasilinear Equations of Parabolic Type*, Trans. AMS **23**, Providence, 1968.

9. Morgan, J., Boundedness and decay results for reaction-diffusion systems, SIAM J. Math. Anal. **21**(5) (1990), 1172–1189.

William E. Fitzgibbon
Department of Mathematics
University of Houston
4800 Calhoun
Houston, TX 77007
fitz@math.uh.edu

Jeff Morgan
Department of Mathematics
Texas A&M University
College Station, TX 77843-3368
Jeff.Morgan@math.tamu.edu

Branch Tree Models of Muscle Sensory Receptors

J. P. A. Foweraker, D. P. Bashor, M. Hulliger and E. Otten

Abstract. Proprioceptive information is transmitted to the central nervous system by two main types of muscle receptors, muscle spindles (MS) and Golgi tendon organs (GTO). A model of how the muscle spindle responds to changes in length is well developed [26,28,36], and a model of the GTO response is being constructed [9,27]. We aim to connect many hundreds of these units to a model of the spinal motor system [5], where interneurones and motoneurones receive input from many different peripheral receptor organs through a two-tier converging afferent tree; one within the muscle receptor and the other integrating inputs from many different muscle receptors. In modelling single MS units, the branch tree within the MS has been simulated by using a set of modified Frankenhauser-Huxley (FH) equations [26] to model the nodal, and hemi-nodal, points. These equations have a very wide range of repetitive firing rates (5-700/sec), although they also have large computational overheads, and are thus unsuitable for the large-scale simulation strategy that we wish to adopt. Our approach to this problem has been to simplify the nodal model, while maintaining an adequate comparison with the results of the more complex model. We have replaced the modified FH equations with a simple point-neurone model based on the work of MacGregor [24]. Further, we have modified the MacGregor code for linking these model nodes in a network. The modified MacGregor neurone exhibits a wide range of firing rates to an applied current, and also has a similar dynamic response to the modified FH equations, to a ramp and hold input. A simple two-neurone modified network can show spike propagation failure and entrainment. Thus, the new models presented here will form a module for integration into our large scale models.

§1. Introduction

1.1. Background and motivation

In the planning of movement, and the perception of limb position, feedback from the peripheral sensory receptors is key. Without feedback from these receptors there is an information deficit, and whilst movement is still possible it becomes relatively uncontrolled and uncoordinated [32,34,35,38]. The

Mathematical Models in Medical and Health Sciences
Mary Ann Horn, Gieri Simonett, and Glenn Webb (eds.), pp. 145–160.
Copyright © 1998 by Vanderbilt University Press, Nashville, TN.
ISBN 0-8265-1310-7.

mechanisms by which feedback, for instance on muscle tension and the rate of change of muscle length, is encoded are not well understood [30]. Further, how such feedback is processed by the central nervous system, is also not clear [30]. There are significant non-linearities in the afferent firing rate of receptors in response to whole muscle force [21] and length [18]. Proprioceptive information is mainly transmitted to the central nervous system by two types of muscle receptors: Muscle spindles (MS) and Golgi tendon organs (GTO). They convey complementary information about the state of the muscle: The muscle spindles mainly signal changes in length, whilst the GTO's mainly signal changes in tension. This information reaches all levels of the nervous system, and at the highest levels is used for the perception of limb position and for planning movements. The MS and GTO are complex structures embedded in the skeletal muscle, and it is very difficult to experimentally study the internal dynamics of these receptors in response to force and length changes at the level of ionic mechanisms of individual receptor compartments, although structural information can be obtained [2]. In particular, the complex nature of the ramifications of an afferent axon are revealed [2,3]. Thus mathematical models based upon the known structural and behavioural properties of the GTO and MS may be useful in understanding the behaviour of those receptors, and so help us to understand the control of movement.

1.2. Role of the afferent branch tree

In the MS and the GTO there are two mechanisms about which little is known; the mechano-ionic transduction process, and the role of the afferent branch tree in integrating trains of action potentials. Here we concentrate on the later mechanism: the afferent branch tree. One theory is that the branch tree serves to collect and integrate currents generated at the most peripheral sites [10,23], and has a single signal generation site in a proximal node near the top of the branch tree. Another view is that action potentials are generated at the most peripheral hemi-nodes, and it is the interaction, at a proximal node, between multiple trains of action potentials generated peripherally, that determines the final firing rate [4,8,19]. Each theory has equal merits, and neither has been proved, or disproved. A recent study [4], utilising physiological, histological and computer modelling techniques, has supplied evidence for multiple encoding sites in afferent branch trees. However, the existence of such sites can only be confirmed by direct experimental evidence, such as the selective lesioning of individual encoding sites, i.e., the sectioning of fine afferent terminal branch trees. Such branch trees are also evident in touch receptors (Figure 1 from [20]), and can thus be seen to be integral to the peripheral processing of somatosensory information.

1.3. Non-linearities of afferent response

Both the MS and the GTO have highly non-linear response patterns. For example, the firing rate of the Ib afferent in the isolated whole GTO has been shown to be approximately linear in response to force, when force is applied to the whole capsule [11]. However, such experiments can be considered non-physiological, and experiments which activate multiple motor units produce significant non-linearities in the force-firing rate relationship [21]. For example, when two different motor units, mu1 and mu2, are activated separately the Ib firing rate might be approximately the same in both cases. However, when the two muscle fibres are activated at the same time, the GTO firing rate is generally neither a summation of the individual firing rates, nor an occlusion of one firing rate by the other, but is some intermediate response (Figure 1).

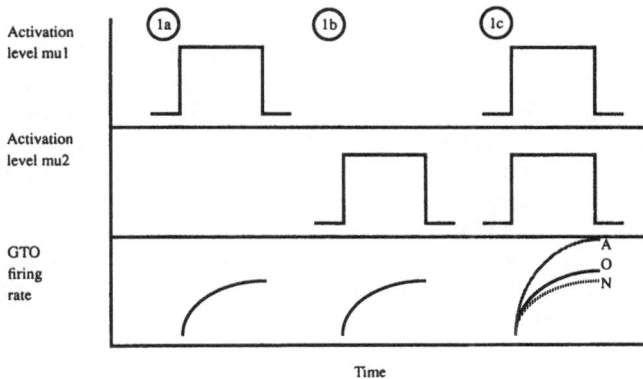

Fig. 1. A schematic representation of the Ib afferent firing rate for a GTO subject to (a) activation of mu1, (b) activation of mu2 and (c) activation of both mu1 and mu2. In 1c the solid line (O) indicates the observed response, the dotted line (N) the response if no summation occurs and the grey line (A) the response if algebraic summation occurs.

There are three mechanisms that are thought likely to play some role in the non-linear properties of the force-firing rate relationship: the mechanical properties of the muscle and the GTO in response to force, the transduction of that response to the generation of receptor potentials at multiple encoding sites, and the competition between action potentials in the encapsulated branch tree of the GTO. However, individually these elements do not account for the observed non-linearities; it is their combination which is thought to be responsible. Such processes have also been shown to be active in the MS branch tree [4] and are thus plausible mechanisms for the extreme non-linearities of response that both the GTO and the MS exhibit.

1.4. Modelling aims and strategies

An understanding of how these organs process sensory information is of practical, as well as theoretical, value. Mathematical models of the GTO and MS will provide a tool to explore the internal mechanisms of these receptors and also provide a module for incorporation into higher order models of sensorimotor circuitry. For the first application the model should include explicit formal descriptions of the model processes, but for the second less analytical detail is required, although models must still be capable of simulating a range of receptor behaviour, including various non-linear properties. The more detailed function and process based model of the GTO will complement the existing model of the MS [26,28,36]. The reasons for developing such models are clear; the GTO and MS are not simple force-, or length-, firing rate transducers, and the inherent non-linearities are a property of the internal structure of the receptors. Further, previous models have been severely limited; in the past quantative description has mostly been limited to approximations by linear transfer functions (e.g. MS: [7,25,29,33], GTO: [1,16,31]), or to more complex, but still limited, power-law descriptions (e.g. MS: [13,15,17,37], GTO: [39]). But these offer little insight into receptor mechanisms and fail to account for the striking non-linearities of receptor responses. The development of such a model for the GTO has been presented elsewhere [9,27]. In this paper we will focus on the simplification of the afferent branch tree as a simpler model element for use in both GTO and MS models. This element will be computationally more efficient, and it will thus be possible to integrate many hundreds of modules into larger scale models of motor systems control at the level of the spinal cord (e.g. [5]). Thus, in this paper we will focus on the simplification of the afferent branch tree.

§2. Methods

2.1. Encoding and the branch tree of the existing model

A key element of both the GTO and MS models is the method of encoding at the most peripheral hemi-nodes, and the integration of such signals in the afferent branch tree. In the MS model of Otten and co-workers [26,28,36], terminal current is fed into a modified Frankenhauser-Huxley (FH) model [26]. The original FH equations are Hodgkin-Huxley type equations, and were developed as a model of an unmyelinated node in a myelinated axon [12]. Thus, they are suitable equations for our modelling project. Both the MS and the GTO exhibit a very wide range of firing rates in their afferent axon, from as low as 5/sec in both GTO and MS, to 700/sec in the MS, and 200/sec in the GTO. The original FH equations, and many subsequent modifications (see [26] for summary), were unable to exhibit such a property. However Otten et al. adapted the FH equations, mainly by reducing the leakage component and adding a slow potassium conductance with a time constant of about 70 ms, to display repetitive firing at extremely low firing rates, as well as pronounced firing rate adaptation and a long-lasting post-stimulus silence. In Otten's model both nodes, and peripheral hemi-nodes, have encoding capability which can dynamically vary, and thus all nodal sites in the axonal branch tree are modelled by the modified FH equations. Signals propagate though the branch tree network by a simple potential gradient method, where current transfer from one node to the other is determined by the difference in the membrane potential of the two nodes concerned. Further, anatomical evidence indicates that the conduction time between afferent branch points can be as little as 0.005 ms.

The existing model of the axonal branch tree has several important characteristics, which have been reported on elsewhere [4,28]. These include response saturation (where an increase in input leads to no further increase in output), sub-linear summation (in principle accounted for by electrotonic coupling of receptor potentials), and an occlusion component (attributed to simple pacemaker competition). Further, model simulations of a simple 3-node branch tree indicate that short node-node conduction times are feasible. Thus it is reasonable to conclude that the development of a plausible branch-tree model for the sensory receptors is possible, and that such a model will have realistic properties.

The model described above is too complex to be included in large scale simulations with models of the motor systems circuitry in the spinal cord. Thus an alternative model needs to be developed. Description of encoding at the heminodes, and the more proximal nodes, of the axonal branch tree both use the modified FH equations. Although the number of sets of modified FH equations that are needed is dependent upon the complexity of the branch tree being modelled, the key computational effort is in solving these equations. Thus, a simplified model needs to be considered. The simplified model nodes will need to exhibit similar current-firing rate properties over a physiologically plausible range, including the very low rates that the modified FH equations exhibit, but with less computational effort. This will thus allow larger network simulations to be studied.

2.2. Development of the simplified model

The neuroscience community understands much of the power of the Hodgkin-Huxley modelling paradigm, and such models have been extensively investigated. However, the power of the point-neurone approach is much underestimated. This power lies first in the algorithmic strength: there is a very wide range of dynamic behaviour which is available from a very few adjustable parameters, and a very long integration interval. Secondly, there is the conceptual power, which has been noted by Hill [14] and Kernell [22], and also MacGregor [24], namely that the physiologically important events in neurones are those which happen when the neurone is near its resting and threshold potentials, not during the action potential itself. So, unless one is investigating the ionic events of the action potential (which has a rise time on the order of 1000 mV/ms) one can ignore its ionic details. Furthermore, much of systems neurophysiology is probably working in the time domain of the interspike interval, where changes are possibly a thousand times slower than those of the action-potential generating currents. Thus for modelling studies in systems neurophysiology a point neurone model is often satisfactory.

Thus for our afferent branch tree model we considered the point neurone model of repetitive firing of MacGregor [24] as a replacement for the modified FH equations of Otten et al. This model is conceptually simple, and it is computationally faster than an equivalent simulation of the modified FH equations, but still has many realistic properties. Thus, we are considering a network of model neurones (MacGregor) to simulate a network of branch tree nodes. This approach equates the behaviour of a node in a branch tree to that of a single neurone. Whilst there are clearly many differences, both structural and ionic, the underlying principle is that both the model neurone, and the branch tree node, integrate inputs from a number of sources and generate an action potential output. Further, the input to the neurone model, in terms of an applied current, represents the inputs from receptor channels in the branch tree.

$$\frac{dE}{dt} = \frac{-E + SC + Gk(Ek - E)}{TMEM},$$

$$\frac{dTH}{dt} = \frac{-(TH - TH0) + cE}{TTH},$$

$$\frac{dGk}{dt} = \frac{-Gk + bS}{TGk},$$

$$S = \begin{cases} 1, & \text{if } E \geq TH, \\ 0, & \text{otherwise}, \end{cases}$$

$$P = E + S(50 - E).$$

b	= level of refractoriness	S	= firing variable
c	= level of accommodation	SC	= applied current
Ek	= transmembrane potential	TH	= time-varying firing threshold
E	= equilibrium potential	$TH0$	= resting threshold
Gk	= potassium conductance	$TMEM, TGK, TTH$	
P	= membrane potential		=time constants

2.3. The MacGregor model

The MacGregor model (above, taken from [24]) for repetitive firing in a point neurone consists of three differential equations, with the input SC reflecting the applied current. Note that the function P is a cosmetic output function, whose output is similar to that which would be recorded by an intracellular electrode. MacGregor [24] formulates and comments on these equations, and provides Fortran code for their stepwise solution in 1 ms steps. His integration approach is an approximation whereby the parameters of each equation are taken to be constant over each time step. The solution of each equation is thus in the form of an exponential decay of the variable in which the equation is formed, combined with an additive term dependent upon other variables. Clearly this method of solving the equations loses some accuracy, but it is very efficient computationally. However, for our application of these equations it was necessary to consider high firing rates (up to 500/sec) for which the 1 ms stepsize gives inaccurate results. Simulations using the differential equation form of the equations were rejected, as the results are sensitive to the step size of the numerical integration being used: The step size affects the time for which $E > TH$, and thus the dynamics of the system through the bS term in the differential equation determining Gk. Thus the code that MacGregor supplies for this model, PTNRN10, was modified to allow for a change in the stepsize. Further, the code which MacGregor gives for the networking of these model neurones (POOL12) was also modified (see below).

2.4. Modification of the MacGregor equations for a single model neurone

The code that MacGregor supplies was modified so that the duration of a model action potential, defined by the time that $S = 1$, is constant, and thus independent of the step-size used in the numerical integration. This modified model exhibits different behaviour to the original equations in response to an applied current, although it still exhibits many features of the original model, and also of the modified FH equations. These include a wide range of steady-state firing rates, spike frequency adaptation and a long-lasting rebound period following stimulus release. A detailed analysis of this parameter space (unpublished) then allowed us to define a small subset of the parameter space where the point-neurone model exhibits the same types of behaviour as the modified FH equations ($b = 10$, $c = 0.5$, $Ek = -10$, $TGk = 70$, $TH0 = 10$, $TMEM = 10$, $TTH = 90$,).

2.5. Modification of the MacGregor network code

The MacGregor code that links the point-neurone models together to form a network, POOL12, was used, in an adapted form, for our network simulations. The original code allows for model neurones to interact via a synaptic mechanism and/or by extracellular field coupling. The "synaptic mechanism" allows for the time delayed increase of the input current to a model neurone by a fixed amount when an adjacent neurone fires, whilst the "extracellular field coupling" allows for an increase in the input current to a model neurone, dependent upon the transmembrane potential of an adjacent neurone. The results generated by a network using these mechanisms did not compare well with the results generated by a network of modified FH equations, linked by a potential difference method. This approach was thus used for the network of modified MacGregor neurones, with the change in input current to a neurone from an adjacent neurone being dependent upon the difference in the membrane potentials, P, rather than E, the transmembrane potentials. This is scaled by a parameter, AC, in effect reflecting the strength of connection between two neurones. Further, the "synaptic mechanism" was dropped from the model to allow for direct comparison with previous, electrotonically coupled, networks. A further modification to the MacGregor network is the introduction of a refractory period to each neurone; thus, if a neurone has fired in one time step, its input current cannot be increased by an adjacent neurone firing in the next time step.

§3. Results

3.1. Single neurone responses

Figure 2 shows the response of a single model neurone, in terms of spikes per second, in response to a range of levels of applied current. The simulation is run for 1500 ms, before sampling occurs for 1000 ms, the simulation thus approaching steady state conditions. Note that the neurone does not fire until $SC = 19.96$ and, after a small initial non-linear response, the firing rate increases in a linear manner with SC.

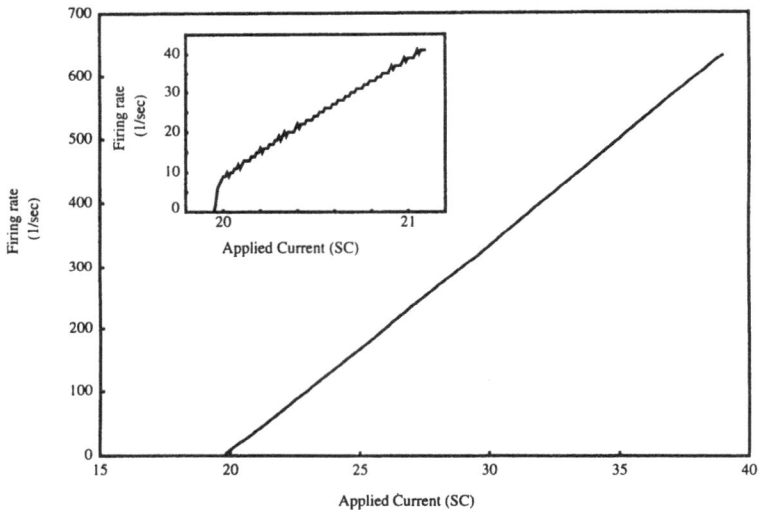

Fig. 2. The firing rate of the modified MacGregor equations as a function of the applied current SC. Inset: detail of low firing rate response.

Such steady state responses are useful, but do not reveal anything about the dynamic response of the model. Thus both a modified MacGregor neurone, and a system of modified FH equations, were subjected to a similar input scheme. The applied current was held at a level sufficient to produce a firing rate of approximately 50/sec for 1000 ms. The current was then increased linearly for 125 ms to a level which gives a steady state firing rate of approximately 120/sec, and held at that level for 500 ms. The applied current was then reduced, instantaneously to its initial level. The results are shown in Figure 3: membrane potential against time for (a) the modified FH equations,

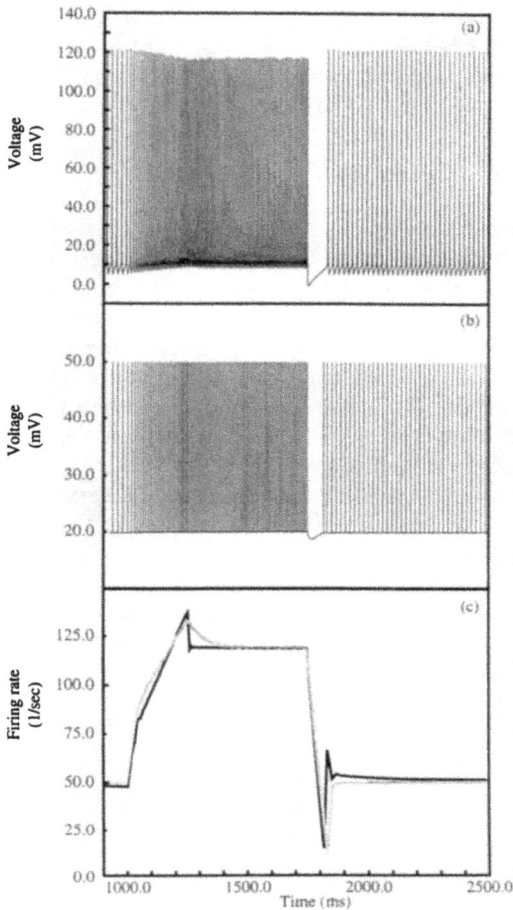

Fig. 3. Response of the modified FH equations [(a) and grey line in (c)], and the modified MacGregor equations [(b) and solid line in (c)], to a ramp and hold applied current (see text). (a) and (b) show action potentials, (c) is an instantaneous firing rate plot.

(b) the modified MacGregor equations, and (c) a plot of the instantaneous firing rates.

It is difficult to discern accurately the similarities, and differences between the two models from the membrane-potential plot. However, the firing rate plot is more revealing and shows that the response of the modified MacGregor model (solid line) and the modified FH equations (grey line) are very similar; both firing rates increase from their base firing rate to a maximum at about 1250 ms. This is followed by a decline to the 120/sec plateau. When the stimulus is reduced at 1750 ms both neurones fall to a firing rate below that at t=1000 ms of approximately 15/sec. There is a quick recovery to the initial firing rate for both neurones, with the point neurone model exhibiting a dynamic overshoot, and evidence of some oscillation in the firing rate, before returning to the base level.

3.2. Node-node interactions

To study node-node interactions the simplest possible network was chosen; two identical nodes with identical connections between them. This gives three parameters which can be varied, the strength of the connectivity between the nodes, and the two currents applied, one to each node. The currents were set at 30 for node 1 (equal to a single neurone firing rate of 333/sec) and 20 for node 2 (equal to a single neurone firing rate of 9/sec). The network connectivity parameter, AC, was then varied between 0 and 8 in steps of 0.025. Data collection was as for the single neurone simulations. Figure 4 shows one example of a time course ($AC = 2.25$) where the two neurones are locked in a 2:1 firing rate relationship; every second action potential at node 1 fails to propagate to node 2; there is an increase in the action potential at node 2, but it is not supra-threshold.

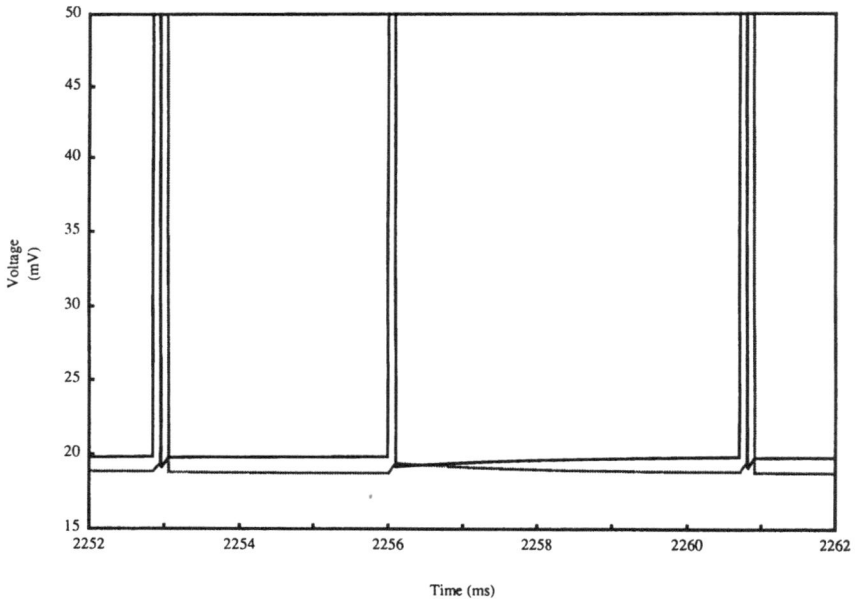

Fig. 4. Evidence of signal propagation failure in a simple modified network. The driving node (node 1, solid line) fires at regular intervals but every other pulse fails to propagate to the secondary node (node 2, grey line).

Figure 5a plots the firing rates of node 1 (solid line) and node 2 (grey line) over the range of AC given above. As AC increases from 0 there is a reduction in the firing rate of node 1, and an increase in that of node 2. Note that for $AC \geq 2.675$ the two traces are identical, showing exact phase locking. Further, there is a stepwise decrease in the firing rate of the two nodes as AC increases above 2.675. This is due to the increased current flow between the two nodes with increases the refractory period between action potentials. Figure 5b shows the ratio of the two firing rates, ρ (=Firing rate node 1/Firing rate node 2). The reduction in ρ as AC increases appears to be of a negative exponential form, with an asymptote at $\rho = 1$. The inset to Figure 5b shows the same data, but on a reduced scale, which allows some of the more interesting features to be revealed, namely that as AC is decreased there are plateaux regions of (moving from right to left) 1:1, 2:1, 5:2, 3:1, 7:2, 4:1, 9:2 and 5:1. Many more may be revealed if investigated on a finer scale.

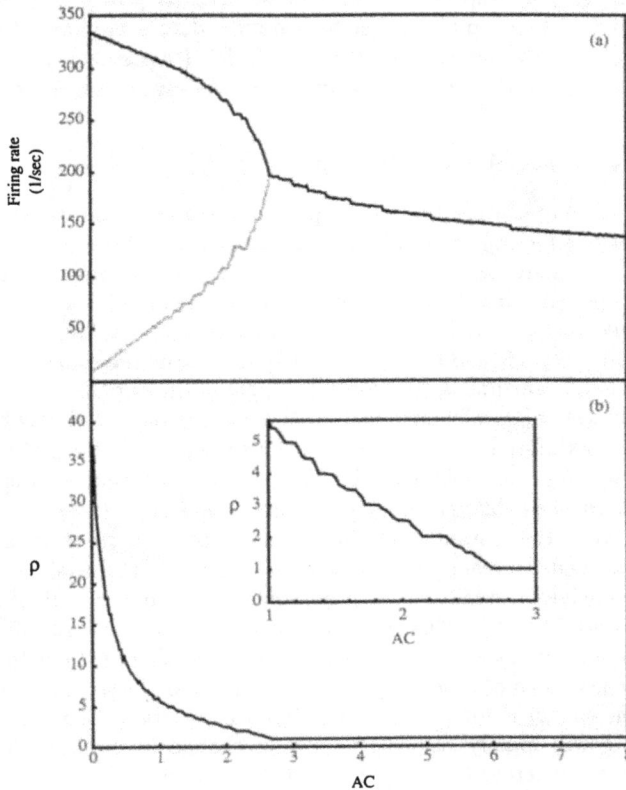

Fig. 5. (a) Firing rate of node 1 (solid line) and node 2 (grey line) as the strength of connection between the nodes (AC) is increased. (b) ρ (the ratio of the two firing rates) vs AC -inset shows "steps" in the apparently smooth curve.

§4. Discussion

4.1. Conceptual change

In making these modifications, and thus adapting the modified MacGregor code as a basis for our larger scale network simulations, we have made an important conceptual change from the initial network model. In that model we have, to all intents and purposes, a time-continuous system of differential equations representing each model neurone, and a time-continuous linkage between the model neurones to form the afferent branch tree. In the modified network model outlined above we now have time-discrete model neurones, with a time-discrete linkage system. There are also a number of logical statements involved in the simulation process, meaning that conventional mathematical analysis of the equations is difficult. The effect of the conceptual change involved here can, however, be seen to be minimal. In simulations of the discrete model a time step of 0.01 ms can be used to give highly accurate results, whilst still being much faster to compute than a similar integration of the original network model using the modified FH equations. Further, we have a model network that exhibits similar behavioural properties to the full network.

4.2. Validity of model simplification

The simulation results using the modified model neurone, and network, that have been presented above are similar in many respects to those obtained using the modified FH equations. From Figure 2 there is a clear linear relationship between the applied current to an isolated model neurone, covering a wide range of frequencies. This is comparable in range to that found by Otten et al. (Fig 4 in [26]), although there is a stronger linear relationship for this model. This is not surprising given the complex nature of the modified FH equations they use. Figure 3 indicates that there is a strong similarity between the behaviours exhibited by the new model neurone, and the modified FH equations to a ramp and hold stretch. Whilst the time courses (Figures 3a and 3b) show marked differences in pulse shape and size, there is a strong similarity between the instantaneous firing rate plots (Figure 3c). The new model neurone tends to react less smoothly to changes in the applied current. Further there are larger overshoots, and no slow decay from the peak of 138/sec to the plateau at 118/sec. This behaviour is due, in part, to the difference equation formulation of the model, which ensures that there is little 'memory' of previous events when determining the next event, and a more rapid response to any system changes; for example a difference equation formulation of a model neurone will mostly respond to a step change in input with a step change in output, whereas the output of a differential equation model will be more like that of a step input passed through a low pass filter. However, since the phenomenon of slow decay of the firing rate is such a characteristic feature of the MS and GTO response to mechanical stimulation, it might be desirable to add a slow conductance, similar to Otten's slow potassium current, to the modified MacGregor model. This would preserve the relative simplicity of our approach, whilst re-introducing the slow, potassium mediated, time-scale of the modified FH equations.

Figures 4 and 5 demonstrate that the simple network model can exhibit properties seen in the original modified FH network. There is a short delay time, using this model, between an action potential occurring at one node, and an action potential occurring at an adjacent node. In the example shown the delay is 0.07 ms. This can be altered by changing the parameter, AC, that scales the potential difference. Figure 4 also shows that spike propagation failure occurs in this network model. This is a phenomenon seen in both the original modified FH model, and also in many experimental preparations.

The same simple two-node network has been used to investigate the effect of changing AC, which reflects the strength of the connectivity between two nodes. The change in firing rates, as AC increases, is initially smooth (within the limits of experimental error), but for $AC > 2$ becomes more irregular. This, perhaps, indicates the existence of more complex dynamics than would be expected from such a model. However, these irregularities appear to be smoothed out when considering the plot of ρ in Figure 5b. By considering only a partial range of the connectivity parameter ($AC \in [1,3]$, inset) we see that this transition is, in fact, not smooth, and there is step-wise phase-locking of a type seen in many other models (e.g.[6]).

Thus, the initial simulation experiments with the modified MacGregor models indicate that we have developed a suitable replacement for the modified FH equations. The new model neurone, and its network formulation, have behaviour patterns close enough to those of the original model elements, are much simpler, and have solutions that are many times faster to compute.

4.3. Further model development

The next stage in the model development is a comprehensive analysis of the parameters determining the strength of the network connections. At present the connections are all of the same strength. Clearly this will not be the case in the afferent branch tree; the connectivity strength will change as the position in the branch tree changes due to changes in the axon diameter and the thickness of the myelin sheath. Further, there is no evidence to that the 'forward' and 'backwards' connections between two nodes need be the same. Model behaviour will change as these are altered.

Larger branch tree models will also be considered. Structural studies of the GTO (R.W. Banks, personal communication) indicate that there are not many levels of bifurcation in a Ib afferent branch after the initial split in the axon. Here the axon may divide into 5 or 6 different branches. For these larger simulations a terminal input strategy will have to be developed which replicates that which might occur in the GTO, i.e., the activation of a single muscle fibre will not necessarily stimulate every terminal encoding site on the Ib axon, and those that it does, may be subject to different levels of stimulation. Simulation results for the MS also need to be recreated with the simpler branch tree model, and other types of complexity need to be addressed. These include, larger branch trees, with more levels in the branching hierarchy, and also with a greater incidence of simple bifurcation in the afferent.

4.4. Summary

The models presented in this paper form part of a much larger modelling scheme. We need models which simulate the behaviour of more detailed function and process based models, yet are simpler in formulation and more efficient to compute. The work presented in this paper is a key step in the development of such models, as well as being of interest to the wider neural modelling community. There are many Hodgkin-Huxley type models in existence, with many different behaviour patterns. The models presented in this paper demonstrate that, for many applications, discrete models may be a simpler, more efficient, replacement. Further, the properties of the new network of modified neurones appear, from the evidence to hand, to be complex and worthy of further investigation. The exact details of pulse formation, and current fluxes, are often lost in presentations of neural network models. Whilst cellular mechanisms are important in many applications, firing rates and network firing patterns are often more important to the systems physiologist.

Acknowledgments. J. P. A. Foweraker is supported by the AHFMR.

References

1. Anderson, J. H., Dynamic characteristics of Golgi tendon organs, Brain Research **67** (1974), 531–537.

2. Banks, R. W., The motor innervation of mammalian muscle spindles, Progress in Neurobiology **43** (1994), 323–362.

3. Banks, R. W., D. Barker and M. J. Stacey, Form and distribution of sensory terminals in cat hindlimb muscle spindles, Philosophical Transactions of the Royal Society of London B **299** (1982), 329–364.

4. Banks, R. W., M. Hulliger, K. A. Scheepstra and E. Otten, Pacemaker activity in a sensory ending with multiple encoding sites: The cat muscle-spindle primary ending, Journal of Physiology **498** (1997), 177–199.

5. Bashor, D. B. and S. Merkel, Simulation of spinal segmental reflexes: the alternate Golgi reflex, Neuroscience Abstracts **22** (1996), 543.2.

6. Chay, T. R., Y. S. Lee and Y. S. Fan, Appearance of phase-locked Wenckebach-like rhythms, devil's staircase and universality in intracellular calcium spikes in non-excitable cell models, J. Theor. Biol. **174** (1996), 21–44.

7. Chen, W. J. and R. E. Poppele, Small-signal analysis of response of mammalian muscle spindles with fusimotor stimulation and a comparison with large-signal responses, Journal of Neurophysiology **41** (1978), 15–27.

8. Eagles, J. P. and R. L. Purple, Afferent fibers with multiple encoding sites, Brain Research **77** (1974), 187–193.

9. Foweraker, J. P. A. and M. Hulliger, Development of a mathematical model of the Golgi tendon organ, Abstracts of 6th Annual Computational Neuroscience Meeting (1997), 54.

10. Fukami, Y., Responses of isolated Golgi tendon organs of the cat to muscle contraction and electrical stimulation, Journal of Physiology **318** (1981), 429–443.

11. Fukami, Y. and R. S. Wilkinson, Responses of isolated Golgi tendon organs of the cat, Journal of Physiology **265** (1977), 673–689.

12. Frankenhaeuser, B. and A. F. Huxley, The action potential in the myelinated nerve fibre of Xenopus laevis as computed on the basis of voltage clamp data, Journal of Physiology **171** (1964), 302–315.

13. Hasan, Z., A model of spindle afferent response to muscle stretch, Journal of Neurophysiology **49** (1983), 989–1006.

14. Hill, A. V., Excitation and accommodation in nerve, Proceedings of the Royal Society London B **119** (1936).

15. Holm, W., D. Padeken and S. S. Schäfer, Characteristic curves of the dynamic response of primary muscle spindle endings with and without gamma stimulation, Pflügers Archiv, European Journal of Physiology **391** (1981), 163–170.

16. Houk, J., A viscoelastic interaction which produces one component of adaptation in responses of Golgi tendon organs, Journal of Neurophysiology **30** (1967), 1482–1493.

17. Houk, J. C., W. Z. Rymer and P. E. Crago, Dependence of dynamic response of spindle receptors on muscle length and velocity, Journal of Neurophysiology **46** (1981), 143–166.

18. Hulliger, M., The mammalian muscle spindle and its central control, Reviews of Physiology, Biochemistry and Pharmacology **101** (1984), 1–110.

19. Hulliger, M. and J. Noth, Static and dynamic fusimotor interaction and the possibility of multiple pace-makers operating in the cat muscle spindle, Brain Research **173** (1979), 21–28.

20. Iggo, A. and R. A. Muir, The structure and function of a slowly adapting touch corpuscle in hairy skin, Journal of Physiology **200** (1969), 763–796.

21. Jami, L., Golgi tendon organs in mammalian skeletal muscle: Functional properties and central action, Physiological Reviews **72** (1992), 623–666.

22. Kernell, D, The repetitive impulse discharge of a simple neuron model compared to that of spinal motorneurones, Brain Research **11** (1986), 685–687.

23. Kröller, J., O.-J. Grüsser and L. R. Weiss, A study of the encoder properties of the muscle-spindle primary afferent fibres by a random noise disturbance of the steady stretch response, Biological Cybernetics **63** (1990), 91–97.

24. MacGregor, R. J., *Neural and Brain Modelling*, Academic Press, New York, 1987.

25. Matthews, P. B. C. and R. B. Stein, The sensitivity of muscle spindle afferents to small changes of length, Journal of Physiology **200** (1969), 723–743.

26. Otten, E., M. Hulliger and K. A. Scheepstra, A model study on the influence of a slowly activating potassium conductance on repetitive firing patterns of muscle spindle primary endings, Journal of Theoretical Biology **173** (1995), 67–87.

27. Otten, E., M. Hulliger and P. Sjölander, Towards a mathematical model of the Golgi tendon organ, in *Alpha and Gamma Motor Systems*, A. Taylor, M.H. Glad-den and R. Durbaba (eds.), Plenum, London, 1995, 322–324.

28. Otten, E., K. A. Scheepstra and M. Hulliger, An integrated model of the mammal-ian muscle spindle, in *Alpha and Gamma Motor Systems*, A. Taylor, M. H. Glad-den, and R. Durbaba (eds.), Plenum, London, 1995, 294–301.

29. Poppele, R. E. and R.J. Bowman, Quantitative description of linear behavior of mammalian muscle spindles, Journal of Neurophysiology **33** (1970), 59–72.

30. Prochazka, A., Proprioceptive feedback and movement regulation, in *Integration of Motor, Circulatory, Respiratory and Metabolic Control during Exercise*, American Handbook of Physiology, L. Rowell and J. Shepard, Oxford University Press, New York, 1996.

31. Rosenthal, N. P., T. A. McKean, W. J. Roberts and C. A. Terzuolo, Frequency analysis of stretch reflex and its main subsystems in triceps surae muscles of the cat, Journal of Neurophysiology **33** (1970), 713–749.

32. Rothwell, J. C., M. M. Traub, B. L. Day, J.A . Obeso, P. K. Thomas and C. D. Marsden, Manual motor performance in a deafferented man, Brain **105** (1982), 515–542.

33. Rudjord, T. A second order mechanical model of muscle spindle primary endings, Kybernetik **6** (1970), 205–213.

34. Sainburg, R. L., H. Poizner and C. Ghez, Loss of proprioception produces deficits in interjoint coordination, Journal of Neurophysiology **70** (1993), 2136–2147.

35. Sanes, J. N., K.- H. Mauritz, M. C. Dalakas, and E. V. Evarts, Motor control in humans with large-fiber sensory neuropathy, Human Neurobiology **4** (1985), 101–114.

36. Schaafsma, A., E. Otten and J. D. Van Willigen, A muscle spindle model for primary afferent firing based on a simulation of intrafusal mechanical events, Journal of Neurophysiology **65** (1991), 1297–1312.

37. Schäfer, S. S. The characteristic curves of the dynamic response of primary muscle spindle endings in the absence and presence of stimulation of fusimotor fibres, Brain Research **59** (1973), 395–399.

38. Taub, E., Movement in nonhuman primates deprived of somatosensory feedback, Ex-er-cise Sports Sci. Rev. **4** (1976), 335–374.

39. Wilkinson, R. S. and Y. Fukami, Responses of isolated Golgi tendon organs of cat to sinusoidal stretch, Journal of Neurophysiology **49** (1983), 976–988.

Key Dynamics from a Simple Model
of HIV Infection

Faustino Sánchez Garduño, Denise Kirschner
and Janelle Reynolds

Abstract. There have been many models to date describing the interaction of the immune system with HIV. Each presents some aspect or aspects of the immune system believed to play a key role in the disease dynamics. In this study, we again explore the immune interactions; however from a very basic perspective. Our focus is the key first order effects which are necessary for a model of HIV-immune interaction to explain the different stages of disease progression. Our model is a non-linear autonomous ODE system; dependent on several biological parameters. We analyze the global dynamics of the system for different sets of parameters varied within the proper parameter space. We also include numerical simulations of the relevant phase portraits.

§1. Introduction

Over the past decade a number of mathematical models have been developed to describe the interaction of the immune system with the human immunodeficiency virus (HIV). For example, see [4,5,6,8,9,10,11,12,14]. Different phenomenon are explained by the different models, but none of the models exhibit all of what is observed clinically. This is partly due to the fact that much about this disease's mechanics is still unknown. However, many of the major features can be simulated with even the simplest of models.

Thus, the main focus of the model we present is to explore the simplest mathematical descriptions of the interaction of HIV and the human immune system necessary to capture the first order effects seen clinically. Namely, the three major outcomes are: an uninfected state, where the body clears HIV (no infection present); an infected state, where the T cells and virus have high turnover rates on a daily basis, but the overall appearance is of a steady state with low levels of free virus in the blood and a significantly reduced T cell count (from normal which is approx. 1000 per mm^3); and then a progression to AIDS state, where the T cells significantly decline and the virus population

Mathematical Models in Medical and Health Sciences
Mary Ann Horn, Gieri Simonett, and Glenn Webb (eds.), pp. 161–196.

expands. The immunological understanding of these different stages of disease progression are still not well understood, but we hope to gain insight into the processes through the modeling endeavors.

In this work, we present a simple model for the interaction of the immune system with HIV and then carry out a non-dimensionalization. On this nondimensionalized version, we do an extensive global analysis using both numerical and analytical techniques to analyze the rich behavior arising in the dynamical system. Finally, we discuss the implications of mathematical results for the biological problem of HIV disease progression.

§2. The Model and Its Non-Dimensional Version

HIV destruction of the immune system works mainly by infecting CD4$^+$ T cells, the cells responsible for the governing of the immune system. Therefore, we create a model incorporating only these two populations and their interactions and effects. More detailed models incorporating different classes of cells and virus have been studied as well (e.g. [4,5,6,8,9,10,11,12,14,16]), but our aim is to create a simple model capturing the rich clinical behavior. Define $T(t)$ to be the CD4$^+$ T cell population at time t. Define $V(t)$ to be the free virus population at time t. We assume only one strain of virus. A simple model describing the interaction of HIV with the immune system is then as follows:

$$\frac{dT}{dt} = \sigma - \mu T(t) + T(t)\frac{pV(t)}{C + V(t)} - K_{V,T}T(t)V(t), \tag{1}$$

$$\frac{dV}{dt} = \hat{N} \cdot K_{V,T}T(t)V(t) - K_{T,V}T(t)V(t) + G_V V(t). \tag{2}$$

Initial conditions are $T(0) = T_0$, and $V(0) = V_0$. (We assume the initial innoculum is free virus and not infected cells.)

The model is explained as follows. The terms of (1), $\sigma + \frac{pV(t)}{C+V(t)}T(t)$, represent the source of new T cells. This incorporates T cells from the bone marrow, thymus and general production. It also includes proliferative production (whether direct or indirect) due to the presence of antigen. This production changes over the course of infection, which is accounted for in the choice of terms. This is followed by a natural death term, because cells have a finite life span; the average of which is $\frac{1}{\mu_T}$. The last term of (1) represents the infection of CD4$^+$ T cells by virus. This term is a mass action type term with constant rate of infectivity $K_{V,T}$. We assume the law of mass action applies here based on the large numbers of cells and virion involved. In (2), the first term is the source for the virus population. Newly produced virion are produced by infected CD4$^+$ T cells (hence it follows from (1)), whereby new virion are produced at the rate $\hat{N} \cdot K_{V,T}T(t)$. There is a high clearance rate of virus, on a daily basis, [14], and this is reflected in the next term $-K_{T,V}T(t)V(t)$. As there is much evidence to support the major production of virus taking place in the external lymphoid system (LS), we account for this phenomenon as a major contributor of virions, other than the small amount produced in the blood [7]. The input rates of lymphoid system virus is $G_V(t)$.

This is a simple possible model representing the interactions of T cells and virus. This model was studied in a 3 equation form (with a separate equation for the infected T cells) and the parameter values were all estimated there [4,5,6]. We summarize those results in Table 1, which gives a list of all parameters along with their estimated numerical values.

If we first examine the system for steady-state values, we find there are three possible steady states in the positive cone depending on the parameter space. Hence, we define the different steady states for the system as follows: *Uninfected steady state* (where the virus population and infected cells are $\bar{V} = 0$ and $\bar{T} = \frac{s}{\mu}$), and an *Infected Steady State* (both virus and T cells exist at some positive level). This corresponds to the extended latent period of the disease. Another limiting behavior for the system is *Progression to AIDS* (the T cell population goes to 0, and V grows without bound - which is consistent with the Center for Disease Control's definition for AIDS).

Before further analysis, we performed a non-dimensionalization. Define the new variables as:

$$T^{\text{new}} = T/T_{\max}, \quad V^{\text{new}} = V/C, \quad t^{\text{new}} = pt,$$

$$\frac{dT^{\text{new}}}{dt^{\text{new}}} = \frac{d(T/T_{\max})}{d(pt)} = \frac{\frac{1}{T_{\max}}}{p} \frac{dT}{dt}. \tag{3}$$

Substituting (3) into (1) and (2) and suppressing the "new" notation, the equations are transformed into:

$$\frac{dT}{dt} = s - mT + \frac{TV}{1+V} - k_1 VT, \tag{4}$$

$$\frac{dV}{dt} = NTV - k_2 VT + gV, \tag{5}$$

with

$$s = \frac{\sigma}{T_{\max} \cdot p}, \quad m = \frac{\mu}{p}, \quad k_1 = \frac{K_{V,T} K}{p} \quad N = \frac{\hat{N} K_{V,T} T_{\max}}{p},$$

$$k_2 = \frac{K_{T,V} T_{\max}}{p} \quad \text{and} \quad g = \frac{G_V}{p}.$$

One advantage of this new system (4-5) is that the number of parameters has been reduced from 9 to 6.

§3. The Phase Portrait Analysis

Define the right hand sides of (4-5) to be the functions $f_1(V,T)$ and $f_2(V,T)$, respectively, as shown:

$$\dot{V} = NTV - k_2 TV + gV \equiv f_1(V,T),$$

$$\dot{T} = s - mT + \frac{TV}{1+V} - k_1 TV \equiv f_2(V,T), \tag{6}$$

where all the parameters are positive.

Before we begin analysis of this system, we wish to point out a transformation. Let $V = e^x$ and $T = e^y$. Then this system is transformed into:

$$\dot{x} = -ke^y + g,$$

$$\dot{y} = se^{-y} - m + \frac{e^x}{(1 + e^x)} - k_1 e^x.$$

This system is well-known from Lotka-Volterra theory. It is easy to show that the divergence of the vector field is $div = -se^{-y}$ which is always negative, thus by Bendixson's negative criterion, there are no periodic solutions, and all bounded trajectories converge. We will however, be concerned directly with the dynamical behavior of the phase portrait in the VT-plane, and what the implications are to the biological problem of HIV-T cell dynamics. Therefore, we will perform the remainder of the analysis on the original system given in (6). Future work could examine how our original VT-plane and trajectories are changed via this transformation. For example, the $V = e^x$ and $T = e^y$ transformation maps the positive orthant into the whole plane. It would be of interest to see how closed trajectories are mapped into closed trajectories, etc.

The dynamics of the system (6) depends strongly on the behavior of the nullclines. These are given by the set $\{(V,T) \mid f_1(V,T) = f_2(V,T) = 0\}$. The horizontal nullcline has two branches: $V \equiv 0$ and the horizontal line

$$T_{hor} = \frac{g}{k_2 - N} \equiv T^*. \tag{7}$$

Hereafter we will assume $(k_2 - N) > 0$, as negative cell populations do not make biological sense. The vertical nullcline is the graph of the function

$$T_{vert}(V) = \frac{s + sV}{k_1 V^2 + rV + m}, \tag{8}$$

where $r = m + k_1 - 1$. Note that $T_{vert}(0) = s/m$, $T_{vert}(-1) = 0$, $T_{vert}(V) \to 0$ as $V \to +\infty$ or as $V \to -\infty$.

Given that the vertical nullcline (8) depends on three parameters: k_1, m and s, its geometric features will also depend on them; particularly, whether or not the denominator, $D(V)$,

$$D(V) = k_1 V^2 + rV + m, \tag{9a}$$

has roots. If they exist, the roots of $D(V)$ are

$$V_1, V_2 = \frac{-r \pm \sqrt{r^2 - 4k_1 m}}{2k_1}. \tag{9b}$$

Clearly, the signs of V_1 and V_2 are of concern for biological feasibility as well. Let us write the discriminant, $d = r^2 - 4k_1 m$, explicitly

$$d = [(m - k_1)^2 - 2(m + k_1) + 1]. \tag{10}$$

We note that in the mk_1-parameter plane the graphs of the functions

$$k_1^1(m) = (1+m) + 2\sqrt{m} \quad \text{and} \quad k_1^2(m) = (1+m) - 2\sqrt{m} \qquad (11)$$

are the boundaries between the regions on which the function $D(V)$ has none or two real roots, corresponding to $d < 0$ and $d > 0$, respectively. Figure 1 illustrates the space of the parameters in the mk_1-plane.

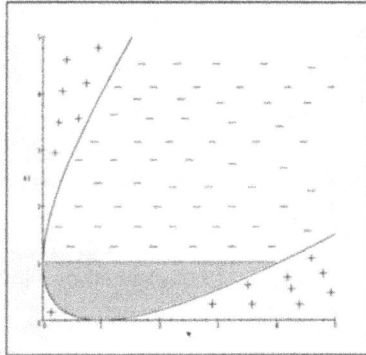

Fig. 1. Space parameters for the roots of $D(V) = k_1 V^2 + rV + m$. On the region $(+)$ D has two real roots, on $(-)$ there are not real roots and on the graph of k_1^1 and k_1^2, D has one real root.

Depending on the sign of d we will divide the analysis in three major cases. Case 1 is $d < 0$; Case 2 is $d = 0$; and Case 3 is $d > 0$. The results are summarized in Table 2 and the analysis follows in the next subsections.

3.1. Phase Portrait Analysis in Case 1:

$$d = [(m - k_1)^2 - 2(m + k_1) + 1] < 0.$$

Here the function $D(V)$, (9a), has no real roots. This situation corresponds to the region marked with negative $(-)$ signs in Figure 1, i.e.

$$m + 1 - 2\sqrt{m} < k_1 < m + 1 + 2\sqrt{m}. \qquad (12)$$

First we need to determine the qualitative profile of T_{vert} (8). One can verify that, provided $[k_1 V^2 + (m + k_1 - 1)V + m] \neq 0$, T_{vert} has a maximum at $V = \tilde{V}_1 = -1 + 1/\sqrt{k_1}$ whose value is $T_{vert}(\tilde{V}_1) = s/(2\sqrt{k_1} + m - k_1 - 1)$ and one minimum at $V = \tilde{V}_2 = -1 - 1/\sqrt{k_1}$ whose value is $T_{vert}(\tilde{V}_2) = s/(m - 1 - 2\sqrt{k_1} - k_1)$. For the set of parameters m and k_1 given in (12), $T_{vert}(\tilde{V}_1) > 0$ and $T_{vert}(\tilde{V}_2) < 0$.

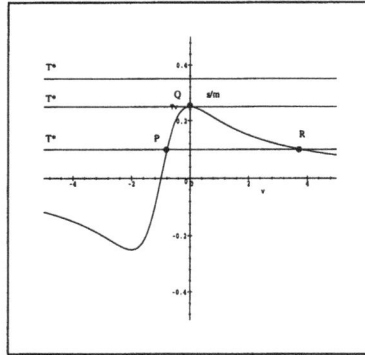

Fig. 2. Case **1.a.i**: $d < 0$. There are at most three steady states as the value of $T^* = T_{hor}$ varies.

Depending on the value of the parameters, providing the inequality (12) holds, we have three Sub-Cases.

Before the phase portrait analysis we first define the region of biological interest, namely

$$\Omega = \{(V, T) \mid 0 \leq V < \infty; 0 \leq T < \infty\}.$$

Case 1.a: $k_1 = 1$.

Here $\widetilde{V}_1 = 0$ and $\widetilde{V}_2 = -2$. The condition $d = [(m - k_1)^2 - 2(m + k_1) + 1] < 0$, implies $0 < m < 4$. In addition we have $T_{vert}(0) = s/m = \max T_{vert}(V) \equiv M$. For the parameter values in Table 1, the value of $M = \frac{1}{3}$ in this scaled form. The graph of T_{vert} is the curve shown in Figure 2. Depending on T^*, we have there possible cases (see Figure 2):

  i) $0 < T^* < M$. Here the system (6) has three equilibria: P, Q and R. Given the biological interpretation of the variables, the point P is not feasible.
 ii) $T^* = M$. Here the points P and R collapse into Q, thus the system (6) has only one equilibrium: Q.
iii) $T^* > M$. Here the nullclines have no intersection. Thus the system (6) has one equilibrium point: Q.

Now we will determine the qualitative behavior of the trajectories of (6) for each one of the above cases. Particularly we will focus on the existence of trajectories of (6) connecting pairs of equilibria (when it makes sense) i.e. on the existence of heteroclinic trajectories of (6).

Case 1.a.i.

The coordinates, (V^*, T^*), of the equilibrium R are $T^* = \frac{g}{k_2 - N}$ and V^* is the positive root of

$$T^* V^2 + (mT^* - s)V + T^* m - s = 0, \tag{13}$$

i.e.

$$V^* = \frac{-(mT^* - s) + \sqrt{(mT^* - s)^2 - 4T^*(T^* m - s)}}{2T^*}. \tag{14}$$

This results from the condition $T^* < s/m$. The other equilibrium is Q. Our analysis starts by considering the local phase portrait of (6) around each equilibrium. Thus the Jacobian matrix of (6) at all points (V, T) is given by

$$
J[f_1, f_2]_{(V,T)} = \begin{bmatrix} \frac{\partial f_1}{\partial V} & \frac{\partial f_1}{\partial T} \\ \frac{\partial f_2}{\partial V} & \frac{\partial f_2}{\partial T} \end{bmatrix}_{(V,T)}
$$

$$
= \begin{bmatrix} NT - k_2 T + g & NV - k_2 V \\ -\dfrac{VT(2+V)}{(1+V)^2} & \dfrac{-m - mV - V^2}{(1+V)} \end{bmatrix}. \tag{15}
$$

Evaluating (15) at Q we obtain

$$
J[f_1, f_2]_{(0, s/m)} = \begin{bmatrix} \frac{s}{m}(N - k_2) + g & 0 \\ 0 & -m \end{bmatrix}, \tag{16}
$$

which implies the trace is: $tr(J[f_1, f_2](0, s/m)) = \frac{s}{m}(N - k_2) + g - m$ and the determinant is $det\ J[f_1, f_2]_{(0, s/m)} = s(k_2 - N) - mg$. Because of the condition $T^* = \frac{g}{(k_2 - N)} < \frac{s}{m}$, $det\ J[f_1, f_2]_{(0, s/m)} > 0$ and $tr(J[f_1, f_2]_{(0, s/m)}) < 0$. Since the roots of the characteristic polynomial $\mathcal{P}(\lambda) = \left[\frac{s}{m}(N - k_2) + g - \lambda\right](-m - \lambda)$, of (16) are λ_1 and λ_2,

$$\lambda_1 = \left[\frac{s}{m}(N - k_2) + g\right] < 0 \quad \text{and} \quad \lambda_2 = -m < 0.$$

Then Q is a locally asymptotically stable node. Given that the element $a_{12} = 0$ in the Jacobian matrix (16), then except for the trajectory approaching Q through the line spanned by the eigenvector $\vec{v}_2 = (\lambda_1, \lambda_2)^T$, all the trajectories of (6) tend to Q tangential to the vertical axis. Moreover, in a neighborhood of Q, the variables T and V are related by the equality

$$T(V) = aV^{\lambda_2/\lambda_1},$$

where a is any real number.

Now we evaluate (15) at $R = (V^*, T^*)$, from which we have

$$tr(J[f_1, f_2]_{(V^*, T^*)}) = \frac{-m - mV^* - V^{*2}}{(1 + V^*)} < 0, \text{ and}$$

$$det\ J[f_1, f_2]_{(V^*, T^*)} = -\frac{V^{*2} g(2 + V^*)}{(1 + V^*)^2} < 0.$$

Thus R is a hyperbolic saddle point.

The characteristic polynomial has the following roots:

$$\lambda_1, \lambda_2 = -\frac{(m + mV^* + V^{*2}) \pm \sqrt{(m + mV^* + V^{*2})^2 + 4gV^{*2}(2 + V^*)}}{2(1 + V^*)},$$

with $\lambda_1 > 0$ and $\lambda_2 < 0$. The eigenvectors corresponding to each eigenvalue are

$$\vec{v}_1 = (1 + p_1^2)^{-1/2} \begin{bmatrix} 1 \\ p_1 \end{bmatrix} \quad \text{and} \quad \vec{v}_2 = (1 + p_2^2)^{-1/2} \begin{bmatrix} 1 \\ p_2 \end{bmatrix},$$

where

$$p_1 = \frac{\lambda_1}{(N - k_2)V^*} < 0 \quad \text{and} \quad p_2 = \frac{\lambda_2}{(N - k_2)V^*} > 0.$$

The local phase portrait of (6) around Q and R is illustrated in Figure 3.

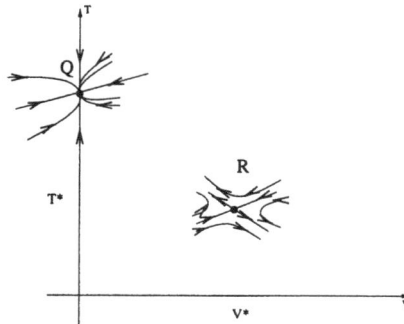

Fig. 3. Local phase portrait of (6) for the Sub-Case **1.a.i** with $0 < T^* < M$. Notice that Q is the locally asymptotic stable node and R is the saddle point.

Now we will determine the global behavior of the trajectories of (6) in the region of biological interest, namely Ω. First, note that the vector field defined by (6) is as in Figure 4(a). Second, note the left unstable manifold of (6), $W^u(R)$, at R leaves this equilibrium below the graph of the nullcline with slope $M^u(R) = \frac{\lambda_1}{(N-k_2)V^*} < 0$. Once $W^u(R)$ leaves R, the vector field (6) pushes it towards the shaded region $\mathcal{R}$ of Figure 4(b). Again, because of the vector field, this trajectory never goes outside of the region $\mathcal{R}$ as time increases. Moreover, given that

$$\frac{\partial f_1}{\partial V} + \frac{\partial f_2}{\partial T} = \left[(N - k_2)T + g - \frac{m - mV - V^2}{(1 + V)}\right] < 0 \quad \forall\, (V, T) \in \mathcal{R},$$

then, by the Dulac's Test, the system (6) has no closed trajectory there. Since the system (6) has an equilibrium in $\mathcal{R}$, thus by the Poincaré-Bendixon Theorem [3], $W^u(R)$ must end at Q as time t goes to infinity.

This proof can be now summarized in the following proposition:

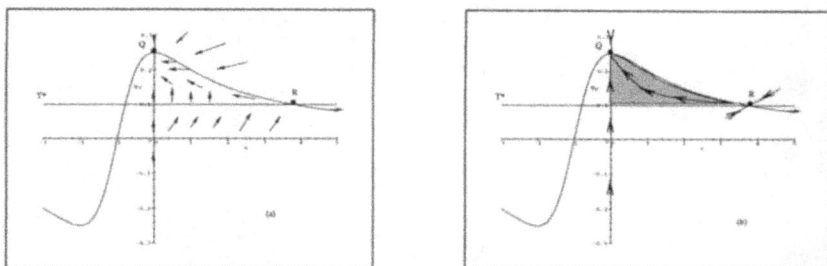

Fig. 4. Global behavior of the trajectories of (6) for the Case **1.a.i:** (a) Vector Field. (b) The trajectory $W^u(R)$ approaches Q as $t \to +\infty$.

Proposition 1.1. *For $k_1 = 1$ and for each m such that $0 < m < 4$ with $\frac{g}{k_2 - N} < \frac{s}{m}$, the trajectory $W^u(R)$ tends to Q as $t \to +\infty$.*

Case 1.a.ii.

Here $T^* = \frac{s}{m} = \frac{g}{k_2 - N}$ and the system (6) has just one equilibrium: $Q = (0, s/m)$. The Jacobian matrix (15) yields the $tr(J[f_1, f_2]_{(0,s/m)}) = -m < 0$ and $det\ J[f_1, f_2]_{(0,s/m)} = 0$. Thus, the equilibrium Q is a *non-hyperbolic* point of *co-dimension one* i.e., the Jacobian has eigenvalues $\lambda_1 = 0$ and $\lambda_2 = -m$. The corresponding eigenvectors are $\vec{v_1} = (m, 0)^T$ and $\vec{v_2} = (0, 1)^T$, respectively.

According to the Centre Manifold Theorem [1], the system (6)

i) has a unique one-dimensional invariant stable manifold locally tangent to the eigenvector $\vec{v_2}$,

ii) has a one-dimensional invariant center manifold locally tangent to the eigenvector $\vec{v_1}$,

iii) except on the stable manifold, all other trajectories tend to the center manifold.

More detailed qualitative information on the local phase portrait of (6) around Q can be obtained by calculating an approximation to the center manifold of (6) at Q. (According with theorems from [1] this approximation of the center manifold of the normal form of the non-linear approximation of (6) at Q can be obtained with a sufficient degree of accuracy.) For this we need higher order terms in the Taylor Series, but for our present purpose, we do not need these technical details. It is enough to say that Q is a *saddle-node bifurcation point* and that the trajectories of (6) leaving Q through the center manifold travels away from Q tending to $(+\infty, 0)$ as time t increases. This follows from the vector field of (6). The phase portrait for this Sub-Case is shown in Figure 5.

The above analysis can be stated as the following proposition:

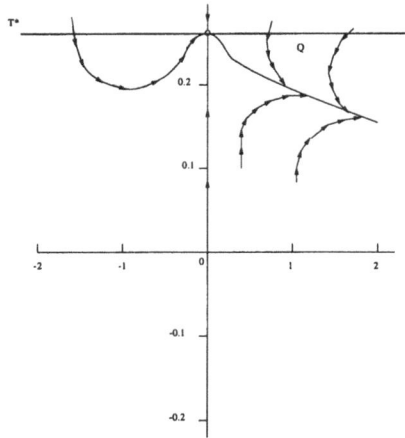

Fig. 5. Case **1.a.ii:** The saddle-node bifurcation point. The center manifold of (6) at Q runs away to $(\infty, 0)$, as $t \to +\infty$.

Proposition 1.2. *For* $k_1 = 1$, $0 < m < 4$ *and* $\frac{s}{m} = \frac{g}{k_2 - N}$, *the system (6) has a unique equilibrium point of saddle-node bifurcation type. Moreover the trajectory of (6) leaving* Q *through the center manifold tends to* $(+\infty, 0)$ *as* $t \to +\infty$.

Case 1.a.iii: $T^* > \frac{s}{m}$.

Here the system (6) has just one equilibrium: Q. The Jacobian matrix at Q yields:

$$det(J[f_1, f_2]_{(0, s/m)}) = -m \left[\frac{s}{m}(N - k_2) + g \right], tr(J[f_1, f_2]_{(0, s/m)})$$
$$= \frac{s}{m}(N - k_2) + g - m. \qquad (17)$$

Because of the condition $\frac{g}{(k_2 - N)} > \frac{s}{m}$, we have $det\, J[f_1, f_2]_{(0, s/m)} < 0$, thus Q is a saddle point. The eigenvalues are $\lambda_1 = \left[\frac{s}{m}(N - k_2) + g \right] > 0$ and $\lambda_2 = -m < 0$. The stable manifold is on the vertical axis, while the unstable manifold has (at Q) a tangent vector (λ_1, λ_2). Again, because of the vector field, the unstable manifold of (6) at Q goes away from Q and tends to $(+\infty, 0)$ as $t \to +\infty$. Figure 6 illustrates the phase portrait.

We have proved the following proposition for Case (iii):

Proposition 1.3. *If* $k_1 = 1$, $0 < m < 4$ *and* $\frac{g}{(k_2 - N)} > \frac{s}{m}$, *the system (6) has only one equilibrium point which is a hyperbolic saddle point. The right unstable manifold of (6) tends to* $(+\infty, 0)$ *as* $t \to +\infty$.

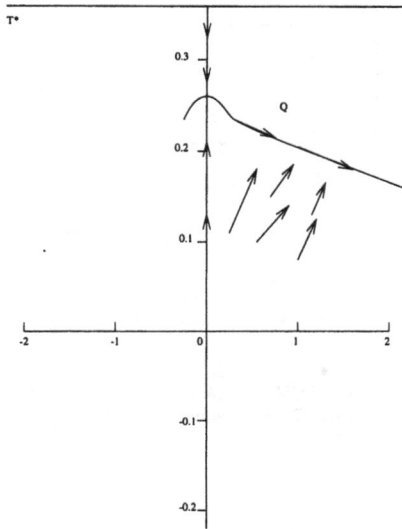

Fig. 6. Case 1.a.iii: The unstable manifold at Q.

Case 1.b: $m + 1 - 2\sqrt{m} < k_1 < 1$ with $0 < m < 4$.

Here the qualitative behavior of T_{vert} is illustrated in Figure 7 which also shows the different locations of T^*. There are rich dynamics in this Case.

Let $\max T_{vert}(V)$ be the maximum value of T_{vert}. There are five Sub-Cases to be considered:

i) $0 < T^* < s/m$, the system (6) has two equilibria.

ii) $T^* = s/m$, here the system (6) has two equilibria.

iii) $s/m < T^* < \max T_{vert}(V) = T_{vert}(\widetilde{V}_1)$, the system (6) has three equilibria.

iv) $T^* = \max T_{vert}(V) = T_{vert}(\widetilde{V}_1)$, here the system (6) has two equilibria.

v) $T^* > \max T_{vert}(V) = T_{vert}(\widetilde{V}_1)$, the system (6) has one equilibrium point.

Before analyzing each possibility separately, let us write the Jacobian matrix of (6) for $k_1 \neq 1$. This is

$$J[f_1, f_2]_{(V,T)} = \begin{bmatrix} (N - k_2)T + g & (N - k_2)V \\ \dfrac{T - k_1 T(1 + V)^2}{(1 + V)^2} & -\dfrac{D(V)}{(1 + V)} \end{bmatrix}, \tag{18}$$

where $D(V) = k_1 V^2 + rV + m$.

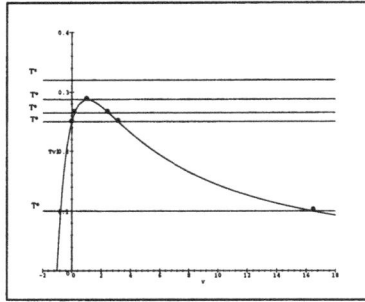

Fig. 7. Case **1.b**: This figure shows the relevant portion of the graph of T_v for $m + 1 - 2\sqrt{m} < k_1 < 1$ with $0 < m < 4$ and the different possibilities for T^*.

Case 1.b.i.

The system (6) has two equilibria: $Q = (0, s/m)$ and R. (Actually there are three, see Figure 8, but one of them is not in Ω, the region of biological interest.)

To obtain the local phase portrait around each equilibrium we evaluate (18) at Q, from which we determine

$$tr(J[f_1, f_2]_{(0,s/m)}) = \left[(N - k_2)\frac{s}{m} + g - m\right] < 0,$$

$$det(J[f_1, f_2]_{(0,s/m)}) = -m\left[(N - k_2)\frac{s}{m} + g\right] > 0.$$

Moreover, given that the eigenvalues, λ_1 and λ_2, of (18) are

$$\lambda_1 = \left[(N - k_2)\frac{s}{m} + g\right] < 0 \quad \text{and} \quad \lambda_2 = -m < 0,$$

then $Q = (0, s/m)$ is a locally asymptotically stable node. Now we obtain the abscissa of the points of intersection of the horizontal line $T^* = \frac{g}{(k_2 - N)}$ with the graph of the function T_{vert}. These are the roots of the quadratic polynomial

$$T^* k_1 V^2 + (rT^* - s)V + (T^*m - s) = 0,$$

i.e.,

$$V_1^*, V_2^* = \frac{-(rT^* - s) \pm \sqrt{(rT^* - s)^2 - 4T^* k_1(T^*m - s)}}{2T^* k_1}. \tag{19}$$

Following from the condition $T^* < s/m$, we have $V_1^* > 0$ and $V_2^* < 0$ as shown in Figure 8.

Thus, we evaluate (18) at $R = (V_1^*, T^*)$ from which

$$tr(J[f_1, f_2]_{(V_1^* T^*)}) = -\frac{D(V_1^*)}{(1 + V_1^*)} < 0 \text{ and}$$

$$det(J[f_1, f_2]_{(V_1^*, T^*)}) = \frac{V_1^* g}{(1 + V_1^*)^2}[1 - k_1(1 + V_1^*)^2].$$

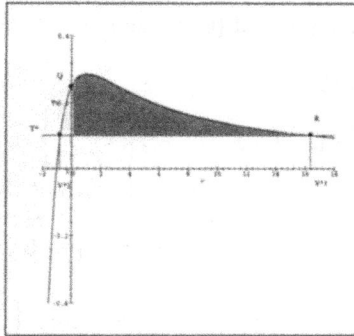

Fig. 8. Case **1.b.i:** Here the system (6) has three equilibrium points, but just two of them (Q and R) are biologically reasonable.

Because of the large number of parameters involved, it is not easy to determine the sign of $det\ J[f_1, f_2]_{(V_1^*, T^*)}$. In order to save work (particularly for the global analysis), the ideal approach then is the use the parameter values known in Table 1, to determine the sign of $det\ J[f_1, f_2]_{(V_1^*, T^*)}$. This would allow us to discriminate two behavior families: Saddle and non-saddle points.

Case 1.b.ii.

Here the system (6) has two equilibria: Q and R. Because of the condition $T^* = s/m$, V_1^* and V_2^* in (19) reduce to

$$V_1^* = 0 \quad \text{and} \quad V_2^* = -\frac{(rT^* - s)}{T^* k_1} = \left(\frac{1 - k_1}{k_1}\right) > 0.$$

Thus $Q = (0, s/m)$ and $R = (V_2^*, T^*)$. The graph of T_{vert} is sketched in Figure 9.

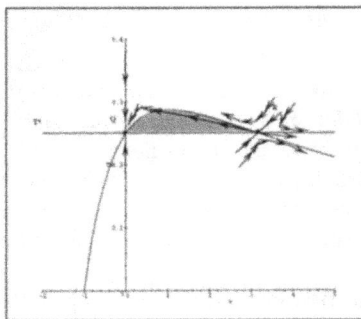

Fig. 9. Case **1.b.ii:** Here, $T^* = M$.

The positivity of V_2^* comes from the condition $m + 1 - 2\sqrt{m} < k_1 < 1$. In order to get the local dynamics of (6) around each equilibria we evaluate the Jacobian at each.

At Q, (18) reduces to

$$J[f_1, f_2]_{(0, s/m)} = \begin{bmatrix} 0 & 0 \\ 0 & -m \end{bmatrix}. \tag{21}$$

Given that $tr\ J[f_1, f_2]_{(0, s/m)} = -m \neq 0$ and $det\ J[f_1, f_2]_{(0, s/m)} = 0$, Q is a non-hyperbolic point of co-dimension one. Moreover it is a saddle-node bifurcation point of (6). The eigenvalues are $\lambda_1 = 0$ and $\lambda_2 = -m$ and the corresponding eigenvectors are

$$\vec{v}_1 = \begin{bmatrix} 1 \\ \frac{s}{m^2}(1 - k_1) \end{bmatrix} \quad \text{and} \quad \vec{v}_2 = \begin{bmatrix} 0 \\ 1 \end{bmatrix}.$$

Again, the Centre Manifold Theorem ensures us the existence of a positive invariant manifold of (6) containing the point Q and whose tangent vector at Q is $\vec{v}_1$. All the local dynamics of (6) around Q are given in terms of the dynamics around the center manifold.

Evaluating (18) at R, we obtain $det\ J[f_1, f_2]_{(V_2^*, T^*)} = \frac{s}{m}(k_1 - 1)^2(N - k_2) < 0$. Therefore R is a saddle point.

The eigenvalues are

$$\lambda_1, \lambda_2 = \frac{- \left[m + \left(\frac{1-k_1}{k_1} \right) m \right] \pm \sqrt{\left[m + \left(\frac{1-k_1}{k_1} \right) m \right]^2 - \frac{4s}{m}(k_1 - 1)^2(N - k_2)}}{2}$$

with $\lambda_1 > 0$ and $\lambda_2 < 0$. The associated eigenvectors are

$$\vec{v}_1 = (1 + p_1^2)^{-1/2} \begin{bmatrix} 1 \\ p_1 \end{bmatrix} \quad \text{and} \quad \vec{v}_2 = (1 + p_2^2)^{-1/2} \begin{bmatrix} 1 \\ p_2 \end{bmatrix},$$

where

$$p_1 = \frac{\lambda_1}{(N - k_2)\left(\frac{1-k_1}{k_1}\right)} < 0 \quad \text{and} \quad p_2 = \frac{\lambda_2}{(N - k_2)\left(\frac{1-k_1}{k_1}\right)} > 0.$$

Let us denote by $M(Q)$ the slope of the path of the center manifold of (6) at Q i.e.,

$$M(Q) = \frac{s}{m^2}(1 - k_1) > 0.$$

Evaluating $T'_{vert}(V)$ at $V = 0$, we deduce $M(Q) = T'_{vert}(0)$.

We address the global analysis of the phase portrait of (6). The left unstable manifold, $W^u(R)$, of (6) at R leaves this point and enters the shaded region of Figure 9. Once there, the vector field pushes it up towards the graph of the nullcline T_{vert}, which it must cross with horizontal tangent vector. As time increases, $W^u(R)$ leaves the graph of T_{vert}, but again, the vector field pushes it down toward the center manifold of (6) ending at Q, as time goes to infinity.

The right unstable manifold of R runs away from R. Because of the vector field this tends to $(+\infty, 0)$ as t increases. This global behavior is shown in Figure 9. The analysis of this Case can be summarized in the following proposition.

Proposition 1.5. *If $m + 1 - 2\sqrt{m} < k_1 < 1$, $0 < m < 4$ and $T^* = \frac{g}{k_2 - N} = s/m$, then the system (6) has: One non-hyperbolic point (Q) of co-dimension one and one hyperbolic saddle point (R). Moreover, the left unstable manifold of (6) at R reaches Q through the center manifold of (6) as $t \to +\infty$ and the right unstable manifold of (6) at R tends to $(+\infty, 0)$ as $t \to +\infty$.*

Case 1.b.iii.

Here we have

$$\frac{s}{m} < T^* < \frac{s}{2\sqrt{k_1} - k_1 + m - 1} \equiv \max T_{vert}(V)$$

with $m + 1 - 2\sqrt{m} < k_1 < 1$ and $0 < m < 4$. In this Case, system (6) has three equilibria: $Q = (0, s/m)$, $R = (V_1^*, T^*)$ and $S = (V_2^*, T^*)$, where V_1^* and V_2^* are given by

$$V_1^*, V_2^* = \frac{-(rT^* - s) \pm \sqrt{(rT^* - s)^2 - 4T^* k_1 (T^* m - s)}}{2T^* k_1}. \tag{21}$$

Because of the previous conditions, $V_1^* > 0$ and $V_2^* > 0$ (See Figure 10).

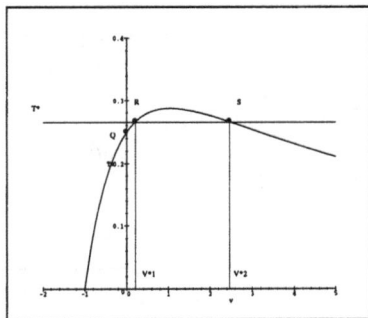

Fig. 10. Case 1.b.iii: Here, $s/m < T^* < \max T_v(V)$.

The local phase portrait analysis follows as with previous arguments, and Q is a saddle node.

Continuing with our phase portrait analysis in a neighborhood of S, evaluating (18) at S yields the Jacobian from which it follows the

$$\text{tr } J[f_1, f_2]_{(V_2^*, T^*)} = -\frac{D(V_2^*)}{(1 + V_2^*)} < 0 \text{ and}$$

$$\det J[f_1, f_2]_{(V_2^*, T^*)} = \frac{V_2^* g}{(1 + V_2^*)^2} [1 - k_1 (1 + V_2^*)^2].$$

Here the *det* has three cases for sign: $i)k_1(1 + V_2^*)^2 - 1 > 0$, $ii)k_1(1 + V_2^*)^2 - 1 = 0$ and $iii)k_1(1 + V_2^*)^2 - 1 < 0$.

Using parameter values from Table 1, including conditions above, we find numerically that Case (iii) is the feasible Case, and hence S is a saddle node.

Case 1.b.iv.

Here we have

$$T^* = \frac{g}{k_2 - N} = T(\tilde{V}_1) = \frac{s}{2\sqrt{k_1} + m - k_1 - 1}$$

with $m + 1 - 2\sqrt{m} < k_1 < 1$ and $0 < m < 4$. Now the equilibria R and S of the previous possibility collapse into one equilibrium: E. It is easy to verify that for T^* as above, $V_1^* = V_2^* = \tilde{V} = \frac{1}{\sqrt{k_1}} - 1$. Thus, the pair of equilibria of (6) are given as follows $Q = (0, s/m)$ and $E = (\frac{1}{\sqrt{k_1}} - 1, T^*)$, as they are shown in the Figure 11(a).

Again, the local phase portrait analysis of (6) starts by evaluating the Jacobian matrix (18) at Q. This gives us

$$\mathrm{tr}\, J[f_1, f_2]_{(0,s/m)} = (N - k_2)\frac{s}{m} + g - m \text{ and} \tag{22}$$

$$\det J[f_1, f_2]_{(0,s/m)} = -m\left[(N - k_2)\frac{s}{m} + g\right]. \tag{23}$$

The condition $\frac{s}{m} < T^* = \frac{g}{k_2-N}$ implies that $[(N - k_2)\frac{s}{m} + g] > 0$. Thus $\det J[f_1, f_2]_{(0,s/m)} < 0$. Therefore Q is a saddle point. The eigenvectors of (23) are

$$\vec{v}_1 = \begin{bmatrix} \frac{[(N-k_2)\frac{s}{m}+g+m]}{(1-k_1)s/m} \\ 1 \end{bmatrix} \quad \text{and} \quad \vec{v}_2 = \begin{bmatrix} 0 \\ 1 \end{bmatrix}.$$

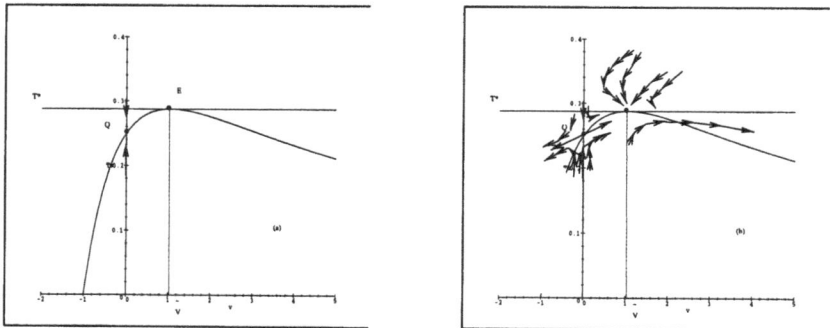

Fig. 11. Case 1.b.iv: The situation for $T^* = \max T_{vert}(V)$. (a) The system (6) has two equilibria. (b) The local phase portrait of (6) around Q and E.

The stable manifold of (6) at Q has as tangent vector $\vec{v}_2$, while the unstable manifold locally has as tangent vector $\vec{v}_1$. See Figure 11(a).

Evaluating (18) at E we get the following

$$tr \; J[f_1, f_2]_{(\frac{1}{\sqrt{k_1}} - 1, T^*)} = [k_1 + 1 - m - 2\sqrt{k_1}] < 0 \text{ and}$$

$$det \; J[f_1, f_2]_{(\frac{1}{\sqrt{k_1}} - 1, T^*)} = 0.$$

Since the eigenvalues are $\lambda_1 = 0$ and $\lambda_2 = (k_1 + 1 - m - 2\sqrt{k_1})$, then the equilibrium E is a non-hyperbolic point of co-dimension one. The associated eigenvectors are

$$\vec{v}_1 = \begin{bmatrix} 1 \\ 0 \end{bmatrix} \quad \text{and} \quad \vec{v}_2 = \begin{bmatrix} \frac{(N-k_2)(\frac{1}{\sqrt{k_1}} - 1)}{k_1 + 1 - m - 2\sqrt{k_1}} \\ 1 \end{bmatrix}.$$

More precise information on the local dynamics of the system (6) around the equilibrium can be obtained by using the Centre Manifold Theorem. For our purposes it is enough to say that E is a saddle-node bifurcation point. The local behavior of the trajectories of (6) can be seen in Figure 11(b).

In order to determine the global phase portrait of (6) in the region Ω, let us denote by $W^u(Q)$ the right unstable manifold of (6) at Q. Let $M^u(Q)$ be the slope of the path of $W^u(Q)$ at Q. To compare $M^u(Q)$ with $T'_{vert}(0)$, we examine the ratio: $\frac{M^u(Q)}{T'_{vert}(0)} = \frac{m}{(N-k_2)s/m+g+m}$. By using the condition $\frac{s}{m} < T^* = \frac{g}{k_2 - N}$, hence it follows $M^u(Q) < T'_{vert}(0)$. The geometric interpretation of this inequality implies that the unstable manifold $W^u(Q)$ leaves the equilibrium Q below the graph of T_{vert} as it is shown in Figure 12(a).

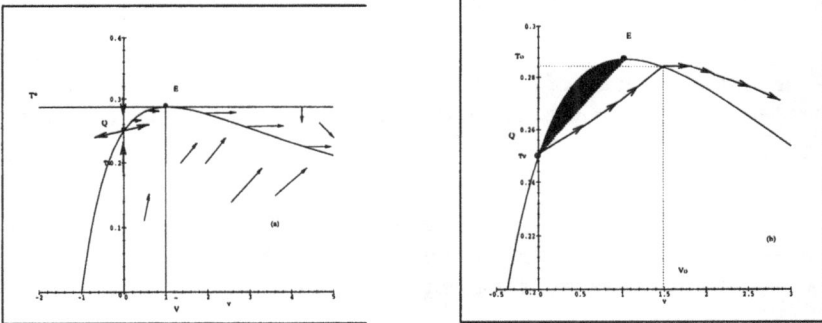

Fig. 12. Case 1.b.iv: Behavior of the trajectories of $T^* = \max T_v$. (a) $W^u(Q)$ leaves Q in this way. (b) The two possible behaviors of $W^u(Q)$.

Once $W^u(Q)$ leaves Q, because of the vector field (6), $W^u(Q)$ initially will have two types of behavior as time t goes to infinity (Figure 12b):

i) $W^u(Q)$ ends at E. The unique way in which $W^u(Q)$ can reach E is through that part of the center manifold of (6) allocated in the nodal sector of E.

ii) $W^u(Q)$ tends to $(+\infty, 0)$. Once $W^u(Q)$ reaches the graph of T_{vert} (which must be at some point (V_0, T_0) with $V_0 > \tilde{V}$ and $T_0 < T^*$) the vector field pushes it down in such a way that as the time increases $W^u(Q) \to (+\infty, 0)$.

In what follows, we will determine which set of parameters such that, in addition to satisfy the conditions of this Sub-Case, the above Cases could occur. For this, we consider the line which connects the points Q and E, i.e., that line whose equation is

$$T(V) = \left(\frac{T^* - s/m}{\tilde{V}}\right) V + s/m, \qquad (24)$$

with $0 \leq V \leq \tilde{V}$. Let $\vec{n}_{out}$ be the normal vector of the above line pointing outward from the shaded region of Figure 12(b). Thus

$$\vec{n}_{out} = (T^* - s/m, -\tilde{V}).$$

Now, we restrict the vector field (6) to the line (24). The resulting system is

$$\dot{V} = (NV - k_2 V)\left[\left(\frac{T^* - s/m}{\tilde{V}}\right) V + s/m\right] + gV \ ,$$

$$\dot{T} = s - m\left[\left(\frac{T^* - s/m}{\tilde{V}}\right) V + s/m\right] + \frac{V}{1+V}\left[\left(\frac{T^* - s/m}{\tilde{V}}\right) V + s/m\right]$$

$$- k_1\left[\left(\frac{T^* - s/m}{\tilde{V}}\right) V + s/m\right].$$

$$(25)$$

Given that on the graph of T_{vert} for $0 < V < \tilde{V}$ the vector field points towards the shaded region of Figure 12(b), then for the set of parameters for which

$$[(\dot{V}, \dot{T}) \cdot \vec{n}_{out}] \leq 0 \qquad \forall \ V \in [0, \tilde{V}], \qquad (26)$$

where $(\dot{V}, \dot{T})$ is given in (25), we have proved that such a region is a positive invariant set of (6). Thus the unstable manifold $W^u(Q)$ ends at E as time t goes to infinity. Conversely, if for certain sets of parameters, we have

$$[(\dot{V}, \dot{T}) \cdot \vec{n}_{out}] > 0 \qquad \forall \ V \in (0, \tilde{V}), \qquad (27)$$

for $(\dot{V}, \dot{T})$ as in the system (25), then the shaded region of Figure 12(b) is not a positively invariant set of (6), resulting in $W^u(Q)$ crossing the graph of T_{vert} as shown in Case 1.b.ii. Now note that in that region of the first quadrant contained below the graphs of $T \equiv T^*$ and T_{vert}, both $\dot{V}$ and $\dot{T}$ are positive. In other words,

$$(\dot{V}, \dot{T}) \cdot \vec{n}_{out} = (T^* - s/m)\dot{V} - \tilde{V}\dot{T}.$$

The inequality (26) implies

$$[(T^* - s/m)\dot{V}] \leq \tilde{V}\dot{T}; \qquad (28)$$

however, (27) yields:

$$[(T^* - s/m)\dot{V}] > \tilde{V}\dot{T}. \qquad (29)$$

To verify which situation is biologically feasible, we again turn to a numerical analysis using conditions of Case 1.b.iv and values from Table 1. We find that (29) holds true, and hence the shaded region is not a positively invariant of (6).

Case 1.b.v.

Here, $T^* > \max T_{vert}(V)$. In this Case, the system (6) has only one equilibrium: Q, which, according with previous analysis, is a hyperbolic saddle point. The right unstable manifold $W^u(Q)$ of (6) at Q crosses the graph of T_{vert} at the point (V_0, T_0) with $V_0 > \tilde{V}$ and $T_0 < \max T_{vert}$. The vector field then pushes it down towards $(+\infty, 0)$ as time t goes to infinity (Figure 13).

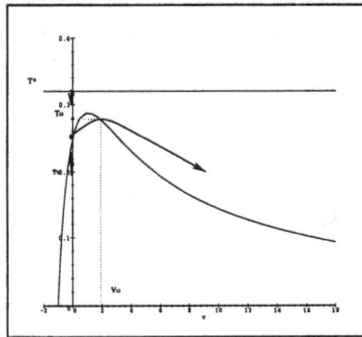

Fig. 13. Case **1.b.v:** This is the global phase portrait of (6) for $T^* > \max T_v(V)$.

Case 1.c.

Here $\tilde{V}_1$ and $\tilde{V}_2$ both are negative. The graph of T_{vert} is illustrated in Figure 14.

Again, depending on the value of T^* we have the following possibilities:

   i) $0 < T^* < s/m$, the system (6) has two equilibria: R and Q. Note that there is a third equilibrium, but this not in the region of biological interest, hence, we leave it.

  ii) $T^* = s/m$, the system (6) has just one equilibrium: Q.

 iii) $T^* > s/m$, again here the system (6) has only one equilibrium.

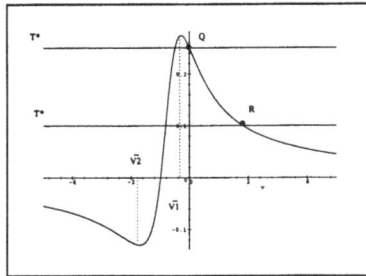

Fig. 14. Case **1.c:** This figure shows the graph of T_v for $1 < k_1 < m + 1 + 2\sqrt{m}$ with $0 < m < 4$ and the different possibilities for T^*.

Case 1.c.i.

Here, $1 < k_1 < m + 2\sqrt{m} + 1, 0 < m < 4$. The system (6) has two equilibria: $Q = (0, s/m)$ and $R = (V_1^*, T^*)$, where V_1^* is given in (21). For the local behavior of the trajectories of (6) we evaluate (18) at Q. By using some straightforward calculations one easily concludes that Q is a locally asymptotically stable node. The local analysis around R is not immediate. Numerically, we find it is a saddle node.

Case 1.c.ii.

System (6) has just one equilibrium $Q = (s/m, 0)$. The Jacobian matrix (18) at Q yields eigenvalues $\lambda_1 = 0$ and $\lambda_2 = -m$, with $det\ J[f_1, f_2]_{(s/m,0)} = 0$ and $tr\ J[f_1, f_2]_{(s/m,0)} = -m \neq 0$. The equilibrium Q is thus a saddle-node bifurcation point of (6). The corresponding eigenvectors are

$$\vec{v}_1 = \begin{bmatrix} \frac{1}{s(1-k_1)} \\ 1 \end{bmatrix} \quad \text{and} \quad \vec{v}_2 = \begin{bmatrix} 0 \\ 1 \end{bmatrix}.$$

Given the conditions on k_1 in this Sub-Case, we have $(1 - k_1) < 0$. Thus the trajectory of (6) which leaves Q through the center manifold of (6) tends to $(+\infty, 0)$ as time goes to infinity (Figure 15).

Case 1.c.iii: Q is a hyperbolic saddle point.

The right unstable manifold $W^u(Q)$ leaves Q and the vector field pushes it down towards $(+\infty, 0)$ where it ends as time t tends to $+\infty$.

This completes the main Case 1.

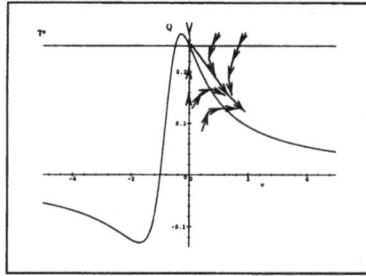

Fig. 15. Case **1.c.ii:** Global phase portrait of (6). See the text for details.

3.2. Phase Portrait Analysis in Case 2:

$$d = [(m - k_1)^2 - 2(m + k_1) + 1] = 0.$$

Here the denominator $D(V) = k_1 V^2 + (k_1 + m - 1)V + m$ of the vertical nullcline (9) has just one real root V^*. In the mk_1-plane this occurs on the graph of the functions

$$k_1(m) = m + 1 - 2\sqrt{m} \quad \text{and} \quad k_2(m) = m + 1 + 2\sqrt{m} ,$$

as it is shown in Figure 1.

Again, the dynamics of (6) depend on both the profile of the vertical nullcline and the relative position of the horizontal null-cline (7) and (8). The first depends on which of the branches of the parabola in Figure 1 is under consideration. We analyze each Case separately.

Case 2.a: $k_1 = m + 1 - 2\sqrt{m}.$

Because of the condition $d = 0$, this implies that the root of D is

$$V^*(m) = \frac{\sqrt{m} - m}{m + 1 - 2\sqrt{m}}, \tag{30}$$

from which one can verify the following properties of V^*: i) $V^*(0) = 0$, ii) $V^* > 0 \Leftrightarrow m \in (0, 1)$, iii) $V^* < 0 \Leftrightarrow m > 1$, iv) $V^* \to +\infty$ as $m \to 1^-$ and v) $V^* \to -\infty$ as $m \to 1^+$. The graph of V^* as a function of m, is shown in Figure 16.

Since D is a second order polynomial and V^* is its unique root, it can be written as $D(V) = A(V - V^*)^2$, where $A = \frac{m}{V^{*2}}$. Then the vertical nullcline (7) takes the form

$$T_{vert}(V) = \frac{V^{*2}}{m} \frac{(s + sV)}{(V - V^*)^2}. \tag{31}$$

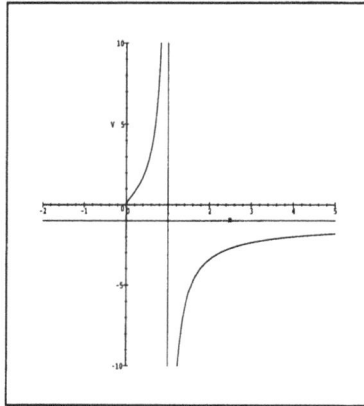

Fig. 16. Case **2.a:** Behavior of V^* as a function of m.

The graph of this function is sketched in Figure 17 for different parameter ranges. If we compare the qualitative behavior of the graphs in Figures 17(a)-(c) on the region Ω, one can see that the above profiles of T_{vert} coincide with those given in Figures 14, 2 and 7, respectively. Thus, for dynamical purposes of the system (6), the behavior is essentially the same.

Figure 17(d) is the new Case. Thus, we will focus on analyzing the phase portrait of (6) for each one of the possibilities illustrated in Figure 18. To do this, we first compute the abscissas of the intersections of T^* with the graph of T_{vert}. Thus, we seek the values of V such that

$$T_{vert}(V) = T^* \Leftrightarrow \frac{V^{*2}}{m} \frac{(s + sV)}{(V - V^*)^2} = T^* = \frac{g}{(k_2 - N)}.$$

These are roots of the quadratic polynomial

$$mT^*V^2 - (2V^*mT^* + sV^{*2})V + mV^{*2}T^* - V^{*2}s = 0, \qquad (32)$$

or

$$V_1^*, V_2^* = \frac{(2V^*mT^* + sV^{*2}) \pm V^*\sqrt{4V^*smT^* + s^2V^{*2} + 4mT^*s}}{2mT^*}, \qquad (33)$$

where V^* is given by the equality (30), with $m \in (0, 1)$. Now we begin the phase portrait analysis for each of the three Cases depicted in Figure 18.

Case 2.a.i: $0 < T^* < s/m$.

In the region of biological interest Ω, the system (6) has two equilibria: $Q = (0, s/m)$ and $R = (V_1^*, T^*)$, where V_1^* is the positive root of (32) (Figure 18). A similar analysis can be used in this case to verify Figure 19 is indeed the behavior of the phase portrait. The following proposition summarizes that analysis.

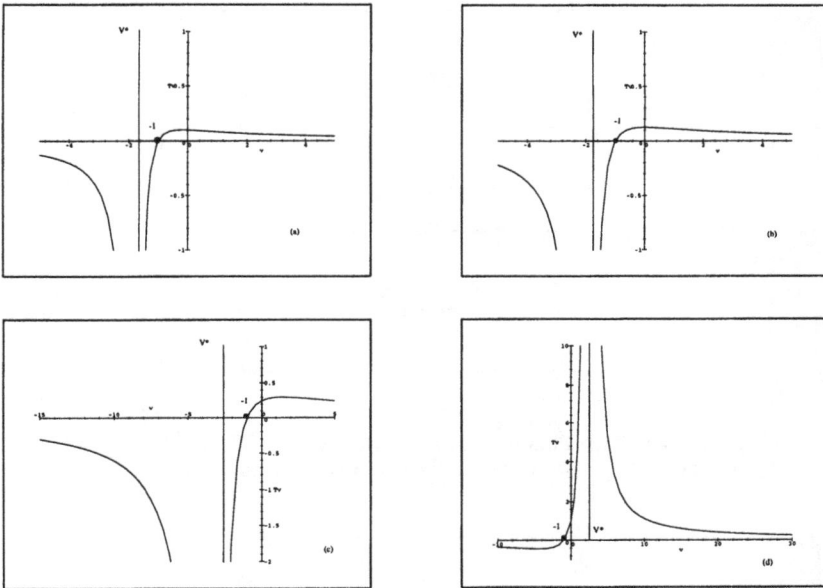

Fig. 17. Case **2.a:** Behavior of T_{vert} for different values of m (i.e of $k_1 = m + 1 - 2\sqrt{m}$) (a) for $m > 4$ (i.e. for $k_1 > 1$). (b) $m = 4$ and $k_1 = 1$. (c) For $m \in (1, 4)$ (i.e. $0 < k_1 < 1$). (d) For $m \in (0, 1)$.

Proposition 2.1. *If $k_1 = m + 1 - 2\sqrt{m}$ with $m \in (0, 1)$, then for each T^* such that $T^* = g/(k_2 - N) < s/m$, the system (6) has two equilibria: One locally asymptotically stable node (Q) and a saddle point (R). Moreover, the left unstable manifold $W^u(R)$ of (6) at R ends at Q as $t \to +\infty$, i.e., $W^u(R)$ is a saddle (R)-node (Q) heteroclinic trajectory of (6).*

Case 2.a.ii: $T^* = s/m$.

From the equality (33), we have $V_1^* = V^*(2 + V^*)$ and $V_2^* = 0$. Here, the system (6) has two equilibria: $Q = (0, s/m)$ and $R = (V^*(2 + V^*), s/m)$. As in the Case 2.a.1, we can prove the behavior shown in Figure 20. The result is summarized in the following proposition.

Proposition 2.2. *If $k_1 = m + 1 - 2\sqrt{m}$ with $m \in (0, 1)$, then for each $T^* = g/(k_2 - N) = s/m$, the system (6) has two equilibria: A saddle-node bifurcation point (Q) and a hyperbolic saddle point. Moreover, the left unstable manifold of Q connects the equilibria R and Q.*

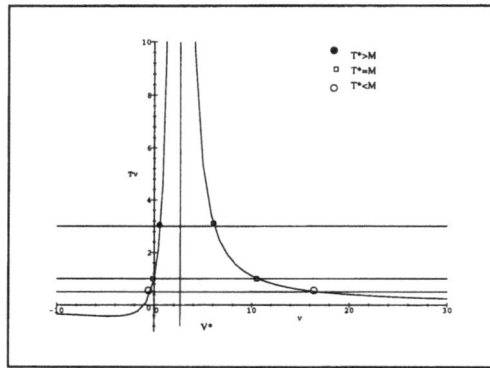

Fig. 18. Case **2.a:** This figure shows the graph of T_v for $k_1 = m + 1 - 2\sqrt{m}$ with $m \in (0, 1)$ and the different possibilities for T^*.

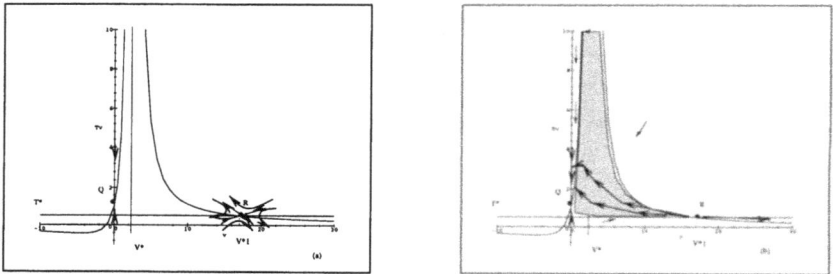

Fig. 19. Case **2.a.i:** Dynamics of (6) for $k_1 = m + 1 - 2\sqrt{m}$ with $0 < T^* < M$. (a) Local phase portrait. (b) Global phase portrait.

Case 2.a.iii.

Figure 18 shows the three equilibrium points of system (6) in Ω: $Q = (0, s/m)$, $R = (V_1^*, T^*)$ and $S = (V_2^*, T^*)$, where V_1^* and V_2^* are given in (33) with V_1^* and V_2^* both positive and $V_1^* > V_2^*$.

The Jacobian matrix at Q is written as follows

$$J[f_1, f_2]_{(0, s/m)} = \begin{bmatrix} (N - k_2)\frac{s}{m} + g & 0 \\ -s + \frac{2s}{\sqrt{m}} & -m \end{bmatrix}, \quad \text{such that}$$

$$tr \ J[f_1, f_2]_{(s/m, 0)} = \left[(N - k_2)\frac{s}{m} + g - m \right] \text{ and}$$

$$det \ J[f_1, f_2]_{(s/m, 0)} = -m \left[(N - k_2)\frac{s}{m} + g \right].$$

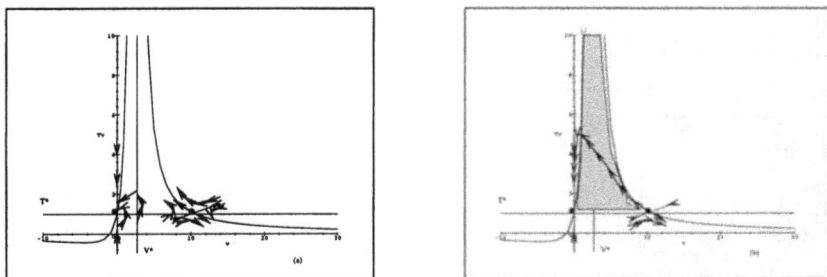

Fig. 20. Case **2.a.ii:** Dynamics of the system (6) for (a) Local behavior of the trajectories (b) Global dynamics in the region of biological interest.

The inequality $\frac{g}{(k_2-N)} > \frac{s}{m}$ implies $det\ J[f_1, f_2]_{(s/m,0)} < 0$, therefore Q is a hyperbolic saddle point. The eigenvalues are $\lambda_1 = \left[(N - k_2)\frac{s}{m} + g\right] > 0$ and $\lambda_2 = -m < 0$. The corresponding eigenvectors are

$$\vec{v}_1 = \begin{bmatrix} \frac{(N-k_2)\frac{s}{m}+g+m}{-s+\frac{2s}{\sqrt{m}}} \\ 1 \end{bmatrix} \quad \text{and} \quad \vec{v}_2 = \begin{bmatrix} 0 \\ 1 \end{bmatrix}.$$

The analysis of R and S are similar to Case 1.b.ii. Thus R is a saddle and S is a locally asymptotically stable node. This is also verified numerically.

Case 2.b: $k_1 = m + 1 + 2\sqrt{m}.$

Here the real root of D can be written as follows

$$V^* = -\frac{\sqrt{m} + m}{m + 1 + 2\sqrt{m}} < 0, \qquad \forall\ m > 0,$$

and $V^* = 0$ for $m = 0$. From the above expression for V^* is straightforward to conclude that $-1 < V^* \leq 0$. Thus, the graph of the vertical nullcline is as in Figure 21.

If we observe Figure 21(a) we note that the tail of the graph of T_{vert} in the region Ω has the same features as that part of the graph of T_{vert} in the same region in Figure 14. For this reason the results given in Case 1.c.i and ii hold here.

In Figure 21(b) we have an extreme situation whose main feature is that the equilibrium of (6) which comes from the intersection of the graph of T_{vert} with the vertical axis runs away to $(0, +\infty)$. Thus, for finite values of the variables V and T, whatever the value of T^* is, the system (6) has just one equilibrium.

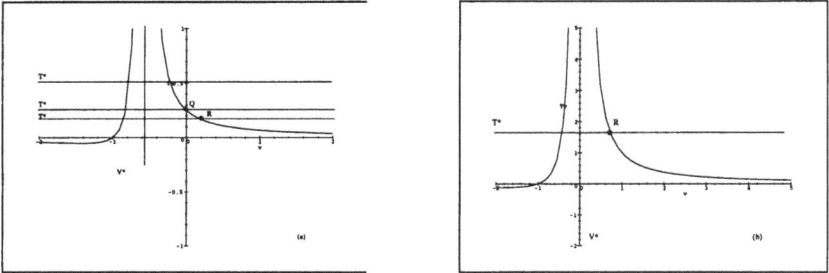

Fig. 21. Case **2.b:** Qualitative behavior of T_v for $k_1 = m + 1 + 2\sqrt{m}$ and for different values of m. (a) $m > 0$. (b) $m = 0$.

3.3 Phase Portrait Analysis in Case 3:

$$d = [(m - k_1)^2 - 2(m + k_1) + 1] > 0.$$

Here the denominator $D(V) = k_1 V^2 + (k_1 + m - 1)V + m$ has two real roots, V_1 and V_2. Hence D can be written as $D(V) = A(V - V_1)(V - V_2)$, where $A = m/V_1 V_2$. The vertical nullcline takes the form

$$T_{vert}(V) = \frac{V_1 V_2 s(1 + V)}{(V - V_1)(V - V_2)}.$$

For $k_1 > 0$ and $m > 0$, neither V_1 or V_2 is zero. Depending on the sign of $(m + k_1 - 1)$ we have different Cases.

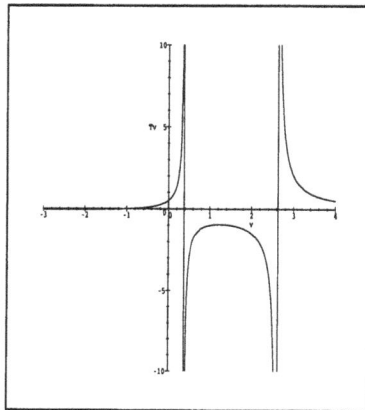

Fig. 22. Case **3.a:** The qualitative behavior of T_v.

Case 3.a.

If $(m + k_1 - 1) < 0$, both V_1 and V_2 are positive. The qualitative behavior of T_{vert} is shown in Figure 22.

Again, depending on $T^* = \frac{g}{k_2 - N}$, we have three Sub-Cases:

Sub-Case 3.a.i: $0 < T* < s/m$.

Here system (6) has two equilibria in the region Ω: $Q = (0, s/m)$, and $R = (V_1^*, T^*)$, where V_1^* is given by the equality (19). By using the linear approximation of (6) around Q one conclude that this equilibrium is an asymptotically stable node.

Although the local phase portrait analysis of (6) around R must be analyzed, our numerical simulations suggest that R is a hyperbolic saddle point. The local phase portrait is shown in Figure 23(a).

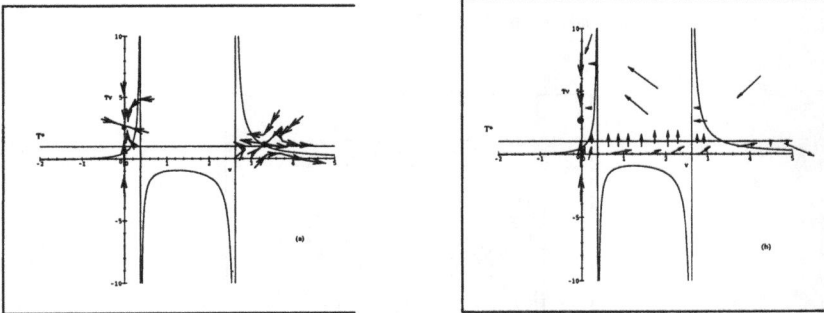

Fig. 23. Case **3.a.i:** The local phase portrait of (6) around Q and R (a). The direction field plot for (6) (b).

For the global analysis we note that the vector field defined by (6) is shown in Figure 23 (b). Hence, once the left unstable manifold, $W^u(R)$ leaves R the vector field pushes it up towards the equilibrium Q where it ends as $t \to +\infty$. The left stable manifold, $W^s(R)$, of R comes from some point on the vertical and reaches R for $t + \infty$. In Figure 24 we have done a numerical simulation to illustrate this.

Sub-Case 3.a.ii: $T^* = s/m$.

Here the system (6) has two equilibria in the region Ω: $Q = (0, s/m)$ and $R = (V_1^*, s/m)$.

The linear analysis of (6) around Q implies that this point is a nonhyperbolic equilibrium of saddle-node type and R is a saddle hyperbolic point. The global analysis follows the same reasoning as that given in the previous Sub-Case. Thus one conclude that $W^u(R)$ tends to Q as t increases. The way in which $W^u(R)$ approaches Q is as is illustrated in Figure 25.

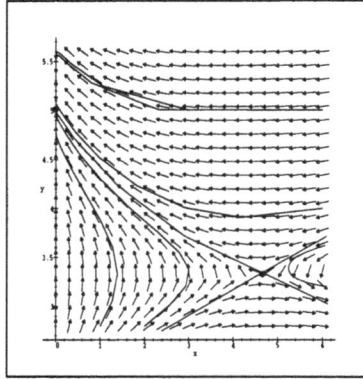

Fig. 24. Case **3.a.i:** Numerical simulations.

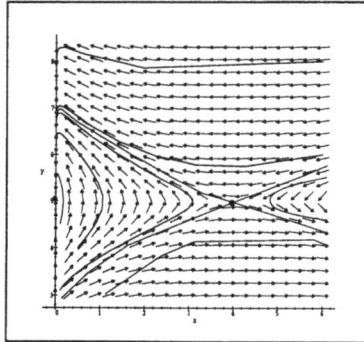

Fig. 25. Case **3.a.ii:** Numerical simulations.

Sub-Case 3a.iii.: $T^* > s/m.$

Here, in addition to $Q = (0, s/m)$ and $R = (V_1^*, T^*)$, a third equilibrium point $S = (V_2^*, T^*)$ of (6), emerges.

The local analysis of (6) around Q tells us that this equilibrium is a saddle node. The numerical phase portrait lends insights on the dynamics associated with the system in the region Ω. In particular note the damped oscillatory behavior of the trajectories of (6) around the equilibrium S, which leads to the left unstable manifold, $W^u(R)$, tending to S as t goes to infinity as is shown in Figure 26.

In Figure 27 we can see a closer picture of the phase portrait of (6) around S and the oscillations are illustrated.

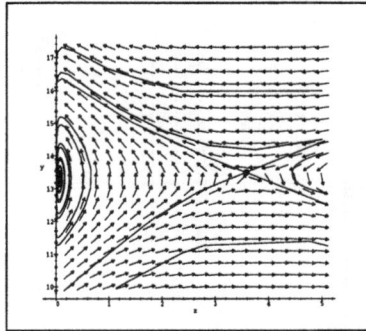

Fig. 26. Case **3.a.iii:** Numerical simulations.

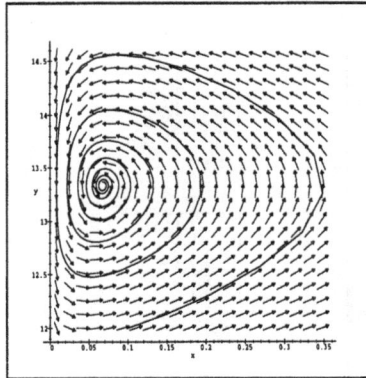

Fig. 27. Case **3.a.iii:** Numerical simulations close-up.

Case 3.b.

If $(m + k_1 - 1) = 0$, the roots V_1^* and V_2^* of the denominator D have opposite signs. The qualitative behavior of the vertical nullcline is as is shown in Figure 28.

Case 3.c.

If $(m + k_1 - 1) > 0$, both V_1^* and V_2^* are negative, hence the vertical asymptotes of the function D are shown in Figure 29.

Given that in the region of biological interest we have the same qualitative behavior as that in the Sub-Case 2.b which, in turn, corresponds to that in Figure 14; thus, we avoid the detailed analysis here of these two Cases.

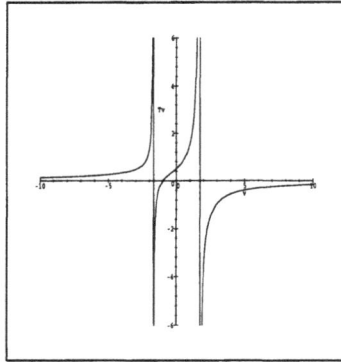

Fig. 28. Case **3.b:** The qualitative behavior of the vertical null-cline.

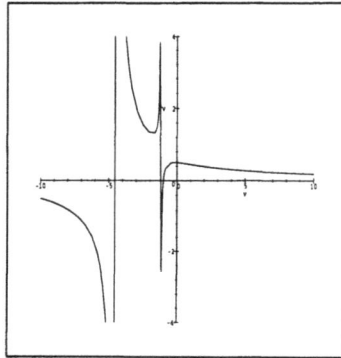

Fig. 29. Case **3.c:** The qualitative behavior of the vertical null-cline.

§4. Discussion

We have presented a very simple model of HIV and the immune system. The model accounts for many of the key dynamical behavior seen in the clinical investigations of HIV infection. In particular, the possibility of multiple steady states which are feasible by this model can allow for a wide range of clinical outcomes. In examining these steady states, we can directly tie the mathematical results to the observed biological phenomena, as follows.

The fixed point $Q = (0, \bar{T})$ represents an uninfected individual. We first want the model to make biological sense in the absence of HIV. This steady state accounts for this, i.e. and *uninfected steady state*. Secondly, the model should encompass the possible scenario that HIV can be cleared after introduction into a host. This may happen due to a low initial innoculum, in which case HIV may get cleared by a natural immune response. Or, whether by drug therapy or enhanced immune environment, the potential for clearance should be possible. There are a few documented cases of this which are mostly pediatric infections, since vertical transmission can be monitored. However, since most initial infection in adults are not traceable to the moment of HIV transferral, (except maybe via blood transfusions), these data are difficult to gather.

This steady state would be expected to be stable up to a certain point (this point could be based on a number of individual features) at which time it would loose stability to one of the infected steady states.

There are two main non-zero steady states (referred to as R and S). These are the *infected steady states*. What is of key interest here is that both of these steady states have the same ordinate i.e. in that the horizontal nullcline T^* (which is a straight line) crosses the vertical nullcline (which is parabolic shaped in that region) twice. Hence, for a given value of the T steady state, there are two possibilities for the viral load value. We distinguish $R = (V_1, \bar{T})$ and $S = (V_2, \bar{T})$ by the fact that $V_2 > V_1$.

In the analysis, every case points to R as an unstable node, and S as a stable node. The idea then is as follows. When only R is present with Q, Q is the stable steady state and R is unstable. This would imply that a small viral load can be cleared. When both infected steady states are present, namely R and S, then Q and R are unstable and S is the stable node. The question then arises, why would the infected steady state with the higher viral load be the stable one? There is now clinical evidence to suggest that the viral loads are very high during latency Ho et al. [2], Wei et al. [16]. There is a high turnover rate for both T cells and virus during the period which traditionally was viewed as a "latent" period. In actuality, there is much taking place during this time. Hence, a higher viral load would make sense in this long infected steady state. We also know there is much antigenic variation within HIV within a given individual. Many strains may comprise the total V population, and since they may be in competition, this may drive the viral population to higher levels. These ideas may explain how the heteroclinic orbit leaving R and going to S is achieved.

Finally, there is a third outcome for the model which was only indirectly addressed in the steady state analysis. It is the *Progression to AIDS state*. This is characterized by the collapse of the CD4$^+$ T cell populations, and the large numbers of virus. Although this is not a steady state, it is a behavior of this system. When all the steady states become unstable, then it is this "state" which is the "stable" one; and hence all the trajectories are drawn to $(V = \infty, T = 0)$.

It should be noted here that in the dynamics of HIV and other diseases, such as cancer, disease progression states are not states of stabilization, but states where there is a rapid physical collapse of the system. In these models, the infected steady state (latency period) is a state of stabilization; however the progression to AIDS is not, since the viral population will eventually, in all infection cases, grow without bound.

TABLE 1
Variables and Parameters

Dependent Variables

		Values
$T(t)$	= CD4$^+$ T cell population	1000 mm^{-3}
$V(t)$	= Infectious virus population (HIV)	1.0×10^{-3}mm^{-3}

Parameters and Constants

		Values
σ	= source of new CD4$^+$T cells	10 d^{-1}
μ	= death rate of CD4$^+$ T cell population	0.02 d^{-1}
$K_{V,T}$	= rate CD4$^+$ T cells becomes infected by free virus	2.4×10^{-5} mm^3 d^{-1}
$K_{T,V}$	= rate HIV is cleared	7.4×10^{-4} mm^3 d^{-1}
p	= maximal proliferation of the CD4$^+$ T cells	0.01 d^{-1}
$\hat{N}$	= production # of virus	10
C	= half saturation constant of the proliferation process	100 mm^{-3}
G_V	= growth rate of external viral source	2 d^{-1}
T_{max}	= Maximal population of T cells	1500 mm^{-3}
s	$= \frac{\sigma}{T_{max} \cdot p}$	
m	$= \frac{\mu}{p}$	
k_1	$= \frac{K_{V,T}K}{p}$	
N	$= \frac{\hat{N}K_{V,T}T_{max}}{p}$	
k_2	$= \frac{K_{T,V}T_{max}}{p}$	
g	$= \frac{G_V}{p}$	

TABLE 2.A
Phase Portrait Analysis in Case 1

CASE I:

Restriction: $d = [(m - k_1)^2 - 2(m + k_1) + 1] < 0$ where d is the discriminant of the roots of the denominator of T_{vert}.

The following are defined for this case: $T_{vert} = \dfrac{s + sv}{k_1 V^2 + rV + m}$, $\max T_{vert} = \dfrac{s}{2\sqrt{k_1} - k_1 + m - 1}$, for Case I.a,

$\max T_{vert} = \dfrac{s}{m} = M$, and $T_{hor} = T^* = \dfrac{g}{k_2 - N}$.

SUB-CASE	SUB-SUB CASE	Steady States (S.S.)	Stability of S.S.	Figure Refrences
Ia. $m + 1 - 2\sqrt{m} < k_1 < m + 1 + 2\sqrt{m}$ $k_1 = 1$ and $0 < m < 4$				Fig. 1
	Iai. $0 < T^* < M$	1. $Q = (0, \frac{s}{m})$ 2. $R = (V^*, \frac{g}{k_2 - N})$ 3. $P = $ negative root	1. locally asymptotically stable node 2. hyperbolic saddle point 3. biologically infeasible, therefore not important	Figs. 2-4
	Iaii. $T^* = M$	1. $Q = (0, \frac{s}{m})$	1. saddle-node bifurcation point	Fig. 5
	Iaiii. $T^* > M$	1. $Q = (0, \frac{s}{m})$	1. saddle-node bifurcation point	Fig. 6
Ib. $m + 1 - 2\sqrt{m} < k_1 < 1$ $0 < m < 4$				Fig. 7
	Ibi. $0 < T^* < M$	1. $Q = (0, \frac{s}{m})$ 2. $R = (V_1^*, T^*)$	1. locally asymptotically stable node 2. saddle node	Fig. 8
	Ibii. $T^* = M$	1. $Q = (0, \frac{s}{m})$ 2. $R = (V_1^*, T^*)$	1. non-hyperbolic point of co-dimension one 2. saddle node	Fig. 9
	Ibiii. $M < T^* < \max T_{vert}$	1. $Q = (0, \frac{s}{m})$ 2. $R = (V_1^*, T^*)$ 3. $S = (V_2^*, T^*)$	1. saddle point node 2. saddle point node 3. locally asymptotically stable node	Fig. 10
	Ibiv. $T^* = \max T_{vert}$	1. $Q = (0, \frac{s}{m})$ 2. $E = (\frac{1}{\sqrt{k_1}}, T^*)$	1. saddle point node 2. saddle-node bifurcation point	Figs. 11,12
	Ibv. $T^* > \max T_{vert}$	1. $Q = (0, \frac{s}{m})$	1. saddle point node	Fig. 13
Ic. $1 < k_1 < m + 2\sqrt{m} + 1$ $0 < m < 4$				Fig. 14
	Ici. $0 < T^* < M$	1. $Q = (0, \frac{s}{m})$ 2. $R = (V_1^*, T^*)$	1. locally asymptotically stable node 2. saddle node	
	Icii. $T^* = M$	1. $Q = (0, \frac{s}{m})$	1. saddle-node bifurcation	Fig. 15
	Iciii. $T^* > M$	1. $Q = (0, \frac{s}{m})$	1. hyperbolic saddle point	

TABLE 2.B
Phase Portrait Analysis in Case 2
Restrictions: $d = [(m - k_1)^2 - 2(m + k_1) + 1)] = 0$.

$$\max T_{vert} = \frac{V^{*2}(s + sv)}{m(V - V^*)^2}$$

$$T^* = \frac{g}{k_2 - N}$$

$$M = \frac{s}{m}$$

$$V^* = \frac{\sqrt{m} - m}{m + 1 - 2\sqrt{m}} \text{ for Case II.a}$$

$$V^* = -\frac{\sqrt{m} + m}{m + 1 + 2\sqrt{m}} < 0 \,\forall\, m > 0 \text{ for Case II.b}$$

SUB-CASE	SUB-SUB CASE	Steady States (S.S.)	Stability of S.S.	Figure References
IIa. $k_1 = m + 1 - 2\sqrt{m}$ $V^*(0) = 0$ $V^* > 0 \Leftrightarrow m \in (0,1)$ $V^* < 0 \Leftrightarrow m > 1$ $V^* \to +\infty$ as $m \to 1^-$ $V^* \to -\infty$ as $m \to 1^+$				Figs. 16,17 There are 4 graphs drawn and a-c show the same type of behavior as previously analyzed, hence, they will be ignored and we'll focus on the d
	IIai. $0 < T^* < M$	1. $Q = (0, \frac{s}{m})$ 2. $R = (V_1^*, T^*)$	1. locally asymptotically stable node 2. hyperbolic saddle pt.	Figs. 18,19
	IIaii. $T^* = M$	1. $Q = (0, \frac{s}{m})$ 2. $R = (V^*(2 + V^*), \frac{s}{m})$	1. saddle-node bifurcation point 2. hyperbolic saddle pt.	Figs. 18,20
	IIaiii. $T^* > M$	1. $Q = (0, \frac{s}{m})$ 2. $R = (V_1^*, T^*)$ 3. $S = (V_2^*, T^*)$	1. hyperbolic saddle pt. 2. saddle node 3. locally asymptotically stable node	Fig. 18
IIb. $k_1 = m + 1 + 2\sqrt{m}$				Fig. 21
	IIbi. $m > 0$ $0 < T^* < M$	1. $Q = (0, \frac{s}{m})$ 2. $R = (V_1^*, T^*)$	1. locally asymptotically stable node 2. saddle point	Fig. 21a
	IIbii. $m > 0$ $T^* = M$	1. $Q = (0, \frac{s}{m})$	1. saddle point	Fig. 21a
	IIbiii $m > 0$ $T^* > M$	1. $Q = (0, \frac{s}{m})$	saddle point	Fig. 21a
	IIbiv $m = 0$	1. $R = (V_1^*, T^*)$	1. saddle point	Fig. 21b

TABLE 2.C
Phase Portrait Analysis in Case 3
Restrictions: $d = [(m - k_1)^2 - 2(m + k_1) + 1] > 0$

SUB-CASE	SUB-SUB CASE	Steady States (S.S.)	Stability of S.S.	Figure References
III.a. $m + k_1 - 1 < 0$				Fig. 22
	III.a.i $0 < T^* < \frac{\ell}{m}$	1. $Q = (0, \frac{\ell}{m})$ 2. $R = (V_1^*, T^*)$	1. asymptotically stable node 2. hyperbolic saddle point	Figs. 23,24
	III.a.ii $T^* = \frac{\ell}{m}$	1. $Q = (0, \frac{\ell}{m})$ 2. $R = (V_1^*, \frac{\ell}{m})$	1. Non-hyperbolic saddle node 2. hyperbolic saddle point	Fig. 25
	III.a.iii $T^* > \frac{\ell}{m}$	1. $Q = (0, \frac{\ell}{m})$ 2. $R = (V_1^*, T^*)$ 3. $S = (V_2^*, T^*)$	1. saddle node 2. saddle node 3. locally asymptotically stable node	Figs. 26,27
III.b. $m + k_1 - 1 = 0$				Fig. 28
III.c. $m + k_1 - 1 > 0$				Fig. 29

Acknowledgments. Part of this work was supported under grant number DMS 9596073 from the National Science Foundation. Part of this paper was carried out during FSG's sabbatical at the Centre for Mathematical Biology at Oxford. He thanks them for the hospitality during his stay. Also he wishes to thank the CONACYT-Mexico and the Facultad de Ciencias-UNAM for their support during this research.

References

1. J. Carr, *Applications of Centre Manifold Theory*, Springer-Verlag, New York, Heidelberg, Berlin, 1981.

2. D. D. Ho et al., Rapid turnover of plasma virions and CD4 lymphocytes in HIV-1 infection, Nature **373** (1995), 123–126.

3. D. W. Jordan and P. Smith, *Nonlinear Ordinary Differential Equations*, Clarendon Press, Oxford, 1994.

4. D. Kirschner and G. F. Webb, A model for treatment strategy in the chemotherapy of AIDS, Bulletin of Mathematical Biology **58**(2) (1996), 367–390.

5. D. Kirschner and G. F. Webb, Qualitative differences in HIV chemotherapy between resistance and remission outcomes, Emerging Infectious Diseases **3**(3) (1997), 273–283.

6. D. Kirschner and G. F. Webb, Understanding drug resistance in the monotherapy treatment of HIV infection, Bulletin of Mathematical Biology **59**(4) (1997), 763–785.

7. D. Kirschner and G. F. Webb, A mathematical model of combined drug therapy of HIV infection, Journal of Theoretical Medicine **1** (1997), 25–34.

8. D. Kirschner and G. F. Webb, Immunotherapy of HIV-1 infection, Journal of Biological Systems, to appear (1998).

9. A. Lafeuillade, C. Poggi, N. Profizi et al., Human immunodeficiency virus type 1 in lymph nodes compared with plasma, J. Infec. Diseases, **174** (1996), 404–407.

10. R. M. May and R. M. Anderson, Transmission dynamics of HIV infection, Nature **326** (1987), 137–42.

11. A. McLean and M. Nowak, Competition between AZT sensitive and AZT resistant strains of HIV, AIDS **6** (1992), 71–79.

12. A. R. McLean and M. A. Nowak, Interactions between HIV and other pathogens, J. Theoret. Biol. **155** (1991), 69–86.

13. M. A. Nowak and R. M. May, AIDS pathogenesis: Mathematical models of HIV and SIV infections, AIDS **7**(supp) (1993), 3–s18.

14. A. Perelson et al., HIV-1 Dynamics in vivo: Clearance rate, infected cell lifespan, and viral generation time, Science **271** (1996), 1582–1586.

15. A. Perelson, D. Kirschner and R. De Boer, The dynamics of HIV infection of CD4$^+$ T cells, Math. Biosciences **114** (1993), 81–125.

16. X. Wei et al., Viral dynamics in human immunodeficiency virus type 1 infection, Nature **373** (1995), 117–122.

Faustino Sánchez Garduño
Departamento de Matemáticas
Facultad de Ciencias, UNAM
Circuito Exterior, Ciudad Universitaria
México, 04510, D.F.
faustino@servidor.unam.mx

Denise Kirschner
Department of Microbiology and Immunology
6730 Medical Science Bldg II
The University of Michigan Medical School
Ann Arbor, MI 49109-0620
kirschne@umich.edu

Janelle Reynolds
Department of Oceanography
University of North Carolina
Chapel Hill, N.C. 27599
janelle@email.unc.edu

Optimal Control of a PDE/ODE System Modeling A Gas-Phase Bioreactor

Naresh Handagama and Suzanne Lenhart

Abstract. Degradation of a contaminant through metabolism of a bacteria in a gas-phase bioreactor is modeled by a system consisting of a parabolic partial differential equation and an ordinary differential equation. The optimal control for the flow rate of contaminant is characterized with the objective to maximize the amount of contaminant degraded less the cost of implementing the control. A numerical simulation and a lab experiment with paraxylene in a gas-phase bioreactor are discussed.

§1. Introduction

In situ bioremediation is a technology using the metabolism of "in situ" bacteria for cleaning subsurface environments contaminated with hazardous materials. Utilizing bioreactors for remediation appears promising [10, 17], and finding the best strategies to control bacteria metabolism in bioreactors is crucial to achieve optimal remediation. We concentrate in this paper on the removal of volatile organic compounds from air emissions in hazardous waste control through biocatalytic processes [11, 15]. We model a new technology of a gas-phase bioreactor [2, 17].

In this paper, optimal control of the flow rate into a gas-phase bioreactor is considered. The feed gas mixture (air/paraxylene) is transported through an annular sand packing where the bacteria (Pseudomonas putida) is immobilized. The bacteria will degrade the toxic paraxylene pollutant in the gas stream producing carbon dioxide and water. See Figure 1 for a diagram of the bioreactor. The flow is radial from an inner core where the feed gas mixture enters the packed bed and flows through the packed bed and into the outer core. The goal of controlling the flow rate is to maximize the amount of contaminant degraded.

Mathematical Models in Medical and Health Sciences
Mary Ann Horn, Gieri Simonett, and Glenn Webb (eds.), pp. 197–212.
Copyright © 1998 by Vanderbilt University Press, Nashville, TN.
ISBN 0-8265-1310-7.

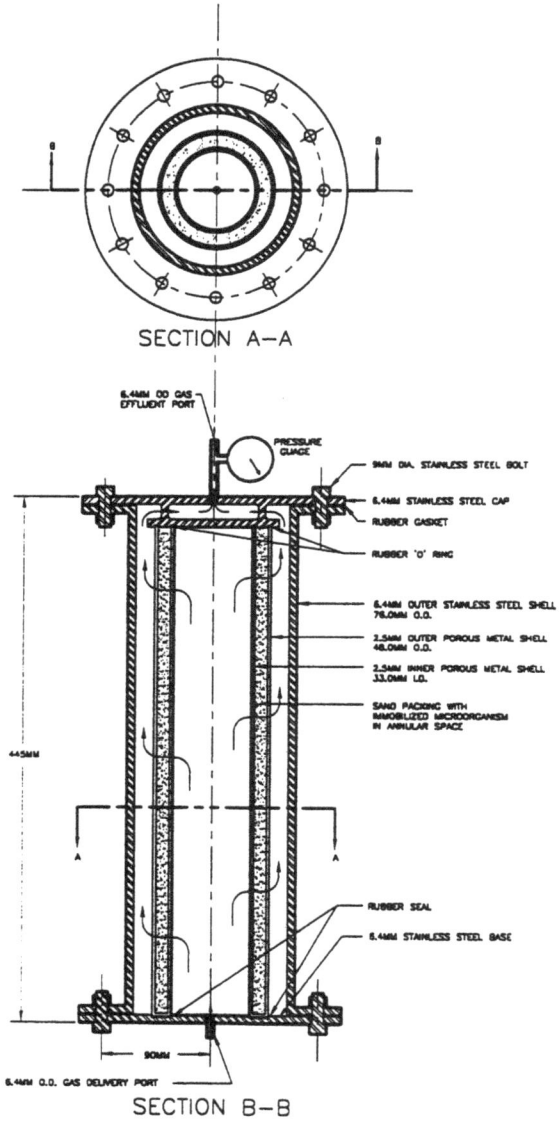

Fig. 1. Diagram of bioreactor.

Our state system consists of a parabolic partial differential equation (PDE) for the concentration of contaminant, $c(r,t)$, and an ordinary differential equation (ODE) in time (with radial parameter r) for the concentration of the immobile bacteria biomass, $b(r,t)$,

$$\frac{\partial c}{\partial t} = \frac{1}{r}\epsilon\frac{\partial}{\partial r}\left(r\frac{\partial c}{\partial r}\right) - f(r)v(t)\frac{\partial c}{\partial r} - \frac{\rho\mu bc}{k+c},$$

$$\frac{db}{dt} = \frac{\mu bc}{k+c} \text{ on } Q = (r_1, r_2) \times (0, T), \tag{1}$$

$$c(r,0) = c_0(r), \quad b(r,0) = b_0(r) \text{ when } t = 0,$$

$$c(r_1, t) = c_1, \text{ a constant,}$$

$$\frac{\partial c}{\partial r}(r_2, t) = 0 \text{ for } 0 < t < T.$$

Note that the interaction term,

$$\frac{-\rho\mu bc}{k+c},$$

is a Monod (or Michaelis-Minton) type term. The flow rate depends on

$$f(r)v(t).$$

Note that this model was developed and validated for this bioreactor by Rouhana [12].

Taking the time varying part of the flow rate as our constrained control, our control set is

$$U = \{v \in L^\infty(0,T) \mid m \le v(t) \le M\}.$$

We seek to maximize the following objective functional:

$$J(v) = 2\pi h \int_0^T v(t)[r_1 f(r_1)c_1 - r_2 f(r_2)c(r_2, t)]dt - \frac{B}{2}\int_0^T (v(t))^2 dt, \tag{2}$$

which represents the amount of contaminant degraded (amount "in" less amount "out"), less the cost of implementing the control. The constant B is the balancing factor between the two terms of the objective functional. We will characterize $v^* \in U$ such that

$$J(v^*) = \sup_{v \in U} J(v).$$

A related work by Chawla and Lenhart [1] considers optimal control of remediation of carbon tetrachloride by controlling the input of acetate nutrient at the inlet. This model contains three PDEs coupled with one ODE. A simpler optimal control problem for a bioreactor using only ODEs in the model is treated in Heinricher et al. [5]. See Rouhana et al. [13] and Davison et al. [2] for background on degradation in gas-phase bioreactors.

In Section 2, the problem is formulated and the existence of an optimal control is proven. In Section 3, the optimal control is characterized in terms of the optimality system, which is the state system coupled with an adjoint system. This optimality system is derived by differentiating the objective functional with respect to the control (in a directional derivative sense) and differentiating the state solution map with respect to the control. Uniqueness of the optimal control is obtained from the uniqueness of solutions of the optimality system for small time T. In the last section, we briefly discuss the successful laboratory implementation of the optimal flow rate on the bioreactor.

§2. Existence of an Optimal Control

We make the following assumptions:

$$0 < r_1 < r_2,$$

$$c_0(r) \geq 0,$$

$$f(r) = \frac{r_1}{r},$$

$$h, M, m, \rho, Y, \mu, k \text{ are positive constants,}$$

$$f(r_2)m - \frac{\epsilon}{r_2} > 0. \tag{3}$$

Assumption (3) means that there is a flow out at radius r_2. To set up a standard solution space for the state system (1), we change variables to get zero boundary conditions at $r = r_1$ by letting

$$\hat{c}(r,t) = c(r,t) - c_1.$$

Our solution space will have zero boundary conditions at $r = r_1$ for the contaminant component. We use the notation $H^1_{r_1}(r_1, r_2)$ to denote the subspace of the Sobolev space $H^1(r_1, r_2)$ with zero boundary condition at r_1. Our solution space is

$$V = L^2(0, T; H^1_{r_1}(r_1, r_2)) \times L^2(Q).$$

Definition 1. $(\hat{c}, b)$ in V is a weak solution of (1) if

(i)

$$\int_0^T < \frac{\partial \hat{c}}{\partial t}, \phi > dt + \int_Q \epsilon D \frac{\partial \hat{c}}{\partial r} \frac{\partial \phi}{\partial r} dr dt - \int_Q \frac{1}{r} \epsilon \frac{\partial \hat{c}}{\partial r} \phi dr dt$$

$$+ \int_Q f(r) v(t) \frac{\partial \hat{c}}{\partial r} \phi dr dt = - \int_Q \rho \frac{\mu b(\hat{c} + c_1)}{k + \hat{c} + c_1} \phi dr dt$$

for $\phi \in L^2(0,T; H^1_{r_1}(r_1,r_2))$;

(ii) $b(r,t) = b_0(r) + \int_0^t \frac{\mu b(\hat{c}+c_1)}{k+\hat{c}+c_1}(s,r)ds$, $r_1 < r < r_2$; and

(iii) $\hat{c}(r,0) = c_0(r) - c_1$,
where $< \cdot, \cdot >$ represents the duality between $(H^1_{r_1}(r_1,r_2))^*$ and $H^1_{r_1}(r_1,r_2)$.

We now give the existence result for the state system.

Theorem 2. *Given $v \in U$, there exists a unique solution of the state system (1).*

Proof: We construct solutions by an iterative scheme [9]. Let U be a solution of

$$\frac{\partial U}{\partial t} = \frac{1}{r}\epsilon\frac{\partial}{\partial r}\left(r\frac{\partial U}{\partial r}\right) - f(r)v(t)\frac{\partial U}{\partial r} \quad \text{in } Q,$$

$$U(r,0) = c_0(r), \ U(r_1,t) = c_1, \ \frac{\partial U}{\partial r}(r_2,t) = 0.$$

Then let V be a solution of

$$\frac{dV}{dt} = \frac{\mu UV}{k+U} \quad \text{in } Q, \ V(r,0) = c_0(r).$$

The bounded functions U, V will serve as supersolutions to our system.
Define $c^0 = 0$, $b^1 = 0$, $c^1 = U$, $b^2 = V$ to start our iterative scheme. Let R be a large positive constant so that

$$Rc - \frac{\rho bc}{k+c}$$

is an increasing function of c for $0 \le c \le \|U\|_\infty$, $0 \le b \le \|V\|_\infty$. Define b^n first and then c^n as solutions of

$$\frac{db^n}{dt} = \frac{\mu b^{n-2}c^{n-1}}{k+c^{n-1}} \text{ on } Q, \qquad b^n(r,0) = b_0(r), \qquad (4)$$

$$\frac{\partial c^n}{\partial t} = \frac{1}{r}\epsilon\frac{\partial}{\partial r}\left(r\frac{\partial c^n}{\partial r}\right) - f(r)v(t)\frac{\partial c^n}{\partial r} - Rc^n + Rc^{n-2} - \frac{\rho\mu b^n c^{n-2}}{k+c^{n-2}} \text{ in } Q \quad (5)$$

$$c^n(r,0) = c_0(r), \ c^n(r_1,t) = c_1, \ \frac{\partial c^n}{\partial r}(r_2,t) = 0.$$

By the comparison principle [6], we obtain the following monotone alternating convergent sequences:

$$b^{2n} \searrow \bar{b}, \ b^{2n+1} \nearrow b, \ c^{2n} \nearrow c, \ c^{2n+1} \searrow \bar{c}$$

for some $c, \bar{c} \in L^2(0,T; H^1(r_1,r_2))$, $b, \bar{b} \in L^2(Q)$. Noting the boundedness of the growth coefficient,

$$\frac{c^{n-1}}{k+c^{n-1}},$$

on the RHS of the b^n in equation (4), Gronwall's Inequality gives an explicit $L^\infty(Q)$ bound on the sequence $\{b^n\}$. Then the equation for b^n gives that b^n is uniformly Lipschitz in t for each r. Using the weak form of the c^n equation (5), and the boundedness of the nonlinear term

$$\frac{\rho\mu b^n c^{n-2}}{k + c^{n-2}},$$

we have

$$\sup_{0 \leq t \leq T} \int_{r_1}^{r_2} (c^n)^2(r,t)dr + \int_0^T \int_{r_1}^{r_2} +(c_r^n)^2 drdt \leq C_1. \tag{6}$$

Then the c^n equation gives

$$\|c_t^n\|_{L^2(0,T;H_{r_1}^1(r_1,r_2)^*)} \leq C_2. \tag{7}$$

We obtain the following weak convergences:

$$c^{2n} \rightharpoonup c, \ c^{2n+1} \rightharpoonup \bar{c} \ \text{in} \ L^2(0,T;H_{r_1}^1(r_1,r_2)),$$

$$c_t^{2n} \rightharpoonup c_t, c_t^{2n+1} \rightharpoonup \bar{c}_t \ \text{in} \ L^2(0,T;H_{r_1}^1(r_1,r_2)^*).$$

By the compactness result [14], inequalities (6) and (7) imply

$$c^{2n} \to c, \ c^{2n+1} \to \bar{c}, \ \text{strongly in} \ L^2(Q).$$

We can pass to the limit in the equations (4), (5). The limiting functions $c, b, \bar{c}, \bar{b}$ satisfy the following system of four equations,

$$\begin{aligned}
\frac{\partial c}{\partial t} &= \frac{1}{r}\epsilon\frac{\partial}{\partial r}\left(r\frac{\partial c}{\partial r}\right) - fv\frac{\partial c}{\partial r} - \frac{\rho\mu\bar{b}c}{k+c}, \\
\frac{db}{dt} &= \frac{\mu bc}{k+c}, \\
\frac{\partial\bar{c}}{\partial t} &= \frac{1}{r}\epsilon\frac{\partial}{\partial r}\left(r\frac{\partial\bar{c}}{\partial r}\right) - fv\frac{\partial\bar{c}}{\partial r} - \frac{\rho\mu b\bar{c}}{k+\bar{c}}, \\
\frac{d\bar{b}}{dt} &= \frac{\mu\bar{b}\bar{c}}{k+\bar{c}},
\end{aligned} \tag{8}$$

in addition to the corresponding boundary/initial conditions. Since $\bar{c}, \bar{b}, c, b$ also satisfies system (8), uniqueness results for that system give $b = \bar{b}, c = \bar{c}$. We conclude that c, b is the desired solution of our state system.

To obtain uniqueness of solutions of the state system, suppose c, b and c^*, b^* are two solutions. For $0 \leq t \leq T$, let $\tilde{c} = c - c^*$, $\tilde{b} = b - b^*$, integrate over $(r_1, r_2) \times (0, t)$ for $0 \leq t \leq T$ to obtain

$$\int_0^t \int_{r_1}^{r_2} \left(\tilde{c}_t\tilde{c} + \tilde{b}_t\tilde{b} + \epsilon(\tilde{c}_r)^2\right) drds$$

$$\leq \frac{\epsilon}{2}\int_0^t \int_{r_1}^{r_2} (\tilde{c}_r)^2 drds + C_1 \int_0^t \int_{r_1}^{r_2} \left(\tilde{b}^2 + \tilde{c}^2\right) drds.$$

Taking the supremum in t for $0 \leq t \leq T_1$ we obtain

$$\sup_{0 \leq t \leq T_1} \left[\frac{1}{2} \int_{r_1}^{r_2} (\tilde{b}^2 + \tilde{c}^2)(r,t)dr + \frac{\epsilon}{2} \int_0^t \int_{r_1}^{r_2} (\tilde{c}_r)^2 drds \right]$$

$$\leq c_3 T_1 \sup_{0 \leq t \leq T_1} \int_{r_1}^{r_2} (\tilde{b}^2 + \tilde{c}^2)(r,t)dr.$$

Taking T_1 small, we obtain

$$\sup_{0 \leq t \leq T_1} \left[\int_{r_1}^{r_2} (\tilde{b}^2 + \tilde{c}^2)(r,t)dr + \int_0^t \int_{r_1}^{r_2} (\tilde{c}_r)^2 drds \right] \leq 0,$$

which gives uniqueness on $(r_1, r_2) \times (0, T_1)$. A second application of the argument on $(r_1, r_2) \times (T_1, 2T_1)$ gives uniqueness on $(r_1, r_2) \times (0, 2T_1)$. Continuation of this iterative process gives uniqueness on $(r_1, r_2) \times (0, T)$. □

Now we have the main result of this section - existence of an optimal control.

Theorem 3. *There exists an optimal control v^* in U which maximizes the functional $J(v)$.*

Proof: Let $\{v^n, n = 1, 2, ...\}$ be a maximizing sequence such that

$$\lim_{n \to \infty} J(v^n) = \sup_v J(v).$$

Denote by $(c^n, b^n) = (c, b)(v^n)$ the corresponding state solution. As in Theorem 2, we have the following a priori estimates:

$$\|c^n\|_{L^2(0,T;H^1(r_1,r_2))} \leq C,$$

and

$$\|b^n\|_{L^2(Q)} \leq C,$$

with

$$b^n(r,t) \text{ is uniformly Lipschitz in } t, \text{ for each } r.$$

Also we have

$$\|c_t^n\|_{L^2(0,T;H^1_{r_1}(r_1,r_2)^*)} \leq C_1.$$

We can extract weakly convergent subsequences, i.e., there exists $c^*, b^* \in V$ such that

$$c^n \rightharpoonup c^* \text{ weakly in } L^2(0,T; H^1(r_1,r_2)),$$

$$b^n \rightharpoonup b \text{ weakly in } L^2(Q),$$

$$b^n \to b \text{ uniformly in } t \text{ for each } r.$$

By an interpolation compactness result [14],

$$c^n \to c^* \text{ strongly in } L^2(Q),$$

$$c^n(r_2, t) \to c^*(r_2, t) \text{ strongly in } L^2(0, T). \tag{9}$$

We obtain
$$(c^*, b^*) = (c, b)(v^*).$$

Using the lower semi-continuity of J with respect to weak convergence and (9) with $r = r_2$, we obtain
$$J(v^*) \geq \limsup_{n \to \infty} J(v^n),$$

which gives that v^* is an optimal control. $\square$

§3. Characterization of the Optimal Control

In order to characterize the optimal control, we must differentiate the maps
$$v \mapsto c(v), b(v)$$

and
$$v \mapsto J(v)$$

in an appropriate directional derivative sense.

Theorem 4. *The solution map*
$$v \in U \mapsto (c, b)$$

is differentiable in the following sense:
$$\begin{cases} \frac{c(v+\delta l)-c(v)}{\delta} \rightharpoonup \psi_1 \\ \frac{b(v+\delta l)-b(v)}{\delta} \rightharpoonup \psi_2 \end{cases} \text{ weakly in } V, \text{ as } \delta \to 0$$

when $v \in U$, $v + \delta l \in U$, δ sufficiently small and $l \in L^\infty(0, T)$. Furthermore, $(\psi_1, \psi_2) \in V$ satisfies the following system in the weak sense,

$$\frac{\partial \psi_1}{\partial t} = \epsilon \frac{\partial^2 \psi_1}{\partial r^2} + \frac{\epsilon}{r} \frac{\partial \psi_1}{\partial r} - f(r)v(t) \frac{\partial \psi_1}{\partial r}$$
$$\qquad - \rho\mu \left(\frac{kb\psi_1}{(k+c)^2} + \frac{c\psi_2}{k+c} \right) - f(r)l(t) \frac{\partial c}{\partial r} \qquad \text{in } (r_1, r_2) \times (0, T)$$

$$\frac{\partial \psi_2}{\partial t} = \frac{\mu k b \psi_1}{(k+c)^2} + \frac{\mu c \psi_2}{k+c} \qquad\qquad\qquad \text{in } (r_1, r_2) \times (0, T) \qquad (10)$$

$$\psi_1 = \psi_2 = 0 \quad \text{at } t = 0$$

$$\psi_1(r_1, t) = 0, \frac{\partial \psi_1}{\partial r}(r_2, t) = 0.$$

Proof: Define $(c^\delta, b^\delta) = (c(v + \delta l), b(v + \delta l))$ and $(c, b) = (c(v), b(v))$. Then the difference quotients satisfy

$$\frac{\partial}{\partial t} \left(\frac{c^\delta - c}{\delta} \right) = \frac{\epsilon}{r} \frac{\partial}{\partial r} \left(r \frac{\partial}{\partial r} \left(\frac{c^\delta - c}{\delta} \right) \right) - fv(t) \frac{\partial}{\partial r} \left(\frac{c^\delta - c}{\delta} \right)$$
$$\qquad - fl(t) \frac{\partial c^\delta}{\partial r} - \rho\mu \left(\frac{c^\delta b^\delta}{k + c^\delta} - \frac{cb}{k+c} \right) \left(\frac{1}{\delta} \right),$$

$$\frac{d}{dt} \left(\frac{b^\delta - b}{\delta} \right) = \mu \left(\frac{c^\delta b^\delta}{k + c^\delta} - \frac{cb}{k+c} \right) \left(\frac{1}{\delta} \right),$$

with zero initial and boundary conditions. We have the following a priori estimates:

$$\left\|\frac{c^\delta - c}{\delta}\right\|_{L^2(0,T;H^1(r_1,r_2))} \leq C,$$

$$\left\|\left(\frac{c^\delta - c}{\delta}\right)_t\right\|_{L^2(0,T;H^1_{r_1}(r_1,r_2)^*)} \leq C,$$

$$\left\|\frac{b^\delta - b}{\delta}\right\|_{L^2((r_1,r_2)\times(0,T))} \leq C.$$

As in the proof of Theorem 2, these estimates justify the existence of $(\psi_1, \psi_2) \in V$ such that

$$\frac{c^\delta - c}{\delta} \rightharpoonup \psi_1 \text{ in } L^2(0,T;H^1(r_1,r_2)),$$

$$\left(\frac{c^\delta - c}{\delta}\right)_t \rightharpoonup (\psi_1)_t \text{ in } L^2(0,T;H^1_{r_1}(r_1,r_2)^*),$$

$$\frac{b^\delta - b}{\delta} \to \psi_2 \text{ uniformly in } t \text{ for each } r$$

and ψ_1, ψ_2 satisfy system (10). $\square$

We can write the ψ_1, ψ_2 system as

$$\mathcal{L}\begin{pmatrix}\psi_1 \\ \psi_2\end{pmatrix} + \mathcal{M}\begin{pmatrix}\psi_1 \\ \psi_2\end{pmatrix} = \begin{pmatrix}-f(r)l(t)\frac{\partial c}{\partial t} \\ 0\end{pmatrix}$$

with $\mathcal{L}$ containing all the derivative terms and

$$\mathcal{M} = \begin{pmatrix} \frac{\rho\mu kb}{(k+c)^2} & \frac{\rho\mu c}{k+c} \\ -\frac{\mu kb}{(k+c)^2} & -\frac{\mu c}{k+c} \end{pmatrix}.$$

We will introduce the adjoint system in the next theorem using the operator

$$\mathcal{L}^*\begin{pmatrix}p \\ q\end{pmatrix} + \mathcal{M}^T\begin{pmatrix}p \\ q\end{pmatrix},$$

where $\mathcal{M}^T$ the the transpose of $\mathcal{M}$ and $\mathcal{L}^*$ is the adjoint operator of $\mathcal{L}$.

Now we use the differentiability of the map $v \mapsto (c,b)$ and adjoint variables to differentiate $J(v)$ with respect to v at v^* which results in a characterization of v^*.

Theorem 5. *Given an optimal control v^* in U and a corresponding state solution c^*, b^*, there exists a solution $(p,q) \in V$ to the adjoint problem:*

$$-\frac{\partial p}{\partial t} = \epsilon\frac{\partial^2 p}{\partial r^2} - \epsilon(\frac{1}{r}p)_r + v^*(t)(f(r)p)_r - \frac{\rho\mu kb^*p}{(k+c^*)^2} + \frac{\mu kb^*q}{(k+c^*)^2},$$

$$-\frac{\partial q}{\partial t} = -\frac{\rho\mu c^*p}{k+c^*} + \frac{\mu c^*q}{k+c^*},$$

$$p(r_1,t) = 0,$$

$$\epsilon\frac{\partial p}{\partial r} + \left(f(r)v^*(t) - \frac{\epsilon}{r_2}\right)p = -v^*(t)2\pi hr_1 \text{ at } r_2,$$

$$p = q = 0 \text{ at } t = T \text{ (transversality condition)}.$$

(11)

Furthermore

$$v^*(t) = \min\left\{\max\left\{\frac{1}{B}\left(2\pi r_1 h(c_1 - c^*(r_2, t))\right.\right.\right.$$
$$\left.\left.\left. - \int_{r_1}^{r_2} f(r)p\frac{\partial c^*}{\partial r}(r, t)dr\right), m\right\} M\right\}. \tag{12}$$

Proof: The existence of p, q follows since the adjoint problem is linear in p, q. For $\delta > 0$, let $v^* + \delta l \in U$ and define

$$(c^\delta, b^\delta) = (c, b)(v^* + \delta l),$$
$$(c^*, b^*) = (c, b)(v^*).$$

The derivative of $J(v)$ with respect to v at v^* in the direction l satisfies

$$0 \geq \lim_{\delta \to 0+} \frac{J(v^* + \delta l) - J(v^*)}{\delta}$$

$$= \lim_{\delta \to 0+}\left\{-\int_0^T 2\pi h r_1 v^*(t)\left(\frac{c^\delta - c^*}{\delta}\right)(r_2, t)dt\right.$$

$$\left. + \int_0^T l(t)2\pi h r_1(c_1 - c^\delta(r_2, t))dt - B\int_0^T\left(lv^* + \frac{\delta l^2}{2}\right)dt\right\}$$

$$= -\int_0^T 2\pi h r_1 v^*(t)\psi_1(r_2, t)dt$$

$$+ \int_0^T l(t)\left[2\pi h r_1(c_1 - c^*(r_2, t)) - Bv^*(t)\right]dt$$

$$= \int_Q\left(-p_t\psi_1 + \epsilon p_r(\psi_1)_r + \epsilon\left(\frac{1}{r}p\right)_r\psi_1 - (f(r)p)_r v^*\psi_1\right)drdt$$

$$+ \int_{r_2 \times (0,T)}(fv^* - \frac{\epsilon}{r_2})p\psi_1 dt + \int_Q\left[\frac{\rho\mu k b^* p}{(k + c^*)^2} + \frac{\mu k b^* q}{(k + c^*)^2}\right]\psi_1 drdt$$

$$+ \int_Q\left[-q_t\psi_2 + \left(\frac{\rho\mu c^* p}{k + c^*} - \frac{\mu c^* q}{k + c^*}\right)\psi_2\right]drdt$$

$$+ \int_0^T l[2\pi h r_1(c_1 - c^*(r_2, t)) - Bv^*(t)]dt$$

$$= \int_Q\left(p(\psi_1)_t + q(\psi_2)_t + \epsilon p_r(\psi_1)_r - \frac{\epsilon}{r}(\psi_1)_r p + f(r)v^*(t)p(\psi_1)_r\right)drdt$$

$$+ \int_Q\left[\rho\mu\left(\frac{kb^*\psi_1}{(k + c^*)^2} + \frac{c^*\psi_2}{k + c^*}\right)p - \mu\left(\frac{kb^*\psi_1}{(k + c^*)^2} + \frac{c^*\psi_2}{k + c^*}\right)q\right]drdt$$

$$+ \int_0^T l[2\pi h r_1(c_1 - c^*(r_2, t)) - Bv^*(t)]dt$$

$$= \int_0^T l(t)\left(2\pi h r_1(c_1 - c^*(r_2, t)) - Bv^*(t) - \int_{r_1}^{r_2} f(r)p\frac{\partial c}{\partial r}dr\right)dt.$$

We use the adjoint system, integration by parts and system (10). By a standard control theory argument, we obtain the characterization of v^* given in (12). $\square$

Substituting for v^* using (12) into the state system (1) and the adjoint system (11) gives the optimality system. We now prove that the solution of the optimality system is unique for small time T. Note that Theorems 3 and 5 imply that v^* and (c^*, b^*) exist and, therefore, (p, q) exists. This gives the existence of solutions to the optimality system. Thus our uniqueness result for the optimality system completes the characterization of the unique optimal control. The uniqueness result holds for T small, due to the opposite time orientations involved.

Theorem 6. *For T sufficiently small, solutions to the optimality system are unique.*

Proof: Suppose c, b, p, q and $\bar{c}, \bar{b}, \bar{p}, \bar{q}$ are both solutions of the optimality system. Let $\tilde{c} = c - \bar{c}$, $\tilde{b} = b - \bar{b}$, $\tilde{p} = p - \bar{p}$ and $\tilde{q} = q - \bar{q}$. Let

$$v = \min\left\{\max\left\{\frac{1}{B}\left(2\pi r_1 h(c_1 - c(r_2, t)) - \int_{r_1}^{r_2} fp\frac{\partial c}{\partial r}(r, t)dr\right), m\right\}, M\right\}$$

$$\bar{v} = \min\left\{\max\left\{\frac{1}{B}\left(2\pi r_1 h(c_1 - \bar{c}(r_2, t)) - \int_{r_1}^{r_2} f\bar{p}\frac{\partial \bar{c}}{\partial r}(r, t)dr\right), m\right\}, M\right\}.$$

We integrate the $\tilde{c}, \tilde{b}$ equations over $(r_1, r_2) \times (0, s)$ and the $\tilde{p}, \tilde{q}$ equations over $(r_1, r_2) \times (s, T)$ for $0 \le s \le T$ to obtain

$$\int_0^s \int_{r_1}^{r_2} (\tilde{c}_t \tilde{c} + \tilde{b}_t \tilde{b})drdt - \int_s^T \int_{r_1}^{r_2} (\tilde{p}_t \tilde{p} + \tilde{q}_t \tilde{q})drdt$$

$$+ \epsilon\left[\int_0^s \int_{r_1}^{r_2} (\tilde{c}_r)^2 drdt + \int_s^T \int_{r_1}^{r_2} (\tilde{p}_r)^2 drdt\right]$$

$$\le \int_0^s \int_{r_1}^{r_2} \left[\frac{\epsilon}{4}(\tilde{c}_r)^2 + C_1(\tilde{c}^2 + \tilde{b}^2)\right] drdt$$

$$+ \int_s^T \int_{r_1}^{r_2} \left[\frac{\epsilon}{4}(\tilde{p}_r)^2 + C_2(\tilde{p}^2 + \tilde{q}^2)\right] drdt \qquad (13)$$

$$- \int_0^s \int_{r_1}^{r_2} f(vc_r - \bar{v}\bar{c}_r)\tilde{c}drdt$$

$$+ \int_s^T \int_{r_1}^{r_2} \left[f(vp_r - \bar{v}\bar{p}_r) - \frac{r_1}{r^2}(vp - \bar{v}\bar{p})\right] \tilde{p}drdt$$

$$+ \int_s^T [2\pi h r_1(\bar{v} - v) + f(\bar{v}\bar{p} - vp)]\tilde{p}(r_2, t)dt$$

$$+ \int_s^T \frac{\epsilon}{r_2}\tilde{p}^2(r_2, t)dt.$$

In the above equation, we have explicitly displayed the terms with $v, \bar{v}$ and the boundary terms. Note that

$$|v - \bar{v}|(t) \leq C_3|c - \bar{c}|(r_2, t) + C_3 \int_{r_1}^{r_2} f|pc_r - \bar{p}\bar{c}_r|dr,$$

which implies

$$\int_0^T |v - \bar{v}|(t)dt \leq C_3 \int_0^T |\tilde{c}|(r_2, t)dt + C_4 \int_0^T \left(\int_{r_1}^{r_2} (\tilde{c}_r)^2 dr\right)^{\frac{1}{2}} dt$$

$$+ C_5 \int_0^T \left(\int_{r_1}^{r_2} (\tilde{p})^2 dr\right)^{\frac{1}{2}} dt.$$

To obtain these estimates, we use the fact that

$$\sup_t \int_{r_1}^{r_2} ((c_r)^2 + (p_r)^2)(r, t)dr$$

is bounded (see [7, 8]). Continuing the estimate from inequality (13), we have

$$\frac{1}{2} \int_{r_1}^{r_2} [\tilde{c}^2 + \tilde{b}^2 + \tilde{p}^2 + \tilde{q}^2](r, s)dr + \epsilon \left[\int_0^s \int_{r_1}^{r_2} (\tilde{c}_r)^2 drdt + \int_s^T \int_{r_1}^{r_2} (\tilde{p}_r)^2 drdt\right]$$

$$\leq \frac{\epsilon}{2} \left[\int_0^s \int_{r_1}^{r_2} (\tilde{c}_r)^2 drdt + \int_s^T \int_{r_1}^{r_2} (\tilde{p}_r)^2 drdt\right]$$

$$+ C_6 \int_0^T \int_{r_1}^{r_2} [\tilde{c}^2 + \tilde{b}^2 + \tilde{p}^2 + \tilde{q}^2]drdt.$$

Taking the supremum in t on both sides yields:

$$\sup_t \int_{r_1}^{r_2} [\tilde{c}^2 + \tilde{b}^2 + \tilde{p}^2 + \tilde{q}^2](r, t)dr \leq TC_7 \sup_t \int_{r_1}^{r_2} [\tilde{c}^2 + \tilde{b}^2 + \tilde{p}^2 + \tilde{q}^2](r, t)dr.$$

Taking T sufficiently small yields the desired uniqueness. □

§4. Lab Implementation of the Optimal Flow Rate

The optimality system was solved numerically with an iterative algorithm coupled with an explicit finite difference scheme. An initial guess for p_0, q_0 was used to solve the state system forward in time for the first iterate c^1, b^1. Using the values of c^1, b^1, we solved the adjoint system backwards in time for p^1, q^1. This procedure was continued until the successive pairs of the iterative scheme were sufficiently close. Such an iterative scheme is needed due to the opposite time orientation of the state system and the adjoint system. See Table 1 for the values of the parameters used in the simulations. See [3] for justification for this iterative method.

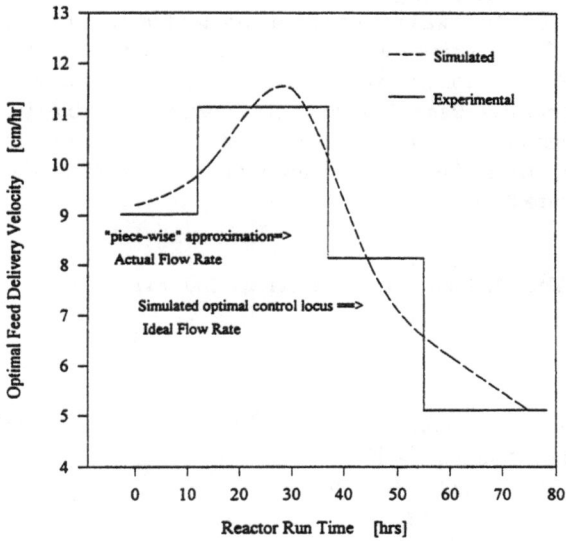

Fig. 2. Simulated optimal flow rates.

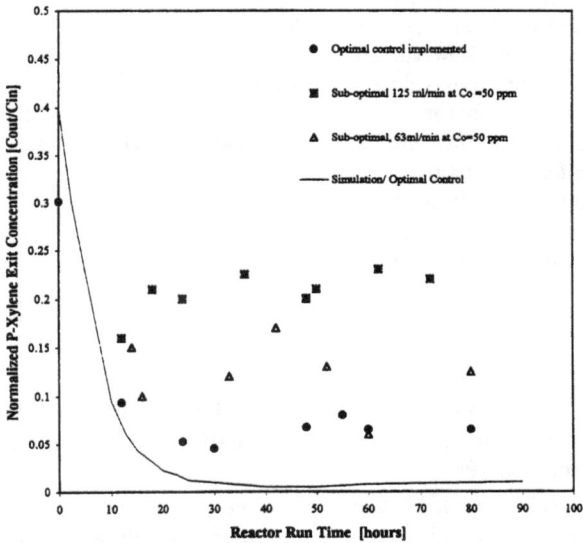

Fig. 3. Optimal flow strategy versus alternative strategies.

The simulated "optimal control" was tested on the bioreactor for two different feed concentrations (para-xylene 50ppm and 100 ppm). A piecewise continuous step function was used to approximate the optimal flow rate since the instrument for adjusting the flow rate could handle such "step" flow rate changes. See Figure 2 for an example illustrating the format of the optimal flow rate. Within this range of feed concentrations, the variable step "optimal" flow rate was demonstrated to be more successful than "constant in time" flow rates. The comparison of our optimal flow strategy with these other flow rates is shown in Figure 3.

Tab. 1. Constants for Model and Lab Experiment.

$\epsilon = \epsilon_1 D$

$\rho = \frac{1}{Y}\rho_1$

$\mu = $ maximum specific growth rate (hr^{-1})	0.437
$k = $ Monod constant (g/l^3)	$6.0E - 6$
$h = $ height of packed bed (cm)	40
$r_1 = $ inner radius (cm)	1.63
$r_2 = $ outer radius (cm)	2.63
$\epsilon_1 = $ void fraction of packed bed	0.3
$\rho_1 = $ specific mass of bed	1.717
(gram of sand/unit volume of packed bed)	
$D = $ effective diffusion coefficient (l^2/t)	2.85
$Y = $ yield coefficient (mass of cell/mass of pollutant)	0.3
$M = $ maximum flow velocity (cm/hr)	10
$m = $ minimum flow velocity (cm/hr)	0.6
$B = $ balancing factor	0.01
$b_0 = $ initial bacteria concentration (G Cells/g sand)	$8.2E - 6$
$(b_0(r) = b_0$, a constant)	
$T = $ upper time limit (hours)	100
$c_0 = $ initial para-xylene concentration (ppm)	$1.8E - 6$
$c_1 = $ para-xylene concentration at r_1	$1.8E - 6$

References

1. Chawla, S and S. Lenhart, Application of optimal control theory to in situ bioremediation, Institute for Mathematics and its Applications, Minnesota, Preprint, 1996.

2. Davinson, B. H. and J. E. Thompson, The removal of alkanes in a liquid-continuous gas-phase bioreactor: Preliminary considerations, Applied Biochemistry and Biotechnology **45/46** (1994), 917–923.

3. Hackbush, W.K., A numerical method for solving parabolic equations with opposite orientations, Computing **20** (1978), 229–240.

4. He, F., A. Leung and S. Stojanovic, Periodic optimal control for competing Volterra-Lotka type system, J. Comp. and Applied Math. **52** (1994), 199–217.

5. Heinricher, A., S. Lenhart and A. Solomon, The application of optimal control methodology to a well-stirred bioreactor, Natural Resource Modeling **9** (1996), 61–80.

6. Krylov, N.V., *Nonlinear Elliptic and Parabolic Equations of the Second Order*, D. Reidel Publishing, Boston, 1987.

7. Ladyzenzskaya, D. A., V. A. Solonnikov and N. N. Ural'ceva, *Linear and Quasilinear Equations of Parabolic Type*, American Math. Society, Providence, 1968.

8. Lenhart, S., Optimal control of a convective-diffusive fluid problem, Math. Models and Methods in Applied Sciences **5** (1995), 225–237.

9. Leung, A. W., *Systems of Nonlinear Partial Differential Equations, Applications to Biology and Egineering*, Kluwer Publishers, Dortrecht/Boston, 1989.

10. Norris, R. D., et al., *Handbook of Bioremediation*, Lewis Publishers, Boca Raton, FL, 1994.

11. Ottengraf, S. P. P. and A. H. C. Van Den Oever, Kinetics of organic compound removal from waste wases with a biological filter, Biotechnology and Bioengineering **25** (1983), 3089–3102.

12. Rouhana-Bhojraj, N., Development and modeling of a radial flow vapor phase bioreactor for the removal of Para-Xylene , Ph.D. Dissertation, University of Tennessee, Chemical Engineering Department (1996).

13. Rouhana-Bhojraj, N., N. B. Handagama and P. R. Bientkowski, Development of a membrane-based vapor phase bioreactor, Applied Biochemistry and Biotechnology **63-65** (1997), 809–821.

14. Simon, J., Compact sets in the space $L^2(0, T; B)$, Annali di Matematica Pura et Applicata **CXLVI** (1987), 65–96.

15. Uchiyama, H., K. Oguri, O. Yagi and E. Kokufuta, Trichloroethylene degradation by immobilized cells of Methylocystis sp. M in a gas-solid bioreactor, Biotechnology Letters **14** (1992), 619–622.

16. Vaugh, B., W. Jones and J. Wolfram, Vapor phase bioreactor evaluated for performance in degrading aromatic compound with novel pseudomas, in *Proceedings of the 48th Industrial Waste Conference 1993*, Purdue Research Foundation, 393–405.

17. Young, L. and M. Haggblom, Biodegradation of toxic and environmental pollutants, Current Opinion in Biotechnology **2** (1991), 429–435.

Naresh Handagama
Pellissippi State Technical Community College
University of Tennessee
Chemical Engineering Department
Knoxville, TN 37993

Suzanne Lenhart
University of Tennessee
Mathematics Department
Knoxville, TN 37996-1300
lenhart@math.utk.edu

Mathematical Analysis for an Evolutionary Epidemic Model

Hisashi Inaba

§1. Introduction

Traditionally mathematical models in epidemiology have dealt with epidemics of diseases such as measles, mumps and rubella, for which one does not need to take into account genetic or evolutionary considerations. However, if we consider epidemics like type A influenza, genetic changes in the virus are thought to play an important role in causing recurrent epidemic.

In the type A influenza epidemic, the virus changes genetically, and hence immunologically from one epidemic to the next. Therefore a descendant virus strain can infect hosts who are immune to the progenitor strain diseases, and hence reinvade communities that recently suffered an epidemic of the progenitor strain. There is some evidence that the probability of reinfection increases almost linearly as the length of time since the last infection increases.

Pease [9] has first proposed a mathematical model which can take into account those gradual changes in the influenza antigens called *drift*, and suggested that a dampening epidemic oscillation could occur under the evolutionary mechanism. In spite of this quite interesting idea, as far as I know, Pease's model has been neglected for a long time in the field of mathematical epidemiology, and its mathematical analysis has not yet been fully established.

Our main purpose in this paper is to understand mathematical aspects of the evolutionary epidemic model proposed by Pease. We first prove the existence and uniqueness of solutions of the evolutionary epidemic model. Next we consider conditions for existence of endemic steady states. Subsequently we introduce a semigroup approach to analyze the stability of endemic steady states. Finally we consider some effects of introduction of vaccination.

§2. Model Formulation

In the model formulated by Pease, it is assumed that only one virus strain circulates in a human community at any one time. Suppose that random drift occurs continually and causes gradual changes in the virus antigens, thereby

Mathematical Models in Medical and Health Sciences
Mary Ann Horn, Gieri Simonett, and Glenn Webb (eds.), pp. 213–236.
Copyright © 1998 by Vanderbilt University Press, Nashville, TN.
ISBN 0-8265-1310-7.

genetic changes in the pathogen from epidemic to epidemic cause previously immune hosts to become susceptible. Moreover we expect that the more a virus has changed genetically from its progenitor, the more easily it will be able to reinfect a host that is immune to its progenitor.

Let $I(t)$ be the number of infected hosts at time t and let $S(t, a)$ be the density of uninfected hosts, so that

$$\int_{a_0}^{a_1} S(t, a)da$$

is the number of uninfected hosts that were last infected by a virus which differed by more than a_0 and less than a_1 amino acid substitution from the virus strain prevailing at time t. We assume that the number of amino acid substitution is a continuous variable, and it is causing the antigenic drift in the virus strain. The host population size $N(t)$ at time t is given by

$$N(t) = \int_0^\infty S(t, a)da + I(t). \tag{2.1}$$

Then the basic model (Pease model) can be formulated by the following integrodifferential equations:

$$\frac{\partial S(t, a)}{\partial t} + \frac{\partial k S(t, a)}{\partial a} = -\gamma(a)S(t, a)I(t), \tag{2.2}$$

$$\frac{dI(t)}{dt} = -vI(t) + I(t)\int_0^\infty \gamma(a)S(t, a)da, \tag{2.3}$$

$$kS(t, 0) = vI(t), \tag{2.4}$$

where v is the rate at which infected hosts recover, k is the rate at which amino acid substitutions occur in the virus population and $\gamma(a)$ specifies how amino acid substitutions affect the probability of reinfection. Note that the demography of the host population is neglected in the above modelling.

It follows immediately from (2.1)-(2.4) that the total size of the host population is constant, $N(t) = N$. Thus we can write

$$I(t) = N - \int_0^\infty S(t, a)da, \tag{2.5}$$

and we arrive at the following single equation for uninfected hosts:

$$\frac{\partial S(t, a)}{\partial t} + \frac{\partial k S(t, a)}{\partial a} = -\gamma(a)S(t, a)\left[N - \int_0^\infty S(t, a)da\right], \tag{2.6}$$

$$kS(t, 0) = v\left[N - \int_0^\infty S(t, a)da\right]. \tag{2.7}$$

Throughout this paper we adopt the following assumption:

Assumption 2.1. *The transmission rate $\gamma(a)$ is a positive monotone increasing continuous function with a finite upper bound, that is, there exists a number $\gamma(\infty) := \lim_{a \to \infty} \gamma(a)$.*

Note that Assumption 2.1 excludes the case considered by Pease when $\gamma(a) = \gamma a$ (γ is a constant coefficient). Though it is biologically questionable whether $\gamma(a)$ could become infinitely large, but it is certain that our assumption will make the mathematical analysis simpler.

Clearly the fact that the transmission rate γ is *not constant* is a crucial point for our modeling, because if γ is constant, the evolutionary mechanism has no effect on the spread of the disease. In fact, if γ is constant, system (2.2)-(2.4) can be reduced to the classical SIS model as

$$\frac{dU(t)}{dt} = vI(t) - \gamma U(t)I(t), \tag{2.8}$$

$$\frac{dI(t)}{dt} = -vI(t) + \gamma U(t)I(t), \tag{2.9}$$

where $U(t)$ denotes the total size of the uninfected hosts;

$$U(t) = \int_0^\infty S(t,a)da.$$

In this simple case, the system can be reduced to the famous *Logistic model,*

$$\frac{dI(t)}{dt} = \gamma\left(\left(N - \frac{v}{\gamma}\right) - I(t)\right)I(t). \tag{2.10}$$

Then if the invasion condition $\frac{N\gamma}{v} > 1$ is satisfied, the number of infected hosts approaches the unique endemic level $N - \frac{v}{\gamma}$.

§3. Existence and Uniqueness of Solutions

In this section let us consider the existence and uniqueness of solutions for our system (2.2)-(2.4). First, by integrating (2.2) along the characteristic line, we obtain the following expression:

$$S(t,a) = \begin{cases} S(t - \frac{a}{k}, 0)e^{-\int_0^{\frac{a}{k}} \gamma(k\sigma)I(t - \frac{a}{k} + \sigma)d\sigma} & t - \frac{a}{k} > 0, \\ S(0, a - kt)e^{-\int_0^t \gamma(a - kt + k\sigma)I(\sigma)d\sigma} & t - \frac{a}{k} < 0, \end{cases} \tag{3.1}$$

where $S(t - \frac{a}{k}, 0)$ is given by

$$S\left(t - \frac{a}{k}, 0\right) = \frac{v}{k}I\left(t - \frac{a}{k}\right).$$

Inserting the above expression (3.1) into (2.5) and using (2.4), we obtain the nonlinear integral equation for $I(t)$,

$$I(t) = N - \frac{v}{k} \int_0^{kt} I\left(t - \frac{a}{k}\right) e^{-\int_0^{\frac{a}{k}} \gamma(k\sigma)I(t - \frac{a}{k} + \sigma)d\sigma} da - \\ - \int_{kt}^{\infty} S_0(a - kt) e^{-\int_0^t \gamma(a - kt + k\sigma)I(\sigma)d\sigma} da, \tag{3.2}$$

where $S_0(a) = S(0, a)$ is a given initial data. It is clear that if we find a positive continuous solution of (3.2), $S(t, a)$ is determined by (3.1) and it gives the solution of (2.6)-(2.7).

Note that equation (3.2) has a trivial solution $I \equiv 0$ if $N = \|S_0\|_{L^1} = \int_0^{\infty} S_0(a)da$. To seek nontrivial solutions for (3.2), we define a subset Ω_T of continuous functions as

$$\Omega_T = \{f \in C[0, T] : 0 \le f(t) \le N\},$$

with norm $\|f\|_T = \sup_{0 \le t \le T} |f(t)|$. Next define a nonlinear operator Φ by

$$\Phi(u)(t) = N - v \int_0^t u(z) e^{-\int_0^{t-z} \gamma(k\sigma)u(z+\sigma)d\sigma} dz - \\ - \int_0^{\infty} S_0(z) e^{-\int_0^t \gamma(z+k\sigma)u(\sigma)d\sigma} dz. \tag{3.3}$$

Then if there exists a positive solution of (3.2), it should be given as a fixed point of Φ in Ω_T.

Lemma 3.1. *Suppose that* $\|S_0\|_{L^1} < N$. *Then for sufficiently small* $T > 0$, *the operator* Φ *maps* Ω_T *into itself and there exists a number* $M > 0$ *such that*

$$\|\Phi^{(n)}(f) - \Phi^{(n)}(g)\|_T \le \|f - g\|_T \frac{M^n T^n}{n!}, \quad for \ u, v \in \Omega_T. \tag{3.4}$$

Proof: If $f \in \Omega_T$, it follows from (3.3) that $\Phi(f) \le N$ and

$$\Phi(f)(t) \ge N - vT\|f\|_T - \|S_0(z)\|_{L^1} \ge N - vTN - \|S_0\|_{L^1}.$$

Then if T is small enough, we have $\Phi(f) > 0$, that is, $\Phi(\Omega_T) \subset \Omega_T$. So we fix a $T > 0$ such that $\Phi(\Omega_T) \subset \Omega_T$. Next observe that for $u, v \in \Omega_T$, we obtain

$$|\Phi(f)(t) - \Phi(g)(t)| \le I + J + K,$$

where

$$I = v \int_0^t |f(z) - g(z)| e^{-\int_0^{t-z} \gamma(k\sigma)f(z+\sigma)d\sigma} dz,$$

$$J = v \int_0^t |g(z)| |e^{-\int_0^{t-z} \gamma(k\sigma)f(z+\sigma)d\sigma} - e^{-\int_0^{t-z} \gamma(k\sigma)g(z+\sigma)d\sigma}| dz,$$

$$K = \int_0^{\infty} S_0(z) |e^{-\int_0^t \gamma(z+k\sigma)f(\sigma)d\sigma} - e^{-\int_0^t \gamma(z+k\sigma)g(\sigma)d\sigma}| dz.$$

Then we can observe that

$$I \leq v \int_0^t |f(z) - g(z)| dz,$$

$$J \leq vN \int_0^t \int_0^{t-z} \gamma(k\sigma)|f(z+\sigma) - g(z+\sigma)| d\sigma dz,$$

$$K \leq \int_0^\infty S_0(z) \int_0^t \gamma(z+k\sigma)|f(\sigma) - g(\sigma)| d\sigma dz,$$

where we use the fact that $|e^{-x} - e^{-y}| \leq |x - y|$ for $x, y \geq 0$. Therefore we have

$$|\Phi(f)(t) - \Phi(g)(t)| \leq M \int_0^t |f(z) - g(z)| dz \leq M\|f - g\|_T t,$$

where

$$M = v + vN\gamma(\infty)T + \|S_0\|_{L^1}\gamma(\infty).$$

By mathematical induction, it is easily verified that

$$|\Phi^{(n)}(f)(t) - \Phi^{(n)}(g)(t)| \leq \|f - g\|_T \frac{M^n}{n!} t^n, \quad (n = 1, 2, ...).$$

This completes our proof. $\square$

Proposition 3.2. *For given initial data $S_0(a) \in L^1_+(0, \infty)$ such that $\|S_0\|_{L^1} < N$, the equation (3.2) has a unique continuous solution such that $0 \leq I(t) \leq N$ for all $t \geq 0$. The solution depends continuously on the initial data.*

Proof: For sufficiently small $T > 0$, it follows from Lemma 3.1 that Φ has a unique fixed point in Ω_T, which is given as the limit of the sequence $u_n = \Phi(u_{n-1}), u_0 \in \Omega_T$. Then we know that (3.2) has a local solution $I(t)$. Let $[0, t_0)$ be the maximal interval of existence for the continuous positive solution of (3.2). Then $t_0 > 0$. Suppose that t_0 is finite. Given any increasing sequence $\{t_n\} \subset [0, t_0)$ with $t_n \to t_0$, it is easily seen that $\{I(t_n)\}$ is a Cauchy sequence and hence $\lim_{t \to t_0 - 0} I(t)$ exists and it is nonnegative. That is, we can extend $I(t)$ to be a continuous function on the closed interval $[0, t_0]$ by defining $I(t_0) = \lim_{t \to t_0 - 0} I(t)$. Since $I(t)$ is differentiable with respect to t, we have

$$I'(t) = -vI(t) + I(t)\left[v \int_0^t I(z)e^{-\int_0^{t-z} \gamma(k\sigma)I(z+\sigma)d\sigma}\gamma(k(t-z))dz \right.$$
$$\left. + \int_0^\infty S_0(z)e^{-\int_0^t \gamma(z+k\sigma)I(\sigma)d\sigma}\gamma(z+kt)dz \right].$$

Then it follows that

$$I(t) = I(0) \exp\left(\int_0^t w(\xi)d\xi \right),$$

where

$$w(t) = -v + v \int_0^t I(z) e^{-\int_0^{t-z} \gamma(k\sigma)I(z+\sigma)d\sigma} \gamma(k(t-z))dz$$
$$+ \int_0^\infty S_0(z) e^{-\int_0^t \gamma(z+k\sigma)I(\sigma)d\sigma} \gamma(z+kt)dz.$$

Hence we can conclude that $I(t) > 0$ for all $t \in [0, t_0]$.

Let us consider the following operator:

$$\Psi(f)(t) = N - v \int_0^{t_0} I(z) e^{-\int_z^{t_0} \gamma(k(\sigma-z))I(\sigma)d\sigma - \int_{t_0}^{t+t_0} \gamma(k(\sigma-z))f(\sigma-t_0)d\sigma} dz$$
$$- v \int_{t_0}^{t+t_0} f(z-t_0) e^{-\int_z^{t+t_0} \gamma(k(\sigma-z))f(\sigma)d\sigma} dz$$
$$- \int_0^\infty S_0(z) e^{-\int_0^{t_0} \gamma(z+k\sigma)I(\sigma)d\sigma - \int_{t_0}^{t+t_0} \gamma(z+k\sigma)f(\sigma-t_0)d\sigma} dz.$$

Then it follows that

$$\Psi(f)(t) \geq N - v \int_0^{t_0} I(z) e^{-\int_z^{t_0} \gamma(k(\sigma-z))I(\sigma)d\sigma} dz$$
$$- v \int_{t_0}^{t+t_0} f(z-t_0) e^{-\int_z^{t+t_0} \gamma(k(\sigma-z))f(\sigma)d\sigma} dz$$
$$- \int_0^\infty S_0(z) e^{-\int_0^{t_0} \gamma(z+k\sigma)I(\sigma)d\sigma} dz$$
$$= I(t_0) - v \int_{t_0}^{t+t_0} f(z-t_0) e^{-\int_z^{t+t_0} \gamma(k(\sigma-z))f(\sigma)d\sigma} dz.$$

Since $I(t_0) > 0$, it is proved in the same way as for Φ that for sufficiently small $\delta > 0$ Ψ maps Ω_δ into itself and has unique fixed point in Ω_δ. Denote the fixed point of Ψ by $J(t)$. If we define $\hat{I}(t) = I(t)$ for $0 \leq t \leq t_0$ and $\hat{I}(t) = J(t-t_0)$ for $t_0 < t < t_0 + \delta$, we can see that $\hat{I}$ satisfies the equation (3.2) on $\Omega_{t_0+\delta}$, that is, we can extend the solution $I(t)$ beyond $t = t_0$. This contradicts the definition of t_0, so we conclude that $t_0 = \infty$.

Subsequently let $I_1(t)$ and $I_2(t)$ be solutions on $[0, T]$ corresponding to initial data S_0^1 and S_0^2, respectively. Then it is easily seen that for $t \in [0, T]$

$$|I_1(t) - I_2(t)| \leq M \int_0^t |I_1(z) - I_2(z)|dz + \|S_0^1 - S_0^2\|_{L^1},$$

where

$$M = v + vN\gamma(\infty)T + \gamma(\infty)\|S_0^2\|_{L^1}.$$

Therefore we have

$$|I_1(t) - I_2(t)| \leq \frac{(e^{MT} - 1)}{M} \|S_0^1 - S_0^2\|_{L^1},$$

which shows the continuous dependence of solutions on initial data. $\square$

§4. Endemic Steady States

Here we seek conditions under which there exist endemic steady states. Let $(S^*(a), I^*)$ be a steady state solution for the system (2.2)-(2.4). That is, we have

$$\frac{dS^*(a)}{da} = -\frac{\gamma(a)I^*}{k}S^*(a),$$ (4.1)

$$kS^*(0) = vI^*.$$ (4.2)

Hence we easily obtain that

$$S^*(a) = \frac{vI^*}{k}e^{-\frac{I^*}{k}\int_0^a \gamma(\sigma)d\sigma}.$$ (4.3)

Then we know that there is no disease-free steady state, which is an important characteristic different from traditional epidemic models. From (2.5), we arrive at the following equation for I^*:

$$N = I^* + \int_0^\infty S^*(a)da = I^* \left(1 + \frac{v}{k}\int_0^\infty e^{-\frac{I^*}{k}\int_0^a \gamma(\sigma)d\sigma}da\right).$$ (4.4)

Since there is no disease-free steady state, the standard threshold argument cannot be applied to our model. However, there is a similar type of criteria for the disease invasion. In fact, if we assume that the initial population is entirely composed by the uninfected hosts $S_0(a)$, then the basic reproduction number at the initial time is given by

$$R_0(S_0) = \frac{1}{v}\int_0^\infty \gamma(a)S_0(a)da.$$

In this case, we can define the maximum and minimum reproduction number, respectively, as

$$R_0^{max} = \frac{\gamma(\infty)N}{v}, \quad R_0^{min} = \frac{\gamma(0)N}{v}.$$

If $R_0(S_0) > 1$, then a very small infected initial population I_0 will grow at the initial stage because $I(t)$ is governed by the linearized equation as $I'(t) = v(R_0(S_0) - 1)I(t)$ in the initial phase. Moreover, in this case the condition $R_0^{max} \geq R_0(S_0) > 1$ is satisfied and we can prove that an endemic steady states will appear as follows:

Proposition 4.1. *For the system (2.2)-(2.4), there is no disease-free steady state. If $R_0^{max} < 1$, then there is no endemic steady state and the disease is eradicated naturally as time evolves. On the other hand, if $R_0^{max} > 1$, then there exists at least one endemic steady state.*

Proof: First it is observed that for all $t > 0$

$$I'(t) \leq v(R_0^{max} - 1)I(t).$$

Since we obtain an estimate, $I(t) \leq I(0)e^{v(R_0^{max}-1)t}$, the infected population will be eradicated if $R_0^{max} < 1$. Next assume that $R_0^{max} > 1$. Let us define a function $F(x)$, $x \in (0, N]$ by

$$F(x) := x\left(1 + \frac{v}{k}\int_0^\infty e^{-\frac{v}{k}\int_0^a \gamma(\sigma)d\sigma}\,da\right).$$

To show the existence of endemic steady states, we need to show that $N - F(x)$ has a zero in $(0, N]$. For this purpose, since $F(N) > N$, it is sufficient to show that $F(+0) < N$. Under the Assumption 2.1, for any small $\epsilon > 0$ there exists a number a_0 such that $\gamma(a) \geq \gamma(\infty) - \epsilon$ for $a \geq a_0$. Then we can observe that

$$\int_0^\infty e^{-\frac{v}{k}\int_0^a \gamma(\sigma)d\sigma}\,da \leq \int_0^{a_0} e^{-\frac{v}{k}\int_0^a \gamma(\sigma)d\sigma}\,da + \int_{a_0}^\infty e^{-\frac{v}{k}\left\{\int_0^{a_0} + \int_{a_0}^a\right\}\gamma(\sigma)d\sigma}\,da,$$

$$\leq a_0 + \int_{a_0}^\infty e^{-\frac{v}{k}(\gamma(\infty)-\epsilon)(a-a_0)}\,da = a_0 + \frac{k}{x(\gamma(\infty) - \epsilon)}.$$

From the above relation, the following estimate is easily obtained:

$$F(x) \leq x\left(1 + \frac{v}{k}a_0 + \frac{v}{x(\gamma(\infty) - \epsilon)}\right).$$

Therefore we have

$$\lim_{x\to+0} F(x) \leq \frac{v}{\gamma(\infty) - \epsilon}.$$

Since $R_0^{max} > 1$, we can choose a small ϵ as $0 < \epsilon < \gamma(\infty) - \frac{v}{N}$ in advance, hence we can conclude that $F(+0) < N$. $\square$

Note that even if $R_0(S_0) < 1$, the threshold condition $R_0(S(t, \cdot)) > 1$ will be satisfied as time evolves if $R_0^{max} > 1$. In fact, we can observe that

$$R_0(S(t, \cdot)) = \frac{1}{v}\int_{kt}^\infty \gamma(a)S_0(a - kt)da$$

$$= \frac{1}{v}\int_0^\infty \gamma(a + kt)S_0(a)da \to \frac{\gamma(\infty)N}{v}, \quad (t \to \infty).$$

That is, a host population isolated from the virus for a long enough time will be able to be invaded by the virus as long as $R_0^{max} > 1$.

On the other hand, if R_0^{min} is not zero, it also plays an important role with respect to the long-run behavior of epidemic. In fact, we can prove the following:

Proposition 4.2. *Assume that $R_0^{min} > 1$. Then the following holds:*

$$I(t) \geq \min\left(I(0), N - \frac{v}{\gamma(0)}\right) \quad for \ all \ t \geq 0. \tag{4.5}$$

That is, the disease does not decay. Moreover, if $R_0^{min} > \frac{\gamma(\infty)}{\gamma(0)}$, then there exists a unique endemic steady state.

Proof: Observe that it follows from (2.3) and (2.5) that the following inequality holds for all $t \geq 0$:

$$I'(t) \geq ((\gamma(0)N - v) - \gamma(0)I(t))I(t). \tag{4.6}$$

Then we obtain the inequality

$$I(t) \geq \frac{I(0)(\gamma(0)N - v)}{(\gamma(0)N - v - \gamma(0)I(0))e^{-(\gamma(0)N - v)t} + \gamma(0)I(0)}.$$

The right hand side of the above inequality is monotone increasing if $I(0) < N - \frac{v}{\gamma(0)}$ and monotone decreasing if $I(0) > N - \frac{v}{\gamma(0)}$, and its limit as $t \to \infty$ is $N - \frac{v}{\gamma(0)}$. Hence we have (4.5)

Next let us define a function $\phi(x), x \in (0, N)$ by

$$\phi(x) := 1 + \frac{v}{k} \int_0^\infty e^{-\frac{x}{k} \int_0^a \gamma(\sigma) d\sigma} da - \frac{N}{x}.$$

From (4.4), we know that our epidemic system has endemic steady states if and only if the equation $\phi(x) = 0$ has solutions in $(0, N)$. By differentiating ϕ, we have

$$\phi'(x) = \frac{N}{x^2} - \frac{v}{k^2} \int_0^\infty e^{-\frac{x}{k} \int_0^a \gamma(\sigma) d\sigma} \int_0^a \gamma(\sigma) d\sigma da.$$

Then it is easily seen from elementary calculation that

$$\phi'(x) \geq \frac{1}{x^2} \left(N - \frac{v\gamma(\infty)}{\gamma(0)^2} \right) = \frac{1}{x^2} \frac{v}{\gamma(0)} \left(R_0^{min} - \frac{\gamma(\infty)}{\gamma(0)} \right).$$

Moreover we can obtain the following estimate

$$\phi(x) \leq 1 + \frac{1}{x} \left(-N + \frac{v}{\gamma(0)} \right).$$

Thus it follows that if $R_0^{min} > \frac{\gamma(\infty)}{\gamma(0)} > 1$, $\phi(x)$ is monotone increasing from $-\infty$ to $\phi(N) > 0$. Then the equation $\phi(x) = 0$ has a unique solution in $(0, N)$, which gives the unique endemic level of the infected hosts. $\square$

§5. Semigroup Approach

Here we will use a semigroup approach to the system (2.6)-(2.7) in order to consider the stability of endemic steady states by using the principle of linearized stability in the following section. So in the following we assume that there exists at least one endemic steady state.

Let us introduce a new variable $x(t, a)$ as

$$S(t, a) = S^*(a) + x(t, a), \tag{5.1}$$

where $S^*(a)$ is a stationary solution of (2.6)-(2.7). Then we can rewrite equation (2.6)-(2.7) as follows:

$$\frac{\partial x(t, a)}{\partial t} + \frac{\partial k x(t, a)}{\partial a}$$
$$= -\gamma(a) I^* x(t, a) + \gamma(a)[S^*(a) + x(t, a)] \int_0^\infty x(t, a) da, \tag{5.2}$$

$$k x(t, 0) = -v \int_0^\infty x(t, a) da, \tag{5.3}$$

where $I^* = N - \int_0^\infty S^*(a) da$.

To construct the semigroup solutions for (5.2)-(5.3), let us define a linear operator A with domain $\mathcal{D}(A)$ as follows:

$$(Af)(a) = \left(-k\frac{d}{da} - \gamma(a) I^*\right) f(a), \tag{5.4}$$

$$\mathcal{D}(A) = \left\{f \in L^1(\mathbb{R}_+) : f \in W^{1,1}, f(0) = -\frac{v}{k} \int_0^\infty f(a) da\right\}. \tag{5.5}$$

Moreover we define a nonlinear operator $F : L^1(\mathbb{R}_+) \to L^1(\mathbb{R}_+)$ by

$$F(f)(a) := \gamma(a)[S^*(a) + f(a)] \int_0^\infty f(a) da. \tag{5.6}$$

Then under Assumption 2.1 it is easy to see that the following holds, though we omit the proof:

Lemma 5.1. The operator F is locally Lipschitz continuous, that is, there exists an increasing function $L(r)$ such that $\|F(f) - F(g)\|_{L^1} \le L(r)\|f - g\|_{L^1}$ for all $f, g \in \{f \in L^1(\mathbb{R}_+) : \|f\|_{L^1} \le r\}$.

Note that from the biological meaning, the value $x(t, \cdot)$ should be included in the following subset:

$$\Omega := \left\{f \in L^1(\mathbb{R}_+) : S^* + f \ge 0, \ N \ge \int_0^\infty S^*(a) da + \int_0^\infty f(a) da\right\}.$$

Under the above setting, the time evolution problem (5.2)-(5.3) can be formulated as an abstract semilinear Cauchy problem in $L^1(\mathbb{R}_+)$,

$$\frac{dx(t)}{dt} = Ax(t) + F(x(t)), \quad x(0) = x_0 \in \Omega. \tag{5.7}$$

Lemma 5.2. *The operator A is a densely defined closed linear operator in $L^1(\mathbb{R}_+)$ and it generates a strongly continuous semigroup.*

Proof: It is not difficult to see that the operator A is a closed linear operator in L^1, so we omit the proof. Let us consider the resolvent equation

$$(\lambda - A)f = g, \ f \in \mathcal{D}(A), \ g \in L^1.$$

Then it is easily verified that for $\Re\lambda > -I^*\gamma(0)$, $(\lambda - A)^{-1}$ exists and it is expressed as follows:

$$(\lambda - A)^{-1}g = J(\lambda)g + K(\lambda)g, \tag{5.8}$$

where $J(\lambda)$ and $K(\lambda)$ are defined by

$$(J(\lambda)g)(a) := \frac{1}{k}\int_0^a e^{-\frac{\lambda}{k}(a-s)-\frac{I^*}{k}\int_s^a \gamma(\sigma)d\sigma}g(s)ds,$$

$$(K(\lambda)g)(a) := -\frac{\frac{v}{k}e^{-\frac{\lambda}{k}a-\frac{I^*}{k}\int_0^a \gamma(\sigma)d\sigma}da}{1+\frac{v}{k}\int_0^\infty e^{-\frac{\lambda}{k}a-\frac{I^*}{k}\int_0^a \gamma(\sigma)d\sigma}da}$$

$$\times \frac{1}{k}\int_0^\infty \int_0^a e^{-\frac{\lambda}{k}(a-s)-\frac{I^*}{k}\int_s^a \gamma(\sigma)d\sigma}g(s)dsda.$$

Then it is easily seen that the following estimates hold for $\lambda > -I^*\gamma(0)$:

$$\|J(\lambda)g\|_{L^1} \le \frac{\|g\|_{L^1}}{\lambda + I^*\gamma(0)}, \tag{5.9}$$

$$\|K(\lambda)g\|_{L^1} \le \frac{v}{(\lambda + I^*\gamma(0))^2}\|g\|_{L^1}. \tag{5.10}$$

Therefore we obtain

$$\|\lambda(\lambda - A)^{-1}g - g\|_{L^1} \le \|\lambda J(\lambda)g - g\|_{L^1} + \|\lambda K(\lambda)g\|_{L^1}.$$

From the estimate (5.10), it follows that $\lim_{\lambda\to\infty}\|\lambda K(\lambda)\| = 0$. On the other hand, note that $J(\lambda)$ is the resolvent of a closed linear operator A_0 given by

$$(A_0 f)(a) = \left(-k\frac{d}{da} - \gamma(a)I^*\right)f(a),$$

$$\mathcal{D}(A_0) = \{f \in L^1(\mathbb{R}_+) : f \in W^{1,1}, f(0) = 0\}.$$

Since it is easily seen that the operator A_0 is the infinitesimal generator of a strongly continuous semigroup, it follows that $\lim_{\lambda \to \infty} \|\lambda J(\lambda)g - g\|_{L^1} = 0$ (see [11, p.92], [3]). This shows that the domain $\mathcal{D}(A)$ is dense in L^1, because $\lambda(\lambda - A)^{-1}g \in \mathcal{D}(A)$ for any $g \in L^1$ and $\lim_{\lambda \to \infty} \lambda(\lambda - A)^{-1}g = g$. Moreover, it follows from the above estimate that if $\lambda > v - I^*\gamma(0)$,

$$
\begin{aligned}
\|(\lambda - A)^{-1}\| &\le \frac{1}{\lambda + I^*\gamma(0)} \left[1 + \frac{v}{\lambda + I^*\gamma(0)}\right] \\
&= \frac{1}{\lambda + I^*\gamma(0)} \frac{\lambda + I^*\gamma(0) + v}{\lambda + I^*\gamma(0)} < \frac{1}{\lambda + I^*\gamma(0) - v}.
\end{aligned}
$$

Therefore we arrive at the following inequality:

$$
\|(\lambda - A)^{-1}\| \le \frac{1}{\lambda - (v - I^*\gamma(0))}, \quad \text{for } \lambda > v - I^*\gamma(0). \tag{5.11}
$$

From the Hille-Yosida Theorem, we know that the densely defined closed operator A is the infinitesimal generator of a strongly continuous semigroup $T(t) = \exp(tA)$ such that

$$
\|T(t)\| \le e^{(v - I^*\gamma(0))t}. \tag{5.12}
$$

This completes our proof. $\square$

Proposition 5.3. For any initial data $x_0 \in \Omega \cap \mathcal{D}(A)$, the semilinear problem (5.7) has a unique global classical solution.

Proof: Since the nonlinear term F is continuously Frechet differentiable on L^1, it is well known that for each $x_0 \in L^1$ there exists a maximal interval of existence $[0, t_0)$ and a unique continuous mild solution $x(t; x_0) \in L^1, t \in [0, t_0)$ for (5.7) such that

$$
x(t; x_0) = e^{tA}x_0 + \int_0^t e^{(t-s)A}F(x(s; x_0))ds, \tag{5.13}
$$

for all $t \in [0, t_0)$ and either $t_0 = \infty$ or $\lim_{t \uparrow t_0} \|x(t; x_0)\| = \infty$. Moreover, if we restrict the initial data as $x_0 \in \mathcal{D}(A)$, then $x(t; x_0) \in \mathcal{D}(A)$ and $x(t; x_0)$ is continuously differentiable and satisfies (5.7) on $[0, t_0)$ (Pazy [8]; Webb [11]). Let $x(t; x_0)$ be a classical solution of (5.7) with $x_0 \in \mathcal{D}(A)$ and let

$$
I(t) := I^* - \int_0^\infty x(t; x_0)(a)da.
$$

Observe that

$$
\frac{dI(t)}{dt} = -\int_0^\infty (Ax(t; x_0) + F(x(t; x_0)))(a)da = I(t)\int_0^\infty \gamma(a)x(t; x_0)(a)da.
$$

Therefore we obtain

$$I(t) = I(0) \exp \left(\int_0^t \int_0^\infty \gamma(a) x(s : x_0)(a) da \, ds \right).$$

Then it follows that if $x_0 \in \Omega$, $I(t) \geq 0$ for all $t \geq 0$. Moreover if we let $S(t, a) := S^*(a) + x(t; x_0)(a)$, it follows that S satisfies the following equation for almost every $a \in \mathbb{R}_+$:

$$\frac{\partial S(t, a)}{\partial t} = \left(-\frac{\partial k S(t, a)}{\partial a} - \gamma(a) I(t) \right) S(t, a),$$

$$S(t, 0) = \frac{v}{k} I(t).$$

Then $S(t, a)$ admits the explicit representation (3.1), hence we obtain that $S(t, a) = S^*(a) + x(t; x_0)(a) \geq 0$ and $I(t) = N - \int_0^\infty S(t, a) da \geq 0$. Therefore $x(t, x_0) \in \Omega$ and the maximal interval of existence is $[0, \infty)$ if $x_0 \in \Omega$. This completes our proof. $\square$

§6. Local Stability

Here we consider the linearized equation at the steady state,

$$\frac{\partial x(t, a)}{\partial t} + \frac{\partial k x(t, a)}{\partial a} = -\gamma(a) I^* x(t, a) + \gamma(a) S^*(a) \int_0^\infty x(t, a) da, \quad (6.1)$$

$$k x(t, 0) = -v \int_0^\infty x(t, a) da. \quad (6.2)$$

Using the abstract setting, (6.1)-(6.2) can be formulated as the linear Cauchy problem in L^1,

$$\frac{d}{dt} x(t) = A x(t) + F'[0] x(t), \quad (6.3)$$

where $F'[0]$ is the Frechet derivative of F at the equilibrium $x = 0$ defined by

$$(F'[0] f)(a) = \gamma(a) S^*(a) \int_0^\infty f(a) da.$$

In order to investigate the stability of the equilibrium $x = 0$, let us consider the resolvent equation for $A + F'[0]$:

$$(\lambda - (A + F'[0])) f = g, \quad f \in \mathcal{D}(A), \ g \in L^1, \ \lambda \in \mathbb{C}. \quad (6.4)$$

Then we obtain

$$k f'(a) + (\lambda + \gamma(a) I^*) f(a) = g(a) + \gamma(a) S^*(a) \int_0^\infty f(z) dz, \quad (6.5)$$

$$f(0) = -\frac{v}{k} \int_0^\infty f(z) dz. \quad (6.6)$$

By formal integration, we have the following expression:

$$f(a) = \frac{1}{k} \int_0^a e^{-\frac{\lambda}{k}(a-s)-\frac{I^*}{k}\int_s^a \gamma(\sigma)d\sigma} g(s)ds \tag{6.7}$$

$$+ \frac{1}{1-\Delta(\lambda)} \frac{1}{k} \int_0^\infty \int_0^a e^{-\frac{\lambda}{k}(a-s)-\frac{I^*}{k}\int_s^a \gamma(\sigma)d\sigma} g(s)dsda$$

$$\times \left\{ -\frac{v}{k} e^{-\frac{\lambda}{k}a-\frac{I^*}{k}\int_0^a \gamma(\sigma)d\sigma} + \frac{1}{k} \int_0^a e^{-\frac{\lambda}{k}(a-s)-\frac{I^*}{k}\int_s^a \gamma(\sigma)d\sigma} \gamma(s)S^*(s)ds \right\},$$

where the mapping $\Delta(\lambda) : \mathbf{C} \to \mathbf{C}$ is defined by

$$\Delta(\lambda) = \frac{1}{k} \int_0^\infty \int_0^a e^{-\frac{\lambda}{k}(a-s)-\frac{I^*}{k}\int_s^a \gamma(\sigma)d\sigma} \gamma(s)S^*(s)dsda \tag{6.8}$$

$$- \frac{v}{k} \int_0^\infty e^{-\frac{\lambda}{k}a-\frac{I^*}{k}\int_0^a \gamma(\sigma)d\sigma} da.$$

We call the complex number λ satisfying the equation $\Delta(\lambda) = 1$ a *characteristic root*.

Here we introduce some notation from functional analysis. For definitions, the reader may refer to Webb [10,11]. Let $\sigma(A)$ be the spectrum of A, let $P_\sigma(A)$ be the point spectrum of A, let $E\sigma(A)$ be the essential spectrum of A and let $\rho(A)$ be the resolvent set of A. In case that the operator A generates a strongly continuous semigroup, $\omega_0(A)$ denotes the growth bound of the semigroup e^{tA} and $\omega_1(A)$ denotes the α-growth bound of e^{tA}.

Lemma 6.1.

(1) $\omega_1(A + F'[0]) \le -\gamma(0)I^*$,

(2) If $\Re\lambda > -\gamma(0)I^*$ and $\Delta(\lambda) = 1$, then $\lambda \in P_\sigma(A + F'[0])$,

(3) If $\Re\lambda > -\gamma(0)I^*$, then $\lambda \in \sigma(A + F'[0])$ if and only if $\lambda \in P_\sigma(A + F'[0])$ if and only if $\lambda \in \{\lambda \in \mathbf{C} : \Re\lambda > -\gamma(0)I^*, \Delta(\lambda) = 1\}$.

Proof: Note that $F'[0]$ is one-dimensional, so it is a compact perturbation. Then it follows that $\omega_1(A + F'[0]) = \omega_1(A)$. If we consider the linear system without perturbation,

$$\frac{d}{dt}x(t) = Ax(t),$$

then it is well known for this type of population operator that $\omega_1(A) \le -\gamma(0)I^*$ (see Webb [10,11]). Hence (1) follows immediately. Next if $\Re\lambda > -\gamma(0)I^*$ and $\Delta(\lambda) = 1$, we can see that

$$f_\lambda(a) = \frac{1}{k} \int_0^a e^{-\frac{\lambda}{k}(a-s)-\frac{I^*}{k}\int_s^a \gamma(\sigma)d\sigma} \gamma(s)S^*(s)ds - \frac{v}{k} e^{-\frac{\lambda}{k}a-\frac{I^*}{k}\int_0^a \gamma(\sigma)d\sigma}$$

is an eigenfunction associated with eigenvalue λ. Then (2) follows. Thirdly suppose that $\lambda \in \sigma(A + F'[0])$ and $\Re\lambda > -\gamma(0)I^*$. Since

$$\omega_1(A + F'[0]) \le -\gamma(0)I^*,$$

we have $\lambda \in \sigma(A + F'[0]) - E\sigma(A + F'[0])$ because

$$\sup_{\lambda \in E\sigma(B)} \Re\lambda \leq \omega_1(B)$$

for an infinitesimal generator B (see Webb [11, Prop. 4.15]). Moreover if $\lambda \in \sigma(A + F'[0]) - E\sigma(A + F'[0])$, then it follows that $\lambda \in P_\sigma(A + F'[0])$ and λ is a pole of $(\lambda - (A + F'[0]))^{-1}$ (Webb [11, Prop. 4.11]). Then we obtain (3), since a pole of the resolvent is a pole of $1/(1 - \Delta(\lambda))$. $\square$

Proposition 6.2. *Assume that $\gamma(0) > 0$ and $\Re\lambda < 0$ for any $\lambda \in P_\sigma(A + F'[0]) \cap \{\lambda \in \mathbf{C} : \Re\lambda > -\gamma(0)I^*\}$. Then the endemic steady state (S^*, I^*) is locally asymptotically stable.*

Proof: First note that there can be only finitely many λ such that $\lambda \in P_\sigma(A + F'[0]) \cap \{\lambda \in \mathbf{C} : \Re\lambda > -\gamma(0)I^*\}$. In fact, if there exists an infinite sequence λ_k $(k = 1, 2, \cdots)$ such that $\lambda_k \in P_\sigma(A + F'[0]) \cap \{\lambda \in \mathbf{C} : \Re\lambda > -\gamma(0)I^*\}$, we can assume that $\lim_{k\to\infty} |\Im\lambda_k| = \infty$, because $1 - \Delta(\lambda)$ is holomorphic for $\Re\lambda > -\gamma(0)I^*$ and its zeros cannot accumulate in this strip. However, by using the Riemann-Lebesgue theorem, we can show that $\lim_{k\to\infty}[1 - \Delta(\lambda_k)] = 1$, which is a contradiction because $1 - \Delta(\lambda_k) = 0$ for all k. Hence under our assumptions it follows that

$$\lambda_0 := \sup_{\lambda \in \sigma(A+F'[0]) - E\sigma(A+F'[0])} \Re\lambda < 0.$$

Therefore it follows from Proposition 4.13 of Webb [11] that

$$\omega_0(A + F'[0]) = \max\{\omega_1(A + F'[0]), \lambda_0\} < 0.$$

Then it follows immediately that $\lim_{t\to\infty} \|e^{t(A+F'[0])}\| = 0$. By the principle of linearized stability (Desch and Schappacher [4]), we can conclude that the endemic steady state (S^*, I^*) is locally asymptotically stable. $\square$

Subsequently we consider concrete conditions under which there is no characteristic root with nonnegative real part, since it guarantees the local stability of the endemic steady state. First we remark the following partial answer:

Proposition 6.3. *Assume that $\gamma(0) > 0$. Let $\lambda \in P_\sigma(A + F'[0]) \cap \mathbb{R}$. If the condition*

$$R_0^{min} > \frac{\gamma(\infty)}{\gamma(0)}, \tag{6.9}$$

holds, it follows that $\lambda < 0$, that is, there is no nonnegative characteristic root.

Proof: Integrating by parts, we can show that the equation $\Delta(\lambda) = 1$ is equivalent to the following equation:

$$N = \Lambda(\lambda) := \frac{vI^*}{k} \int_0^\infty \int_0^a \left[\frac{\lambda + I^*\gamma(z)}{k}\right] e^{-\frac{\lambda}{k}(a-z) - \frac{I^*}{k}\int_0^a \gamma(\sigma)d\sigma} dz\,da. \tag{6.10}$$

In fact, it follows that $\Lambda(\lambda) = N + I^*(\Delta(\lambda) - 1)$. Then if $\lambda \geq 0$, we obtain

$$|\Lambda(\lambda)| \leq \frac{vI^*}{k} \int_0^\infty \int_0^a \left[\frac{\lambda + I^*\gamma(z)}{k} \right] e^{-\frac{\Re e\lambda}{k}(a-z) - \frac{I^*}{k}\gamma(0)a} dzda$$

$$\leq \frac{v}{\gamma(0)} \frac{\lambda + I^*\gamma(\infty)}{\lambda + I^*\gamma(0)}.$$

Then if the condition (6.9) is satisfied, we have

$$|\Lambda(\lambda)| \leq \frac{v}{\gamma(0)} \frac{\lambda + I^*\gamma(\infty)}{\lambda + I^*\gamma(0)} \leq \frac{v\gamma(\infty)}{\gamma(0)^2} < N.$$

Then the equation $\Lambda(\lambda) = N$ has no nonnegative root. This completes the proof. □

Proposition 6.4. *Assume that $\gamma(0) > 0$. If the following condition holds*

$$R_0^{min} > 2 + \frac{\gamma(\infty)}{\gamma(0)}, \tag{6.11}$$

then there exists a unique endemic steady state and it is locally stable.

Proof: The unique existence of an endemic steady state follows directly from Proposition 4.2, because (6.11) implies $R_0^{min} > \frac{\gamma(\infty)}{\gamma(0)}$. In order to show its local stability, we prove that under the assumption (6.11), the characteristic equation $\Delta(\lambda) = 1$ has no root in the right half plane $\Re e\lambda \geq 0$. First we write

$$1 - \Delta(\lambda) = g(\lambda) + f(\lambda),$$

where

$$g(\lambda) := \frac{v}{k} \int_0^\infty e^{-\frac{\lambda}{k}a - \frac{I^*}{k}\int_0^a \gamma(\sigma)d\sigma} da,$$

$$f(\lambda) := 1 - \frac{1}{k} \int_0^\infty \int_0^a e^{-\frac{\lambda}{k}(a-s) - \frac{I^*}{k}\int_s^a \gamma(\sigma)d\sigma} \gamma(s)S^*(s)dsda.$$

Then g and f are entire functions of $\lambda \in \mathbf{C}$. Consider the roots of the equation $f(\lambda) = 0$. By an elementary calculation, we obtain

$$|f(\lambda)| \geq f(\Re e\lambda) \geq 1 - \frac{v\gamma(\infty)}{\gamma(0)(\Re e\lambda + I^*\gamma(0))}, \text{ for } \Re e\lambda \geq 0. \tag{6.12}$$

In particular, it follows that

$$f(0) \geq 1 - \frac{v\gamma(\infty)}{I^*\gamma(0)^2}.$$

Thus under the condition

$$I^* > \frac{v\gamma(\infty)}{\gamma(0)^2}, \tag{6.13}$$

we can conclude that $|f(\lambda)| \geq f(\Re\lambda) \geq f(0) > 0$ in the right half plane $\Re\lambda \geq 0$, that is, $f(\lambda)$ has no zeros in the right half plane. On the other hand, it is easy to see that

$$|g(\lambda)| \leq \frac{v}{\Re\lambda + I^*\gamma(0)}. \tag{6.14}$$

From (6.12) and (6.14), if

$$1 - \frac{v\gamma(\infty)}{\gamma(0)(\Re\lambda + I^*\gamma(0))} > \frac{v}{\Re\lambda + I^*\gamma(0)} \tag{6.15}$$

holds, we have the relation

$$|f(\lambda)| > |g(\lambda)| \tag{6.16}$$

for any λ in the right half plane $\Re\lambda \geq 0$. Then it is easily seen that the following condition is sufficient for the relation (6.15) to hold in the right half plane:

$$I^* > \frac{v(\gamma(\infty) + \gamma(0))}{\gamma(0)^2}. \tag{6.17}$$

Finally note that from (4.3) we have the following estimate:

$$I^* = N - \frac{vI^*}{k} \int_0^\infty e^{-\frac{I^*}{k} \int_0^a \gamma(\sigma)d\sigma} da \geq N - \frac{v}{\gamma(0)}. \tag{6.18}$$

Therefore if the following condition holds

$$N - \frac{v}{\gamma(0)} > \frac{v(\gamma(\infty) + \gamma(0))}{\gamma(0)^2}, \tag{6.19}$$

then the condition (6.17) is satisfied and we can conclude that $|f(\lambda)| > |g(\lambda)|$ in the right half plane. The condition (6.19) can be written as (6.11) and it also implies the condition (6.13). Hence it follows from Rouché's theorem that under the condition (6.11), $f(\lambda) + g(\lambda)$ and $f(\lambda)$ have the same number of zeros in the right half plane, hence the characteristic equation has no root in the right half plane. $\square$

Finally note that since $\lim_{\lambda \to \infty}[1 - \Delta(\lambda)] = 1$, it follows immediately that there exists a positive characteristic root if $1 - \Delta(0) < 0$. That is, a sufficient condition for the instability of the endemic steady state is given as follows:

$$1 + \frac{v}{k} \int_0^\infty e^{-\frac{I^*}{k} \int_0^a \gamma(\sigma)d\sigma} da < \frac{1}{k} \int_0^\infty \int_0^a e^{-\frac{I^*}{k} \int_s^a \gamma(\sigma)d\sigma} \gamma(s)S^*(s)ds\,da. \tag{6.20}$$

§7. Effects of Vaccination

In this section we consider how a vaccination strategy could affect the dynamics of our evolutionary epidemic model. Though there exist many vaccination strategies, we here assume a simple one, that is, uninfected hosts are vaccinated by a constant rate per unit time. Let $\epsilon > 0$ be the rate of vaccination. Since the biological age a of newly vaccinated hosts is reset to be zero, we obtain a new system:

$$\frac{\partial S(t,a)}{\partial t} + \frac{\partial kS(t,a)}{\partial a} = -\epsilon S(t,a) - \gamma(a)S(t,a)I(t), \tag{7.1}$$

$$\frac{dI(t)}{dt} = -vI(t) + I(t)\int_0^\infty \gamma(a)S(t,a)da, \tag{7.2}$$

$$kS(t,0) = vI(t) + \epsilon \int_0^\infty S(t,a)da. \tag{7.3}$$

An important feature different from the original system without vaccination is that a disease-free steady state appears. First we consider the initial invasion phase. Observe that in this case a disease-free steady state is given by

$$S^*(a) = \frac{\epsilon N}{k}e^{-\frac{\epsilon}{k}a}, \quad I^* = 0. \tag{7.4}$$

Then we can define the basic reproduction ratio as

$$R_0 = \frac{1}{v}\int_0^\infty \gamma(a)S^*(a)da = \frac{\epsilon N}{kv}\int_0^\infty e^{-\frac{\epsilon}{k}a}\gamma(a)da. \tag{7.5}$$

Here we should note that R_0 is not monotone decreasing with respect to the rate of vaccination ϵ. However we can prove that

Proposition 7.1. If $R_0^{min} < 1$, then $R_0 < 1$ for sufficiently large ϵ.

Proof: For any $\xi > 0$, there exists a $\delta > 0$ such that $\gamma(a) \leq \gamma(0) + \xi$ for $a \in [0, \delta]$. Then it follows that

$$R_0 \leq \frac{N}{v}\left[\int_0^\delta \phi(a)(\gamma(0) + \xi)da + \int_\delta^\infty \phi(a)\gamma(\infty)da\right],$$

where $\phi(a) := \frac{\epsilon}{k}e^{-\frac{\epsilon}{k}a}$. Therefore we obtain

$$R_0 \leq \frac{N}{v}\left[(\gamma(0) + \xi) + \gamma(\infty)e^{-\frac{\epsilon\delta}{k}}\right].$$

Thus we have

$$\lim_{\epsilon\to\infty} R_0 \leq \frac{N(\gamma(0) + \xi)}{v}.$$

Since $\xi > 0$ can be chosen as any small number, it follows that

$$\lim_{\epsilon\to\infty} R_0 \leq \frac{N\gamma(0)}{v} = R_0^{min}.$$

This shows that if $R_0^{min} < 1$, then R_0 is smaller than the unity for sufficiently large ϵ. $\square$

From the above result, we know that if $R_0^{min} < 1$, the entirely susceptible population could in principle be prevented from the disease invasion by introducing vaccination. But note that since the equation (7.2) is the same as (2.3), Proposition 4.2 again holds for the vaccination model. Then if $R_0^{min} > 1$ the disease is persistent if the host population is once invaded by the virus; it cannot be eradicated by the vaccination as considered here. On the other hand, if $R_0^{max} < 1$ the disease is automatically eradicated as time passes. Let $(S^*(a), I^*)$ be a steady state solution for system (7.1)-(7.3). Then we have

$$\frac{dS^*(a)}{da} = -\frac{\epsilon}{k}S^*(a) - \frac{\gamma(a)I^*}{k}S^*(a), \tag{7.6}$$

$$kS^*(0) = vI^* + \epsilon \int_0^\infty S^*(a)da. \tag{7.7}$$

Therefore we have

$$S^*(a) = S^*(0)e^{-\frac{\epsilon}{k}a - \frac{I^*}{k}\int_0^a \gamma(\sigma)d\sigma}. \tag{7.8}$$

Integrating (7.8) from zero to infinity and using the boundary condition (7.7), we can obtain the following expression:

$$\int_0^\infty S^*(a)da = \frac{\frac{vI^*}{k}\int_0^\infty e^{-\frac{\epsilon}{k}a - \frac{I^*}{k}\int_0^a \gamma(\sigma)d\sigma}da}{1 - \frac{\epsilon}{k}\int_0^\infty e^{-\frac{\epsilon}{k}a - \frac{I^*}{k}\int_0^a \gamma(\sigma)d\sigma}da}, \tag{7.9}$$

where the denominator is positive if $I^* > 0$. Therefore I^* must satisfy the following equation

$$N = I^* + \frac{\frac{vI^*}{k}\int_0^\infty e^{-\frac{\epsilon}{k}a - \frac{I^*}{k}\int_0^a \gamma(\sigma)d\sigma}da}{1 - \frac{\epsilon}{k}\int_0^\infty e^{-\frac{\epsilon}{k}a - \frac{I^*}{k}\int_0^a \gamma(\sigma)d\sigma}da}. \tag{7.10}$$

Proposition 7.2. *Assume that the following condition holds:*

$$R_1 := \frac{N\epsilon^2}{vk^2}\int_0^\infty e^{-\frac{\epsilon}{k}a}\int_0^a \gamma(\sigma)d\sigma da > 1. \tag{7.11}$$

Then the epidemic model with vaccination term (7.1)-(7.3) has at least one endemic steady state. In particular, if $R_0^{min} > 1$, there exists at least one endemic steady state.

Proof: Let us consider a function $\psi(x)$ defined by

$$\psi(x) = x\left(1 + \frac{v}{\epsilon}\frac{\phi(x)}{1 - \phi(x)}\right),$$

where

$$\phi(x) := \frac{\epsilon}{k} \int_0^\infty e^{-\frac{\epsilon}{k}a - \frac{x}{k}\int_0^a \gamma(\sigma)d\sigma}\, da.$$

Then it is clear that the positive solutions of equation $\psi(x) = N, x \in (0, N)$ correspond to the possible endemic levels of infected hosts. Observe that $\psi(N) > N$ and

$$\lim_{x \to +0} \psi(x) = \frac{v}{\epsilon}\lim_{x \to +0} \frac{x\phi(x)}{1 - \phi(x)} = \frac{v}{\epsilon}\frac{\phi(0)}{-\phi'(0)} = \frac{N}{R_1}.$$

Therefore if $R_1 > 1$, then $\psi(+0) < N$, and hence we can conclude that there exists at least one positive root $x \in (0, N)$ for the equation $\psi(x) = N$. Finally it is easy to see that $R_1 \geq R_0^{min}$. Then it follows that if $R_0^{min} > 1$, there exists at least one endemic steady state. $\square$

Let $x(t, a)$ be a small perturbation from the endemic steady state $S^*(a)$. Then the linearized equation at the endemic steady state is easily derived as follows:

$$\frac{\partial x(t, a)}{\partial t} + \frac{\partial k x(t, a)}{\partial a} = -(\epsilon + \gamma(a)I^*)x(t, a) + \gamma(a)S^*(a)\int_0^\infty x(t, a)da, \quad (7.12)$$

$$x(t, 0) = \frac{\epsilon - v}{k}\int_0^\infty x(t, a)da. \quad (7.13)$$

In order to investigate the stability of the equilibrium $x = 0$, let us again consider the resolvent equation for $A_\epsilon + F'[0]$:

$$(\lambda - (A_\epsilon + F'[0]))f = g, \quad f \in \mathcal{D}(A_\epsilon), \ g \in L^1, \ \lambda \in \mathbb{C}, \quad (7.14)$$

where the operator A_ϵ is defined by

$$(A_\epsilon)(a) := \left(-k\frac{d}{da} - (\epsilon + \gamma(a)I^*)\right)f(a), \quad (7.15)$$

$$\mathcal{D}(A_\epsilon) = \left\{f \in L^1(\mathbb{R}_+) : f \in W^{1,1}, f(0) = \frac{\epsilon - v}{k}\int_0^\infty f(a)da\right\}. \quad (7.16)$$

Then we obtain

$$kf'(a) + (\epsilon + \lambda + \gamma(a)I^*)f(a) = g(a) + \gamma(a)S^*(a)\int_0^\infty f(z)dz, \quad (7.17)$$

$$f(0) = \frac{\epsilon - v}{k}\int_0^\infty f(z)dz. \quad (7.18)$$

By formal integration, we have the following expression:

$$f(a) = \frac{1}{k}\int_0^a e^{-\frac{\epsilon+\lambda}{k}(a-s) - \frac{I^*}{k}\int_s^a \gamma(\sigma)d\sigma}g(s)ds \quad (7.19)$$

$$+ \frac{1}{1 - \Delta_\epsilon(\lambda)}\frac{1}{k}\int_0^\infty \int_0^a e^{-\frac{\epsilon+\lambda}{k}(a-s) - \frac{I^*}{k}\int_s^a \gamma(\sigma)d\sigma}g(s)dsda$$

$$\times \left\{\frac{\epsilon - v}{k}e^{-\frac{\epsilon+\lambda}{k}a - \frac{I^*}{k}\int_0^a \gamma(\sigma)d\sigma} + \frac{1}{k}\int_0^a e^{-\frac{\epsilon+\lambda}{k}(a-s) - \frac{I^*}{k}\int_s^a \gamma(\sigma)d\sigma}\gamma(s)S^*(s)ds\right\},$$

where the mapping $\Delta_\epsilon(\lambda) : \mathbb{C} \to \mathbb{C}$ is defined by

$$\Delta_\epsilon(\lambda) := \frac{1}{k} \int_0^\infty \int_0^a e^{-\frac{\epsilon+\lambda}{k}(a-s)-\frac{I^*}{k}\int_s^a \gamma(\sigma)d\sigma} \gamma(s)S^*(s)dsda \qquad (7.20)$$
$$+ \frac{\epsilon - v}{k} \int_0^\infty e^{-\frac{\epsilon+\lambda}{k}a-\frac{I^*}{k}\int_0^a \gamma(\sigma)d\sigma} da.$$

Proposition 7.3. *Suppose that $\gamma(0) > 0$ and the following condition holds:*

$$R_0^{min} > 1 + \frac{\gamma(\infty)}{\gamma(0)} + \frac{|v - \epsilon|}{v}. \qquad (7.21)$$

Then there exists at least one endemic steady state which is locally asymptotically stable.

Proof: The existence of an endemic steady state follows from Proposition 7.2. In order to show its local stability, we prove that under assumption (7.21), the characteristic equation $\Delta_\epsilon(\lambda) = 1$ has no root in the half plane $\Re\lambda \geq 0$. As in the proof of Proposition 6.4, we write

$$1 - \Delta_\epsilon(\lambda) = g_\epsilon(\lambda) + f_\epsilon(\lambda),$$

where

$$g_\epsilon(\lambda) := \frac{v - \epsilon}{k} \int_0^\infty e^{-\frac{\epsilon+\lambda}{k}a-\frac{I^*}{k}\int_0^a \gamma(\sigma)d\sigma} da,$$
$$f_\epsilon(\lambda) := 1 - \frac{1}{k} \int_0^\infty \int_0^a e^{-\frac{\epsilon+\lambda}{k}(a-s)-\frac{I^*}{k}\int_s^a \gamma(\sigma)d\sigma} \gamma(s)S^*(s)dsda.$$

By an elementary calculation, we obtain

$$|f_\epsilon(\lambda)| \geq f_\epsilon(\Re\lambda) \geq 1 - \frac{v\gamma(\infty)}{\gamma(0)}(\epsilon + \Re\lambda + I^*\gamma(0)), \quad \text{for } \Re\lambda \geq 0. \qquad (7.22)$$

In particular, it follows that

$$f_\epsilon(0) \geq 1 - \frac{v\gamma(\infty)}{I^*\gamma(0)^2}.$$

Thus under the condition

$$I^* > \frac{v\gamma(\infty)}{\gamma(0)^2}, \qquad (7.23)$$

we can conclude that $|f(\lambda)| \geq f(\Re\lambda) \geq f(0) > 0$ in the right half plane $\Re\lambda \geq 0$, that is, $f(\lambda)$ has no zero in the right half plane. On the other hand, it is easy to see that

$$|g_\epsilon(\lambda)| \leq \frac{|v - \epsilon|}{\epsilon + \Re\lambda + I^*\gamma(0)}. \qquad (7.24)$$

From (7.22) and (7.24), if

$$1 - \frac{v\gamma(\infty)}{\epsilon + \gamma(0)(\Re\lambda + I^*\gamma(0))} > \frac{|v - \epsilon|}{\epsilon + \Re\lambda + I^*\gamma(0)} \tag{7.25}$$

holds, we have the relation

$$|f(\lambda)| > |g(\lambda)| \tag{7.26}$$

for any λ in the right half plane $\Re\lambda \geq 0$. Observe that the following condition is sufficient for relation (7.25) to hold in the right half plane:

$$I^* > \frac{v\gamma(\infty)}{\epsilon + \gamma(0)^2} + \frac{|v - \epsilon|}{\epsilon + \gamma(0)}. \tag{7.27}$$

Finally note that from (7.10) we have the following estimate:

$$I^* = N - \frac{\frac{vI^*}{k} \int_0^\infty e^{-\frac{\epsilon}{k} - \frac{I^*}{k} \int_0^a \gamma(\sigma)d\sigma} da}{1 - \frac{\epsilon}{k} \int_0^\infty e^{-\frac{\epsilon}{k} - \frac{I^*}{k} \int_0^a \gamma(\sigma)d\sigma} da} \geq N - \frac{v}{\gamma(0)}. \tag{7.28}$$

Therefore if the following condition holds

$$N - \frac{v}{\gamma(0)} > \frac{v\gamma(\infty)}{\epsilon + \gamma(0)^2} + \frac{|v - \epsilon|}{\epsilon + \gamma(0)}, \tag{7.29}$$

then the condition (7.25) is satisfied and we can conclude that $|f(\lambda)| > |g(\lambda)|$ in the right half plane. The condition (7.21) implies (7.29) and (7.23). Hence it follows from Rouché's theorem that under the condition (7.21) $f(\lambda) + g(\lambda)$ and $f(\lambda)$ have the same number of zeros in the right half plane and $f(\lambda)$ has no zero in the right half plane, hence the characteristic equation has no root in the right half plane also. □

Finally, we show that the classical invasion condition holds for the evolutionary epidemic model with vaccination term:

Proposition 7.4. *If $R_0 < 1$, then the disease-free steady state is locally asymptotically stable and if $R_0 > 1$, it is unstable.*

Proof: To show the local stability, it is sufficient to prove that the characteristic equation $\Delta_\epsilon(\lambda) = 1$ has no root in the right half plane. From (7.20), the characteristic equation for the trivial steady state is given as follows:

$$\Delta_\epsilon(\lambda) = \frac{1}{\epsilon + \lambda} \frac{\epsilon N}{k} \int_0^\infty \gamma(a)e^{-\frac{\lambda}{k}a}da + \frac{\epsilon - v}{\epsilon + \lambda} = 1.$$

Then only one possible characteristic root is given as

$$\lambda_0 = -v + \frac{\epsilon N}{k} \int_0^\infty \gamma(a)e^{-\frac{\lambda}{k}a}da = v(R_0 - 1).$$

Then if $R_0 < 1$, we conclude that there is no nonnegative characteristic root, which implies the local stability of the disease-free steady state. On the other hand, if $R_0 > 1$, the disease-free steady state is unstable because there is a positive characteristic root. □

§8. Discussion

In this paper we have discussed some mathematical aspects of the evolutionary epidemic model. We have established the existence and uniqueness of solutions, and then we have shown a threshold condition for existence of endemic steady states. Next we adopted a semigroup formulation to consider the stability of endemic steady states and proved a sufficient condition to guarantee the local stability of an endemic steady state. Finally, we extended our results to the model with a vaccination term.

Here it should be noted that we have adopted a technical condition such that $\gamma(0) > 0$ to obtain results for local stability. Biologically, this assumption means that recovery from infection by a type of virus does not lead a complete immunity to the same type of virus. This would be a doubtful assumption, at least if we consider influenza virus, because it is normally thought that an individual recovered from influenza infection would not be again infected within the same epidemic. On the other hand, it is reasonable to assume that the immunity led by vaccination would be partial and vaccinated individual could be infected by the same type of virus. Under the above mentioned assumption of partial immunity, our stability analysis suggests that for sufficiently large R_0^{min}, there would exist a unique endemic steady state with local stability, which is similar to the situation of a non-evolutionary epidemic. Investigation of the long term behavior of solutions when $R_0^{min} \approx 0$ is an interesting, but difficult open problem. One of the most important questions would be whether the evolutionary epidemic mechanism could explain the sustained oscillations as observed in influenza. It would also be an interesting problem to loosen our assumption and treat the model in which $\gamma(a)$ could become infinite as a increases.

Throughout this paper we have neglected demography of the host population, but to consider the long-run behavior of the epidemic with reality, we should combine the epidemic process with the demography of the host population. For this purpose, we would have to introduce a new class of subpopulation, that is, a group of individuals who have never been infected. Newborns are the inflow to this new class. This type of model will be investigated in a separate paper.

Another basic assumption adopted here is that the rate of amino acid substitution, k, is constant. If density-dependent selection rather than random drift is causing genetic changes in the virus, the rate of amino acid substitution should be assumed to be a function of the number of infected hosts. In such a case, the evolutionary epidemiological models could show more complicated dynamics and it would be an interesting future challenge.

As was pointed out by Pease, the genetic variations in the pathogen, which is the prerequisite of the evolutionary mechanism, are widely observed among viral diseases. Hence the evolutionary mechanism may work in many viral diseases other than influenza and would make control of infectious diseases more difficult. The reader may find some recent developments in the understanding of the evolutionary mechanism in Andreasen, Levin and Lin

[1,2] for influenza dynamics and in Nowak and May [7] for HIV dynamics. Designing an effective vaccination program will first require more knowledge of the evolutionary mechanism of the viral diseases. This would be important non-mathematical motivation for applying mathematical analysis to the evolutionary epidemic model.

References

1. Andreasen, V., S. Levin and J. Lin, A model of influenza A drift evolution, Z. Angew. Math. Mech. **76,** S2 (1996), 421–424.

2. Andreasen, V., J. Lin and S. A. Levin, The dynamics of cocirculating influenza strains conferring partial cross-immunity, J. Math. Biol. **35** (1997), 825–842.

3. Belleni-Morante, A. and G. Busoni, Some remarks on densely defined streaming operators, Math. Comput. Modelling **21,** No. 8, (1995), 13–15.

4. Desch, W. and W. Schappacher, Linearized stability for nonlinear semigroups, In *Differential Equations in Banach Spaces*, A. Favini and E. Obrecht (eds.), LNM 1223, Springer-Verlag, Berlin, 1986, 61–73.

5. Iannelli, M., *Mathematical Theory of Age-Structured Population Dynamics*, Applied Mathematics Monographs 7, C. N. R., Giardini Editori e Stampatori in Pisa, 1995.

6. Miller, R. M., *Nonlinear Volterra Integral Equations*, W. A. Benjamin, Menlo Park, 1971.

7. Nowak, M. A. and R. A. May, Mathematical biology of HIV infections: antigenic variation and diversity threshold, Math. Biosci. **106**(1) (1991), 1–21.

8. Pazy, A. *Semigroups of Linear Operators and Applications to Partial Differential Equations*, Springer-Verlag, New York, 1983.

9. Pease, C. M., An evolutionary epidemiological mechanism, with applications to type A influenza, Theor. Popul. Biol. **31** (1987), 422–452.

10. Webb, G. F., A semigroup proof of the Sharpe-Lotka theorem, in *Infinite-Dimensional Systems*, F. Kappel and W. Schappacher (eds.), LNM 1076, Springer-Verlag, Berlin, 1984, 254–268.

11. Webb, G. F., *Theory of Nonlinear Age-Dependent Population Dynamics*, Marcel Dekker, New York and Basel, 1985.

Hisashi Inaba
Department of Mathematical Sciences
University of Tokyo
3-8-1 Komaba Meguro-ku
Tokyo 153
Japan
inaba@ms.u-tokyo.ac.jp

A Mathematical Model of the
Time Course of Myelosuppression
Resulting from Cancer Chemotherapy

Paul B. Laub

Abstract. Mathematical derivation of an indirect response model of the time course of myelosuppression from cancer chemotherapy is presented. Concentration of circulating, bone marrow-derived cells, typically neutrophils or platelets, in the blood is described as governed by rates of synthesis and removal (e.g., death) of these cells. Myelosuppression is posited to act through the temporary cessation of progenitor cell proliferation in marrow. The ability of the model to be fit to simulated and actual clinical data is evaluated.

§1. Introduction

Myelosuppression (MYS), that is, temporary depletion of neutrophils and platelets from blood, is a common outcome of cancer chemotherapy, which when extreme leaves the patient susceptible to life-threatening infection and hemorrhage [10]. However, alleviating MYS by reducing subsequent doses leaves the patient at risk from a cancer treated at insufficient dose intensity. For many of the widely used anticancer drugs, such as topotecan, paclitaxel and carboplatin, MYS is a major, often dose-limiting, toxicity [6]. Thus a major challenge for oncology is creating tolerable treatment regimens combining these active, but mutually myelosuppressive, drugs [14].

Administration of colony stimulating factors (CSFs), such as granulocyte-colony stimulating factor, helps manage of neutropenia, one form of MYS. These recombinant protein pharmaceuticals are clinically effective in rapidly stimulating neutrophil production. However, their high cost [1] impedes their use. In addition, their current style of use has yet to translate into practical clinical benefit such as reduced hospitalization [9].

Timing and sequencing of single and multiple drugs are important in clinical studies. Dose-limiting toxicity of paclitaxel changes from hypersensitivity

Mathematical Models in Medical and Health Sciences
Mary Ann Horn, Gieri Simonett, and Glenn Webb (eds.), pp. 237–245.
Copyright © 1998 by Vanderbilt University Press, Nashville, TN.
ISBN 0-8265-1310-7.

reactions and peripheral neuropathy to neutropenia as the duration of infusion is lengthened [6]. When cisplatin and topotecan are administered together, greater MYS is experienced when cisplatin is infused first [16]. CSFs can unexpectedly enhance the severity of MYS when incorrectly combined with other chemotherapeutic drugs [4].

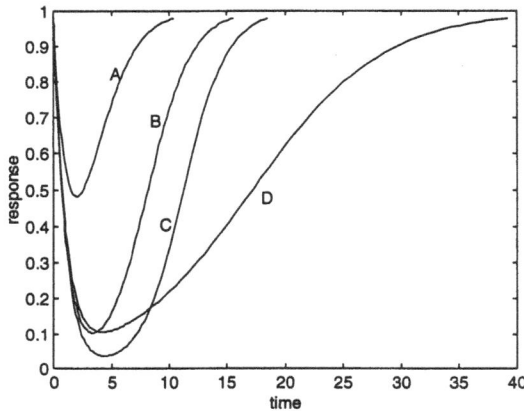

Fig. 1. Hypothetical myelosuppression profiles created by numerical integration of equation (4). Response can represent blood cell concentration. As discussed in the text, these profiles lack an initial lag phase characteristic of myelosuppression. For curves A, B and C, $K = 0.56$ and Q is 3.2, 56, and 316, respectively. For curve D, $K = 0.18$ and $Q = 17.7$.

To better understand how anticancer drugs, as well as CSFs, might be more effectively administered, I have sought to characterize the entire time course of MYS. In clinical trials, MYS is conventionally reported by a single point measure of nadir depth. As an illustration, in Figure 1, patients with hypothetical profiles B and D would be reported as experiencing the same 90% extent of MYS. However, it is visually evident that profile D describes more profound, sustained MYS. Previous models fit to MYS data have been constructed from splines [12] or from piecewise collections of functions [15]. In this paper, I describe the derivation and initial testing of a physiologically based parametric model of the time course of MYS. Designed to be fit to often sparse clinical data, this model has been designed keeping adjustable parameters to a minimum.

§2. Derivation of the Model

The first generation model of myelosuppression derived here is an example of an indirect response model (IRM). These physiologically based models have been applied to describe pharmacodynamic effects as diverse as the effects of warfarin on blood coagulation and of furosemide on urine flow from the kidney [3, 11]. In oncology, IRMs have been fit to the time course of drug-induced glutathione depletion, a targeted therapeutic response [7]. IRMs apply to drugs acting by the inhibition or stimulation of the synthesis or consumption of biochemicals mediating response. In the present model, response (R) is the concentration of blood cells, typically neutrophils or platelets, in circulation. R is governed by the k_{in}, the zero order rate constant at which cells enter the blood, and by k_{out}, the first order rate constant by which cells leave the blood (equation 1),

$$\frac{dR}{dt} = k_{in}I(t) - k_{out}R(t). \tag{1}$$

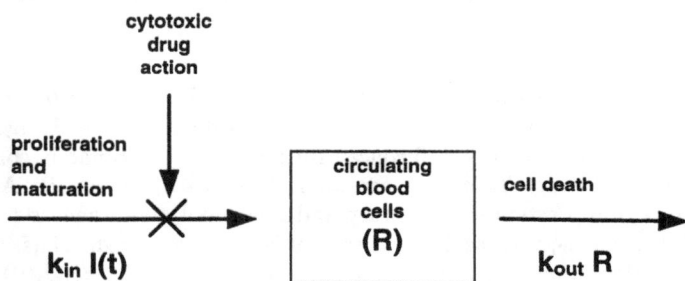

Fig. 2. Schematic representation of myelosuppression described by equation (1). Response (R) is the concentration of circulating blood cells. Drug-induced myelosuppression occurs by inhibition of blood cell synthesis via function $I(t)$ (see equation (2)).

In this model, k_{in} has units of blood cell concentration per unit time and is time-invariant. In a more complex model, k_{in} could be allowed to vary with time, thereby describing (for example) increased hematopoiesis as a homeostatic response to prolonged chemotherapy. Chemotherapy-induced myelosuppression occurs through the inhibition of blood cell synthesis (Figure 2) and is realized as a dimensionless saturable function, $I(t)$, equation (2), of the plasma concentration, C, of the drug. Consequently, IC_{50} is the drug concentration needed to produce a 50 percent inhibition of synthesis.

$$I(t) = \frac{IC_{50}}{C(t) + IC_{50}}. \tag{2}$$

Doses of chemotherapy capable of reducing tumor mass by killing are transiently toxic to normal renewing cells, such as those composing bone marrow and lining the gastrointestinal tract. The sometimes life-threatening depletion of circulating neutrophils and platelets is first noted approximately five days after treatment, reaches nadir at 10 to 20 days and is recovered by 30 days [10]. Depletion is believed to originate from cell cycle arrest of the hematopoietic progenitor cells. DNA damage resulting from chemotherapy halts basal proliferation of these cells long enough for either repair or programmed cell death to occur [5]. Because equation (1) models the concentration of the differentiated, mature progeny of affected progenitor cells, an inhibition of synthesis IRM [3] is used.

Equations (1) and (2) compose a pharmacodynamic (PD) model. A pharmacokinetic (PK) model describing the time course of drug concentration, $C(t)$, must also be specified. For simplicity, drug is administered a short pulse or bolus with its disposition described by a single exponential in equation (3), where k_{el} is the elimination rate and C_0 is the initial concentration of the drug,

$$C(t) = C_0 e^{-k_{el}t}. \tag{3}$$

Equations (1-3) possess five parameters and $R(0)$. These equations can be recast with fewer parameters. As $t \to \infty$, $C(t) \to 0$ and $I(t) \to 1$. Ignoring any diurnal variation in blood cell concentration, R is approximately constant in the absence of drug. Therefore, equation (1) yields $k_{in} = k_{out}R$. Assuming that myelosuppression is temporary and noncumulative, then as $t \to \infty$, $R(t) \to R(0)$, that is, the basal concentration is fully recovered. Thus, nondimensionalization of equation (1) proceeds by replacing k_{in} by $k_{out}R(0)$. Further simplification comes from substituting equations (2) and (3) into equation (1) and recasting it in nondimensional form with the following substitutions: $R^* = R(t)/R(0)$, $t^* = tk_{out}$, $K = k_{el}/k_{out}$, and $Q = C(0)/IC_{50}$. The model then becomes

$$\frac{dR^*}{dt^*} = -R^* + \frac{1}{1 + Q\exp(-Kt^*)}. \tag{4}$$

Solving equation (4) by an integrating factor yields an integral lacking a simple antiderivative,

$$R(t) = \exp(-t)\left[R(0) + \int_0^t \frac{\exp(s)}{1 + Q\exp(-Ks)}ds\right]. \tag{5}$$

For notational simplicity, the asterisks indicating dimensionless variables have been dropped in equation (5) and in all equations below. The four traces in Figure 1 illustrate equation (4) when numerically integrated using the MATLAB ODE Suite [17] for four different (Q,K) parameter combinations with $R(0)$ set to unity.

Equation (4) possesses several interesting properties. In its nondimensional form, the number of adjustable parameters used in fitting is reduced to three: $R(0)$, K and Q. A fourth parameter, t_{lag}, will be introduced below. From the substitutions above, K appears as the ratio of fundamental rate constants, while Q is the ratio of fundamental concentrations. Immediately after administration of a large dose and where $C(0) >> IC_{50}$, the right hand side of equation (4) becomes approximately $-R$ such that blood cell count initially falls exponentially. By definition of the model in equations (1) and (3), both k_{el} and k_{out} and thus K, are positive. Hence, at long times after dosing, $Q \exp(-Kt)$ tends to zero, and the right hand side of equation (4) reduces to $-R+1$. $R(t)$ returns to its dimensionless baseline value of unity exponentially. Thus, at the short and long time extremes, the shape of the IRM resembles the concentration - time profile of an orally administered drug when response is reflected across the time axis. The approach of each profile to their extreme value is at least initially described by a single exponential. After sufficient time, the disposition of the oral drug also shows a single exponential return to baseline.

§3. Fitting the Model to Data

In fitting simulated as well as actual clinical data, I found it necessary to add an adjustable lag parameter, t_{lag}, to the model. Though maximum response lags behind maximum plasma concentration in IRMs (hence, "indirect response"), change in response begins immediately upon dosing, as illustrated by the traces in Figure 1. As DeVita [5] notes, as many as eight to ten days are required for chemotherapeutic toxicity experienced by stem cells and progenitor cells in the bone marrow to be manifest in the peripheral blood, a time during which the model trace would be horizontal, representing an unchanging mean cell concentration. For the fitting of data, the piecewise differential equation (6) is adequate, although the next generation of this model might better incorporate lag into Figure 2 and resulting equations. Using the ADAPT II (release 3) software for PK-PD systems analysis [2], equation (6) is directly fit to the data using the Nelder-Mead simplex algorithm and the maximum likelihood criterion. This algorithm does not require a solution of the ordinary differential equation. In the discussion that follows, the "model" refers specifically to equation (6).

$$\frac{dR}{dt} = \begin{cases} 0 & \text{for } t \leq t_{lag}, \\ -R + \dfrac{1}{1 + Q \exp(-Kt)} & \text{for } t > t_{lag}. \end{cases} \quad (6)$$

Figure 3 illustrates equation (6) fit to the absolute neutrophil count (ANC) of a patient treated with topotecan. Clinical data is often quite noisy as these data are. Equation (6) fits the initial lag (t_{lag}) to about 10 days. It appears as the horizontal segment in Figure 3. Thereafter, MYS is realized with a model-predicted nadir occurring just after three weeks of treatment. To keep the number of parameters small, equation (6) is constructed on the basis of a simple pharmacokinetics, namely, a single bolus dose of a drug having single compartment kinetics. Equation (6) may still be fit to MYS generated by drugs having more complex kinetics or dosing, as is the case in the data in Figure 3. In these cases, the elegant interpretation of Q and K is lost.

Details on testing the model are presented elsewhere [13]. Briefly, in fitting noisy data such as that in Figure 3, the performance of equation (6) in estimating ABEC, the area between effect curves, was evaluated. ABEC is the area bounded by an upper effect curve (the dashed horizontal line in Figure 3)

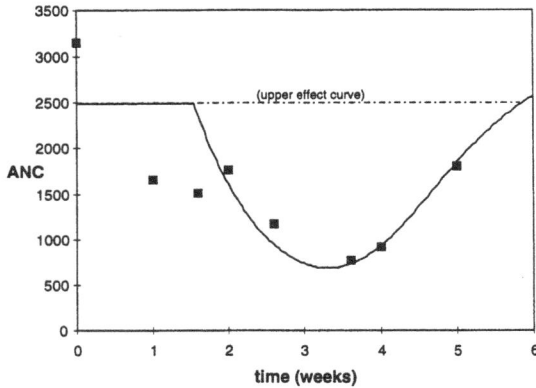

Fig. 3. Absolute neutrophil count (ANC) data fit with equation (6). For the patient whose data is shown, topotecan was administered by 24 hour infusion weekly at 2.0 mg/m^2 body surface area [8]. Dosing was suspended on weeks 3 and 4 because of depression of ANC below 1000 cells / mm^3.

and by a lower effect curve, which is the trace of the model fit. One of many possible quantities numerically determinable from the model fit, ABEC is measure of total myelosuppressive response. ABEC estimation was performed by fitting the model and, in parallel, a spline to simulated noisy data sets to determine whether the mechanistic information (Figure 2) inherent in model permitted better estimation. Data sets composed of nine points equally spaced in time were created with equation (7). These equations R(t) are simple and yield simulated data with shape similar to that seen clinically (Figure 3). They are ad hoc and have no known physiological basis. They were created because parameters A and B control the depth and relative time of nadir, respectively, thereby facilitating systematic sampling of shapes of MYS profiles. $V(t)$ is the variance function producing Gaussian output noise added to each $R(t)$ value.

$$R(t) = 1 \qquad\qquad\qquad \text{for } t \leq t_{lag},$$
$$R(t) = 1 - A\sin[(t - t_{lag})^B] \qquad \text{for } t > t_{lag}, \qquad (7)$$
$$V(t) = (0.15R(t))^2 + 0.05^2.$$

For each of 80 MYS profile shapes, 1000 data sets were simulated from equations (7). The model was superior ($P < 0.01$) to the spline for 59 of the profiles and superior, but not significantly so, for 17 other profiles. Defined as the proportion of data sets with less than 15% error in ABEC, superiority of the model was greatest for profiles with deep nadirs or long lag periods prior to MYS onset. For those MYS profiles with no lag time and deep (90% depression) nadir, the spline is clearly superior. The model failure for these profiles, four out of a total 80 studied, is graphically explained by a lack of flexibility in the model. However, because few myelosuppressive drugs act without some initial lag, inflexibility of the model is unlikely to affect its utility.

§4. Conclusions and Applications of the Model

I sought to develop a physiological model of MYS, one parsimonious in the number of adjustible parameters. The model embodied in equation (6) performs satisfactorily in fitting simulated data. It deserves to be tested further in a larger clinical context. A model of MYS could form a part of a population PK-PD model fitting the concentration-time data as well as response data collected as part of phase I and II clinical trials. One example is Gallo et al.'s model [7] of glutathione depletion by the anticancer drug buthionine sulfoximine. Population modeling is distinguished by fitting data pooled from many individuals and partitioning variability between interindividual sources (e.g., due to age, body size, or renal function) and intraindividual sources (e.g., assay error) [18].

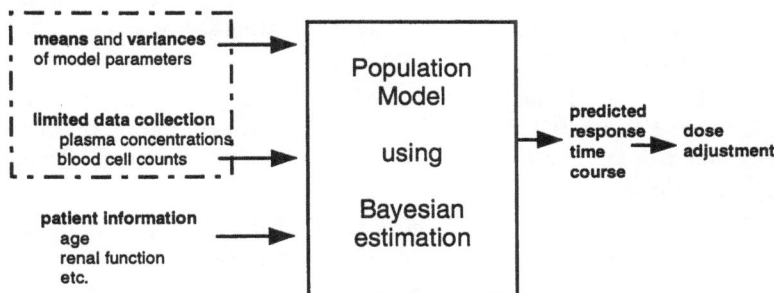

Fig. 4. An illustration of how a model of MYS might be applied to clinical practice.

A major task of model building is accounting for and thus reducing interindividual variability by incorporation of patient information into the model. Thus, parameter K in equation (6), which relates to rate of recovery from MYS, might be cast as a function of age or prior treatment history. Figure 4 illustrates one way such a model might be used. Model development would yield both a best fitting parametric model as well as the population means and variances of its parameters. Outside of the clinical trial setting, data derived from blood sampling is apt to be sparse. However, using parameter means and variances within Bayesian estimation [2], sparsely sampled data could still be modeled to predict the time course of response or clinically useful quantities derived from it. From this information, more informed dose adjustment could be made for subsequent courses of treatment.

Acknowledgments. Supported by NCI Postdoctoral Fellowship CA 72245 and by NIH Core Grant CA-06827 awarded to Fox Chase Cancer Center.

References

1. Anonymous, American Society of Clinical Oncology recommendations for the use of hematapoietic colony-stimulating factors: evidence-based, clinical practice guidelines, Journal of Clinical Oncology **12** (1994), 2471–2508.

2. D'Argenio, D. Z. and A. Schumitzky, *ADAPT II User's Guide, Biomedical Simulations Resource*, University of Southern California, Los Angeles, 1992.

3. Dayneka, N. L., V. Garg and W. J. Jusko, Comparison of four basic models of indirect pharmacodynamic responses, J. Pharmacokin. Biopharm. **21** (1993), 457–78.

4. de Wit, R., J. Verweij, M. Bontenbal, W. H. Kruit, C. Seynaeve, P. I. Schmitz and G. Stoter, Adverse effect on bone marrow protection of prechemotherapy granulocyte colony-stimulating factor support, J. Natl. Cancer Inst. **88** (1996), 1393–1398.

5. DeVita, V. T., Principles of cancer management, in *Chemotherapy in Cancer: Principles & Practice on Oncology* (5th edition), V. T. DeVita, S. Hellman and S. A. Rosenberg (eds.), Lippincott-Raven, Philadelphia, 1997, 333–347.

6. Dorr, R. T. and D. D. Von Hoff, *Cancer Chemotherapy Handbook* (2nd edition), Appleton & Lange, Norwalk, Conn., 1994.

7. Gallo, J. M., J. Brennan, T. C. Hamilton, T. Halbherr, P. B. Laub, R. F. Ozols and P. J. O'Dwyer, Time-dependent pharmacodynamic models in cancer chemotherapy: Population pharmacodynamic model for glutathione depletion following modulation by buthionine sulfoximine (BSO) in a Phase I trial of melphalan and BSO, Cancer Res. **55** (1995), 4507–4511.

8. Haas, N. B., F. P. LaCreta, J. Walczak, G. R. Hudes, J. M. Brennan, R. F. Ozols and P. J. O'Dwyer, Phase I/pharmacokinetic study of topotecan by 24-hour continuous infusion weekly, Cancer Res. **54** (1994), 1220–1226.

9. Hartmann, L. C., L. K. Tschetter, T. M. Habermann, L. P. Ebbert, P. S. Johnson, J. A. Mailliard, R. Levitt, V. J. Suman, T. E. Witzig, H. S. Wieand, L. L. Miller and C. G. Moertel, Granulocyte colony-stimulating factor in severe chemotherapy-induced afebrile neutropenia, New England Journal of Medicine **336** (1997), 1776–1780.

10. Hoagland, H. C., Hematological complications of cancer chemotherapy, in *The Chemotherapy Source Book*, M. C. Perry (ed.),Williams and Wilkins, Baltimore, 1992, 498–507.

11. Jusko, W. J. and H. C. Ko, Physiologic indirect response models characterize diverse types of pharmacodynamic effects, Clin. Pharmacol. Ther. **56** (1994), 406–419.

12. Karlsson, M. O., R. E. Port, M. J. Ratain and L. B. Sheiner, A population model for the leukopenic effect of etoposide, Clin. Pharmacol. Ther. **57** (1995), 325–334.

13. Laub, P. B. and J. M. Gallo, Feasibility and utility of pharmacodynamic models to characterize the time course of myelosuppression, Cancer Research, submitted.

14. Lynch, T., Topotecan today, J. of Clinical Oncology **14** (1996), 3053–3055.

15. Rosner, G. L. and P. Muller, Pharmacodynamic analysis of hematologic profiles, J. Pharmacokinet Biopharm. **22** (1994), 499–524.

16. Rowinsky, E. K., S. H. Kaufmann, S. D. Baker, L. B. Grochow, T. L. Chen, D. Peereboom, M. K. Bowling, S. E. Sartorius, D. S. Ettinger, A. A. Forastiere and R. C. Donehower, Sequences of topotecan and cisplatin: Phase I, pharmacologic and in vitro studies to examine sequence dependence, J. of Clinical Oncology **14** (1996), 3074–84.

17. Shampine, L. F. and M. W. Reichelt, The MATLAB ODE suite, SIAM Journal on Scientific Computing **18** (1997), 1–22.

18. Sheiner, L. B. and T. M. Ludden, Population pharmacokinetics/dynamics, Annu. Rev. Pharmacol. Toxicol. **32** (1992), 185–209.

Paul B. Laub
Incyte Pharmaceuticals, Inc.
3174 Porter Drive
Palo Alto, California 94304
plaub@incyte.com

Modeling the Effects of Angiogenic Factors on Tumor-related Angiogenesis and Vascularization: A Review

Sophia A. Maggelakis

§1. Introduction

Tumor growth begins when a single normal cell is changed to a cancer cell by the activation of oncogenes [1]. The growing tumor passes through an early prevascular (avascular) stage during which the tumor colony grows in three dimensions [30]. During this early developmental phase of growth, the tumor lacks its own network of blood supply so that the transport of nutrients and the removal of waste products must be accomplished by simple diffusion through its host [25]. A tumor in the prevascular stage has a diameter of 1 - 2 mm and consists of approximately 1 million cells [56]. Examples of such prevascular tumors are carcinomas in situ [26]. A prevascular tumor can stay in a dormant state for several months, in which the number of the proliferating cells in the periphery of the tumor balances the number of the dying cells at the center (necrotic core) of the tumor. All living normal tissues, however, need blood supply in order to receive nutrients and oxygen and to get rid of waste products. Malignant tissues have the same or even increased requirements [57]. Thus, at some point in the growth process, *vascularization* must take place, so that the avascular phase of growth is usually followed by a vascular phase. Tumor vascularization is considered to be a *neovascularization* process, which is the development of new blood vessels in tissues in which the blood vessels that existed there before either do not function at all or are not sufficient any longer [56]. This occurs because the vessels that penetrate the tumor, during vascularization, eventually start to break down to the extent that they cannot function as carriers for nutrients and oxygen, and the existing blood vessels are no longer adequate to meet the needs of the tumor. Usually, two layers of cells have been exhibited in histological sections of large solid tumors. An inner layer consisting of dead cells which constitutes the necrotic

Mathematical Models in Medical and Health Sciences
Mary Ann Horn, Gieri Simonett, and Glenn Webb (eds.), pp. 247–266.
Copyright © 1998 by Vanderbilt University Press, Nashville, TN.
ISBN 0-8265-1310-7.

core of the tumor, and an outer layer consisting of proliferating cells. In the outer layer, all types of blood vessels stand out very clearly [56], while in the necrotic part of the tumor, there is hardly any supply of nutrients and oxygen due to the regression of vasculature [22, 29].

After vascularization, rapid tumor growth follows, because the tumor does not depend any longer on diffusion processes in order to receive nutrients and oxygen and to remove wastes. This transport is now accomplished via the blood supply. Initially, the necrotic core of a vascular tumor disappears, and it is penetrated by capillaries. The excessive increase in tumor volume, however, causes the cells at the center of the tumor to die due to insufficient supply of nutrients, and *necrosis* eventually reappears [9]. It is not completely clear why some tumors grow very slowly and remain in a prevascular stage for a long time while others enter the vascular stage rapidly and as a result grow very fast. What is known, however, is that the origin of tumor vascularization lies in the neighborhood of the tumor itself. The tumor cells are capable of inducing the formation of new blood vessels in the neighborhood of the tumor, a process known as *angiogenesis*. These newly formed blood vessels elongate to reach the tumor or form lateral sprouts which eventually grow toward the tumor and try to penetrate it. Angiogenesis is most active during embryonic development and very inactive in adults, except under pathological conditions and in tumors [52]. Two types of angiogenesis processes have been identified [56]: The normal or physiological process and the pathological process. Under normal conditions, the growth of new blood vessels stops as soon as the embryo or the respective organ has fully developed. Under pathological conditions, however, angiogenesis does not stop, but it continues indefinitely for some diseases, such as rheumatoid disease and retinopathy, while it is terminated in other types of diseases as soon as its purpose is fulfilled, such as in wound healing where angiogenesis continues until the wound is closed. In tumors, angiogenesis does not stop. Even after the whole tumor is penetrated, angiogenesis continues since tumor cells can spread through the blood to other parts of the living organism forming secondary tumor masses, a process known as *metastasis,* which in turn must be vascularized [72]. It can, therefore, be concluded that tumor-related angiogenesis never stops until the host is killed [29], but if angiogenesis and vascularization is prevented, an avascular tumor can stay in a dormant state for rather long periods of time during which there is no danger of invasion and metastasis [33, 36].

What triggers the onset of angiogenesis is an angiogenic signal that can originate from a wound fluid, from retinal cells or from tumor cells, and it can activate the *endothelial cells* (EC) in the walls of the neighboring capillaries [21, 61, 62, 71]. The EC then release enzymes and start to migrate into the *extracellular matrix* (ECM). Small sprouts are formed which grow towards the angiogenic stimulus. Mitosis of EC also takes place at some distance from the tips of the sprouts and contributes to the number of the cells that are migrating through the ECM. Adjoining sprouts form loops, called *anastomoses,* and from these loops new sprouts rise, and circulation of blood is realized. It has been observed that during tumor-related angiogenesis, EC and the vast majority of tumor cells interact with each other in a cooperative way to complete angiogenesis [41], and that the first events of angiogenesis are rearrangements of EC rather than mitosis of EC. While migration of EC and proliferation of EC are distinct events, and sprouts can be formed without any cell division [21, 61, 62, 65, 71], the angiogenesis process cannot be complete unless mitosis of EC, which takes place at some distance from the tips of the sprouts, occurs [21, 61, 62].

All the studies so far have shown that the growth of primary tumors and metastasized tumors is dependent on vascularization, and therefore on angiogenesis, and that tumors cannot grow unless they can induce angiogenesis [27]. Very little is known, however, about the genetic aspect of angiogenic signals. What is known is that when the tumor reaches a threshold size, tumor cells eventually start to produce and secrete chemical compounds, called *angiogenic factors,* which have the capacity to stimulate the nearby normal vessels to sprout toward and into the tumor, thus, providing it with the necessary vasculature. It should be noted that the dead tumor cells in necrotic areas contribute nothing to the initiation of angiogenesis, and that there is a major difference between tumor-related angiogenesis and other angiopathies. Normal cells stop sending angiogenic signals as soon as the stimulator has been eliminated, while tumor cells never lose the capacity to produce angiogenic factors [56].

Although some of the known angiogenic factors could be analyzed, the molecular mode of action of all such factors is practically unknown. It has been recognized, however, that angiogenic factors that come from different types of tissues, including tumors, induce three main activities of EC, and angiogenesis is not complete unless all these activities take place in a well-ordered sequence. These activities include: (i) the production of enzymes by EC and their secretion into the extracellular matrix (ECM), (ii) the initiation of EC migration, (iii) and proliferation of EC [56]. While mitosis is not the first response to an angiogenic stimulus, it is a vital event in the angiogenesis process. Angiogenic factors have the ability either to stimulate migration only (mitogens) or to induce both migration and proliferation of EC. A collection of different angiogenic factors have been found and are classified into two main groups. One group consists of factors that act directly on EC, and the other group consists of factors that activate other factors or host cells which then in turn activate EC.

The majority of tumor cells produce the angiogenic factor called *Tumor Angiogenesis Factor* (TAF) which is capable of inducing tumor vascularization by activating directly the EC and not via other factors. Many types of tumor cells also release growth factors that function via an autocrine mechanism, in which a cell secreting the growth factor has also a surface receptor for that factor such that a positive feed-forward control loop may be established. Such growth factors are called *Transforming Growth Factors* or *Tumor Growth Factors* (TGFs), and they can also stimulate angiogenesis in-vivo [31]. Of particular interest are the *Type alpha Transforming Growth Factor* (TGF-α) and *Type beta Transforming Growth Factor* (TGF-β) [8, 23, 24, 51]. There is evidence that human cancer cells produce and release TGF-α which has the characteristic to stimulate cell proliferation [68]. TGF-α has also been shown in a variety of neoplastic tissues, including human placenta, mouse and rat embryos, and it has been tested in the hamster cheek pouch assay [63]. TGF-β, on the other hand, is structurally unrelated to TGF-α, and it has both stimulatory and inhibitory effects on the growth of EC [10, 35, 40]. It has been found that TGF-β induces a strong angiogenic response in the cornea [31] and at subcutaneous sites in newborn mice, but it inhibits the division of endothelial cells in culture [60]. Another major growth factor that regulates vascularization and angiogenesis and is specific to EC is the *Vascular Endothelial Growth Factor* (VEGF) [50]. It has been discovered that this growth factor is produced in parts of the tumor where there is lack of oxygen, and that VEGF production arises when there is a sudden change in the oxygen concentration [58, 66]. In addition to these fairly well-defined angiogenic factors, there exist several other chemical compounds that can stimulate the proliferation of EC or can induce the migration of EC or both of these activities and, therefore, promote angiogenesis [27]. Such compounds are the *Prostaglandins* and in particular PGE1 and PGE2 which are found in increased amounts in tumors, wound fluid, macrophages, and in regions of inflammation [34].

Recently new angiogenic factors have been identified [50], such as *angio-poietin-1* (Ang1) which signals through a tyrosine kinase receptor (Tie2/Tek) that is expressed only on EC and early hemopoietic cells [50]. It has been observed that the absence of Ang1 or its receptor can cause severe vascular abnormalities in developing mouse embryos [50]. A naturally occurring antagonist for Ang1 and its Tie2 receptor is the factor termed *angiopoietin-2* (Ang2). It was suggested that in the presence of plenty VEGF, Ang2 can promote vessel sprouting by blocking an Ang1 signal, while in the absence of VEGF, Ang2 can inhibit an Ang1 signal which in turn can contribute to regression of blood vessels. There is evidence that these angiopoietins and Tie2 receptor play an important role in the maturation and remodeling of blood vessels and in the angiogenic outgrowth, but they do not participate in the initial vascular development [50].

It should also be mentioned that there exist some compounds which are not angiogenic, but can induce angiogenesis when they are combined with other substances. An example of such a compound is *heparin* which alone does not induce neovascularization, but when it is combined with copper ions can act as angiogenic stimulus [59, 69]. Heparin together with tumor cells induces a stronger reaction than the tumor alone. The basic *Fibroblast Growth Factors* (a-FGF, b-FGF [43]) are heparin-binding growth factors. These factors have been shown to stimulate EC proliferation *in-vitro* and angiogenesis *in-vivo*. When a-FGF is combined with heparin, it can induce EC proliferation in a more effective manner than pure a-FGF can [70]. *Tumor Necrosis Factor* (TNF) is yet another important compound which influences both the proliferation and migration of EC [64].

It has been found that some tumor cells, in addition to being able to induce angiogenesis in the tissue around them, also, for some unknown reason, produce angiogenesis factors that act as inhibitors [13]. While the stimulators die off quickly, the inhibitors accumulate in high concentrations so that in the neighborhood of the tumor the balance of inhibitors to inducers benefits the growth of blood vessels, but the vessel growth is inhibited at locations far from the tumor where there are high concentrations of inhibitors [12]. One of these inhibitors is *thrombospondin* which is a protein also found in extracellular protein matrix and in platelets [12]. This inhibitor makes the EC unable to respond to any of the angiogenesis stimulators, but how this is done it is not yet known. Another angiogenesis inhibitor, which was identified by Folkman and O'Reilly, is the inhibitor *angiostatin* [12, 50, 55]. This inhibitor was found to stop experimental tumor growth in mice and shrank the tumors significantly. Recently, a new antiangiogenesis factor, known as *endostatin,* was described. This inhibitor was found to be more effective in shrinking a wide variety of tumors in mice and in keeping primary tumors and metastases in check [55]. The mechanisms of action by which angiostatin and endostatin block angiogenesis have not yet been understood, and it is still unknown whether these inhibitors will produce the same results in humans. Heparin is yet another compound which, as mentioned earlier, when it is combined with some other substances it supports angiogenesis, but when it is combined with cortisone it inhibits the development of new blood vessels and it also induces the regression of new vessels [32].

Cancer research has shown that when a primary tumor is removed it results in growth of metastasized tumors, while the growth, but not the number of metastases, is suppressed when the tumor is present [55]. This is an indication that the primary tumor produces chemical substances, such as angiostatin and endostatin, that can block neovascularization and keep the metastases in control [55]. It was recently proposed [55] that when a primary tumor reaches a threshold size, it produces both angiogenesis stimulators and inhibitors and can inhibit a secondary tumor of a different type. Initially the angiogenic stimulators are in excess of the angiogenic inhibitors, but the angiogenesis inhibitors have longer half-life in the circulation and, therefore, eventually accumulate in higher concentrations relative to stimulators. This results in inhibition of secondary tumors or metastases due to the fact that there is more inhibitor than stimulator present in the vascular bed of a secondary tumor.

To construct a mathematical model, that incorporates all the distinct and not necessarily related events, described in this section, of the complex process of angiogensis, is a very difficult task. Although mathematical models that study the growth of solid tumors exist in the literature, only a small number of these models examine the effects of angiogenic factors on tumor-related angiogenesis and vascularization. In what follows, an effort has been made to discuss and present examples of such models, which can serve as frameworks for developing other models in the area.

§2. Mathematical Models

It is rather difficult to study angiogenesis in detail, because it consists of a series of events that take place within complex organs or organisms. Various mathematical models have been developed in order to investigate this complicated process of tumor-related angiogenesis and vascularization. The main objective of these models has been to quantify the effects of induction or inhibition of angiogenesis, to compare the results, and to design new strategies in order to enhance or to inhibit tumor-related angiogenesis.

Several mathematical models that describe the early stages of tumor growth exist in the literature. Most of these models describe tumor growth in a qualitative manner under various simplifying assumptions. In many cases, one-dimensional deterministic models have been developed to describe the basic physics of diffusion processes that take place during prevascular tumor growth and to provide insight into the nature of growth processes in more realistic goemetries. Models which use three-dimensional spherical geometry can also be found. Such models usually imitate closely the growth of multicellular spheroids *in-vitro*. Multicellular spheroids are spherical prevascular aggregates of cells that are supplied by diffusion of oxygen and substrates from the surrounding medium, and they show many characteristics of solid tumors. Although mathematical models that describe prevascular tumor growth are limited, there has been a substantial interest in them. Since the vascular stage of tumor growth can only occur *in-vivo*, prevascular models can be compared with experimental data and form a framework for further theoretical work on tumor-related angiogenesis and vascularization. A description of several mathematical models of prevascular and vascular tumor growth can be found in a review paper [2].

The present paper is focused on presenting models that have incorporated the effects of angiogenic factors on tumor-related angiogenesis and vascularization. In section 2.1, four mathematical models that examine the effects of Tumor Angiogenesis Factor (TAF) are discussed, and a brief description of some other related models is presented. Section 2.2 is devoted to models that have incorporated the effects of angiogenesis inhibitors on tumor-related angiogenesis and vascularization, and section 2.3 contains a discussion of two models that have incorporated the effects of Tumor Growth Factors (TGFs) on the growth of solid tumors. Also, reference to and a summary of other existing models incorporating TGFs are included in this last section.

2.1. Models Describing the Effects of Angiogenesis Stimulators on Tumor-related Angiogenesis and Vascularization

Several mathematical models have been developed that examine the effects of Tumor Angiogenesis factor (TAF) on angiogenesis and vascularization. Most of these models describe the effects of TAF on blood vessels and endothelial cells after it has been released into the surrounding medium. In [18], two models for the production of TAF within the tumor while in its diffusion limited state and prior to its release into the surrounding host tissue are described. The models are based on the hypothesis that there is a direct association between the size of the tumor and the subsequent release of TAF. Thus, depending on the tumor size, vascularization may or may not occur. In these models, *quenching* is used to describe this direct relationship. Quenching is a phenomenon where the solution of a diffusion equation remains finite, but some derivative of the solution becomes unbounded in finite time. In each of the models, it is assumed that the concentration, $c(x,t)$, of TAF satisfies a diffusion equation. The first model takes into account the proliferation of tumor cells and the production of TAF by using the diffusion equation

$$c_t = c_{xx} + \phi(c), \qquad 0 < x < L, \ t > 0,$$

where the function $\phi(c)$ is used to model the production of TAF by the tumor cells, and L represents the ultimate size of the tumor. The initial and boundary conditions that are used to solve this diffusion equation are

$$\begin{aligned}
c(x,0) &= 0, & 0 < x < L, \\
c(0,t) &= 0, & t \geq 0, \\
c_x(L,t) &= 0, & t \geq 0.
\end{aligned}$$

It was shown that for a tumor size $L_0 > 0$ such that $L < L_0$ there is global existence of the solution $c(x,t)$, and that the solution quenches for $L > L_0$. It was suggested that when the solution quenches, the concentration of TAF reaches a critical level. It was also pointed out that when the activity of TAF reaches a critical level, the solution cannot be continued and TAF is subsequently released into the surrounding tissue.

The second model in [18] takes into account the production of TAF and the activity of cells on the boundary of the tumor. The function $\phi(c)$, which is the same function used in the first model, is now included in the boundary conditions so that the solution depends on the boundary conditions rather than on the production term for TAF. This model was described by the following system:

$$\begin{aligned}
c_t &= c_{xx}, & 0 < x < L, \ t > 0, \\
c(x,0) &= 0, & 0 < x \leq L, \\
c(0,t) &= 0, & t \geq 0, \\
c_x(L,t) &= \phi(c(L,t)), & t \geq 0.
\end{aligned}$$

The function $\phi(c)$ was used, in both models, to represent a type of mutual beneficial relationship between the tumor and the production of TAF. This means that as the production of TAF increases, there is a greater probability that its concentration will reach a critical level. As soon as this critical level is approached, TAF will be secreted into the surrounding host tissue to subsequently attract blood vessels and as a result fresh nutrients. It is, therefore, in the interest of the tumor to produce TAF. It was shown that for a tumor size L_0^* such that $L_0^* > L$ the solution quenches, while for $L_0^* \leq L$ no quenching is possible.

Both models were extended to higher more realistic dimensions, and it was clearly indicated that the size of a tumor plays an important role in predetermining vascularization. This was contributed to the fact that the release of TAF, which eventually leads to vascularization, is dependent on the size of the tumor.

The neovascularization that takes place when a tumor is implanted in the cornea of an animal has been studied in [11]. A model, that considers the diffusion of TAF and the formation of sprouts from pre-existing vessels, was developed. This model is based on the model of Edelstein (1982) for fungal growth, and it describes how the sprouts move to form new capillaries as a chemostatic response to the presence of TAF. One-dimensional growth is assumed with respect to the x-axis, which is taken to be the distance between the edge of the tumor (origin) and the nearest limbal vessels. It is also assumed that the capillary density $\rho(x,t)$, i.e., capillary length per unit area per unit time, increases only by the movement of the tips of the capillaries so that

$$\frac{\partial \rho}{\partial t} = -n(x,t)v(x,t) - \gamma_1 \rho,$$

where $v(x,t)$ is the velocity of the tips, and $\gamma_1 \rho$ represents the death rate of the capillaries with γ_1 being a fixed proportion of branches that break down in each time unit. The number of capillary tips per unit area is represented by $n(x,t)$ such that

$$\frac{\partial n}{\partial t} = -\frac{\partial (nv)}{\partial x} + \sigma,$$

where σ is the number of capillary tips created per unit area per unit time, and is taken to be $\sigma = \alpha_0 c \rho$ with $c(x,t)$ being the concentration of TAF, and α_0 being the rate of appearance of tips per unit area per unit TAF concentration for a unit length of branch per unit area. The concentration of TAF outside the tumor is taken to satisfy the diffusion equation

$$\frac{\partial c}{\partial t} = D \frac{\partial^2 c}{\partial x^2},$$

with D being the diffusion coefficient of TAF in the cornea. The tip extension rate is given by $v = \chi_1(c)\frac{\partial c}{\partial x}$ with $\chi_1(c)$ being the chemotactic coefficient which was assumed to be constant. The above coupled first-order differential equations were solved subject to the conditions that initially there are no vessels or tips in the cornea, that the vessel density at the limbus remains at its initial value, and that both the tip and vessel density tend to zero far from the limbus. The model was applied to the case in which the source of TAF was removed. It was assumed that for some time the concentration of TAF was zero everywhere so that the velocity v of the tips of the capillaries was also zero. The results indicated that after the removal of TAF, angiogenic activity slowed down and eventually stopped, and the decline of vascularization was much slower. The migration of vascular loops, which takes place during the early stages of neovascularization, was not incorporated into this model. It was suggested, however, that high tip density could be interpreted as indicating a large number of capillary loops experiencing migration.

A mathematical model for the diffusion of TAF after it has been secreted into the surrounding host tissue was developed by [19]. This model serves as a complementary level of description for the models described above, and it takes into account several events which are involved during the angiogenesis process. A free boundary problem was formulated in order to monitor the concentration of TAF and its effects on cell migration and proliferation. The model uses two stages. In the first stage, the TAF is assumed to diffuse and be absorbed by the surrounding host tissue. A free boundary, which is allowed to move as TAF progresses or recedes into the tissue, is used to determine the farthest extent of TAF outside the tumor. The following system is used to describe this stage:

$$\frac{\partial c}{\partial t} = D\frac{\partial^2 c}{\partial x^2} - g(c)$$

$$c = c_b \text{ on } x = 0, \qquad c = \frac{\partial c}{\partial x} = 0 \text{ on } s(t),$$

$$c(x, 0) = c_0(x), \qquad s(0) = s_0,$$

where $c(x, t)$ denotes the concentration of TAF, $x = 0$ is taken to be the boundary of the tumor, L is used to represent the distance between the tumor and the capillary vessels, $s(t)$ represents the free boundary, and c_b, which is maintained at a constant level, represents the concentration of TAF on the boundary of the tumor. A decay or sink term, $g(c)$, is used to model the depletion of TAF into the surrounding tissue. The authors concentrated on a simple choice for $g(c) = m$, with m being a constant, to describe the linear decay in time in the absence of the diffusion term. The function $g(c) = kc+m$, which describes exponential decay with time in the absence of the diffusion term is also briefly examined. This stage continues until a steady state has been reached, which occurs when

$$c = \frac{m}{2D}(x - s)^2, \qquad s = (2Dc_b/m)^{1/2}.$$

This means that the concentration of TAF reaches a finite critical distance $L = s$ in the surrounding tissue beyond which it cannot penetrate the tissue any further. It is assumed that once the tumor is within this critical distance from the nearby blood vessels, EC migration and proliferation takes place. The second stage of the model deals with this possibility, and it is described by the following system:

$$\frac{\partial c}{\partial t} = D\frac{\partial^2 c}{\partial x^2} - g(c) - f\left(\frac{x}{s}, c\right),$$

$$c = c_b \text{ on } x = 0, \qquad c = \frac{\partial c}{\partial x} = 0 \text{ on } s(t),$$

$$c(x, 0) = c_0(x), \qquad s(0) = s_0 = L.$$

It is assumed that the proliferating EC act as a sink for the TAF so that a function f is included to model the uptake of TAF by EC. This function is taken to be a product of a function p dependent on the TAF concentration and a function q dependent on the distance from the tumor, i.e., $f(x/s, c) = p(c)q(x/s)$. The Michaelis-Menten kinetics, a logarithmic law, and a receptor kinetic law are used to model the function p. Circular and spherical geometries were also used to solve the problem in two and three dimensions, and the case in which the tumor implant is removed was examined. This qualitative model also provides a possible explanation for anastomosis, which is one of the critical events of the angiogenesis process. It was implied that a change in the concentration of TAF and approaching a second steady state for the TAF concentration profile at a definite distance form the blood vessels could be responsible for anastomosis. This model was later extended to include the chemotactic response of endothelial cells to tumor angiogenesis factor, and such a model is described in [20]. The reader is also referred to a model that examines the effects of tumor-related angiogenesis on tumor invasion [15].

2.2. Models Describing the Effects of Angiogenesis Inhibitors on Tumor-related Angiogenesis and Vascularization

In addition to producing angiogenic factors that stimulate angiogenesis, growing tumors produce angiogenic factors that have the capacity to regulate and inhibit the formation of new blood vessels. Like the stimulators, the inhibitors are released into the bloodstream, but while the stimulators die off quickly, the inhibitors accumulate in high concentrations away from the growing tissue. Thus, nearby the tumor, capillary growth is benefited while at locations far from the tumor it is inhibited. Several mathematical models that examine the effects of the chemical inhibition of mitosis within multicellular spheroids have been developed [6, 7, 17, 38, 39, 47, 48, 49, 67], and the main assumption of all these models is that the growth inhibitor is produced within the tumor in some spatially-dependent fashion.

A model developed by [44] incorporates angiogenic inhibitors and examines their effects on tumor angiogenesis and vascularization. In this model, the concentration of the Tumor Inhibitor Factors (TIFs) is monitored by a diffusion equation given by

$$\frac{\partial C_i}{\partial t} = D\nabla^2 C_i + \lambda S(r) - \gamma C_i - mf(r, C_i),$$

where $C_i(r, t)$ are the chemical substances produced by the proliferating cells of a prevascular tumor with $C_1(r, t)$ being the concentration of angiogenic factors that act as stimulators, such as Tumor Angiogenesis Factor (TAF), and $C_2(r, t)$ being the concentration of angiogenic factors that act as inhibitors, such as angiostatin or endostatin. It is assumed that the chemical substances are produced by the proliferating cells in the outer region, $\hat{R} \le r \le R_0$, of a solid tumor at a rate λ with $S(r)$ being the source term indicating the non-uniform production of these substances so that

$$S(r) = \begin{cases} 0, & 0 \leq r \leq \hat{R}, \\ 1 + \alpha \dfrac{r - \hat{R}}{R_0 - \hat{R}}, & \hat{R} \leq r \leq R_0. \end{cases}$$

The natural loss of the angiogenic factors into the surrounding tissue is modeled using the term γC_i, with γ being the decay or depletion rate. To model the absorption of the chemical substances by the endothelial cells, a sink term, $mf(r, C_i)$, is introduced. The parameter m represents the positive and/or negative effects of the chemical substances on the growth of the new blood vessels. Thus, positive m represents the stimulatory effects of the angiogenic factors and negative m represents their inhibitory effects. The concentrations of the chemical substances are monitored, and the model tracks a free boundary, R_m, which represents the farthest extent of these substances into the surrounding tissue. It is assumed that the external architecture of the tumor consists of an outer peripheral layer which is made up of the growing capillaries, and a layer, squeezed between the capillary boundary, R_c, and the tumor, consisting of the diffusible chemical substances. The growth rate of the capillary boundary which grows toward the prevascular tumor and tries to penetrate it is determined by an integro-differential equation of the form

$$\frac{4\pi}{3} \frac{dR_c^3}{dt} = 4\pi \int_{R_m}^{R_c} r^2 P(C_i)dr,$$

where $P(C_i) = \frac{mpC_i(r)}{C_{max}}$ represents the endothelial cell proliferation rate with p being the normal cell proliferation rate and C_{max} being the critical concentration above which the action of the chemical substances is evident. The solution to this equation provides the consideration of three different cases:

  (i) If $R_0 < R_m < R_c$, then the release of the chemical substances into the blood stream begins (R_0 represents the boundary of the tumor).
 (ii) If $R_m = R_c$, the regulation (stimulation and/or inhibition) of blood vessel growth begins.
(iii) If $R_c = R_0$, the vascularization begins.

Inhibition of tumor metastasis by an angiogenesis inhibitor, such as angiostatin, is discussed in [5]. A model was developed to describe the post-surgical response of the local environment to the "surgical" removal of a spherical tumor in an infinite homogeneous domain. It was assumed that the primary tumor is the source of the growth inhibitor, and the resulting initial value problem was solved in an infinite domain bounded internally by a spherical tumor. The space-time behavior of a "pulse" of growth inhibitor when the tumor is removed was analyzed.

The growth of necrotic tumors in the presence and absence of inhibitors was described in the model by [14]. This model examines tumors that possess a central necrotic core, and it compares the roles of *apoptosis* (natural cell death) and *necrosis* (induced death by changes in cell's environment). The actions of a range of inhibitory mechanisms on tumor growth were compared, and it was suggested that the inhibitor may act either directly, by reducing the cell proliferation rate, or indirectly, by reducing the nutrient concentration, and that cell loss mechanism depends on the tumor's size and structure. An inhibitor-free setting and an inhibitor-present setting was used, and numerical simulations were presented for various parameter values. The effects of nutrients and inhibitors on the existence and stability of the time-independent solutions of the model were studied using a combination of numerical and asymptotic techniques. The nonlinear diffusion of a growth inhibitor factor in multicellular spheroids is described in another model [16].

2.3. Models Describing the Effects of Tumor Growth Factors on Tumor-related Angiogenesis and Vascularization

Growth factors are defined as protein hormones or similar molecules called peptides, and they can affect more processes than just cell growth [37]. Such processes include cell proliferation, cell differentiation, angiogenesis, and response to other growth factors. Normal cells and tumor cells produce growth factors, but while the growth of normal cells is controlled at large by the interplay between several growth factors that are present in tissue fluids, malignant cells may produce increased amounts of growth factors and may require less growth factors supplied to them in order to survive and divide. It has been proposed that malignant cells require smaller amounts of such growth factors in order to break away from normal growth controls [42]. The impact of growth factors in the etiology of cancer is a major one due to their involvement in the control of normal cell growth as well as of malignant cell growth. Of particular interest are the Transforming Growth Factors (TGFs) which were discussed in the introduction section. These growth factors may act either on tumor cells (autocrine pathway) or on the extracellular matrix (paracrine pathway).

One of the first attempts to model the effects of growth factors on a growing tumor was made in [53]. The authors developed a mathematical model which incorporates the autocrine and paracrine pathways as control mechanisms in tumor growth. The tumor is assumed to be a single homogeneous population, and the model is based on the logistic equation of Verhulst,

$$\frac{dV}{dt} = rV\left(1 - \frac{V}{K}\right).$$

The actions exerted by the TGFs are modeled as functions of TGF concentration and receptor activity. In the above equation, V is used to denote the volume of the tissue which consists of a population of tumor cells. The initial population size V_0, the Malthusian growth rate r of the population, and the carrying capacity K of the environment are the basic parameters that describe the system. The term $-rV^2/K$ represents the size of the population at which the growth rates balance the death rates due to the existing competition for resources. This equation was modified to describe autocrine controls as modifiers of the Malthusian growth rate r and paracrine controls as modifiers of the carrying capacity K of the Verhulst model. A set of possible functions for r and K, that represent the control process of TFG-α and TGF-β, are suggested, and three typical growth cases of tissue growth are described. These cases are: (1) normal tissue wound healing, (2) unrestricted and undisturbed tumor growth, and (3) tumor growth in a (ionizing radiation) damaged environment. Computer simulations for a set of biological parameters, that were used to test the model against known phenomena observed *in-vivo*, are presented for each case. Results from this model indicate that paracrine signals, especially TGF-β, are able to induce the expansion of the local stroma to support the growing tumor. An increasing growth rate for the tissue as a whole was observed even when TGF-β did not exert a negative autocrine control. This overall increase was attributed to an expanding carrying capacity. This model was extended to include heterogeneous tumors and growth factor controls such as autocrine, paracrine, and endocrine [54]. The endocrine pathway is similar to the paracrine pathway except that the signal received by the target cells is systematic and it originates far from the population that receives it. The normal endocrine system of the host can be considered as the primary source of this signal.

A diffusion model which takes into account the concentration-dependent behavior of TGF-α and TGF-β was developed in [45]. This model incorporates the effects of the autocrine and paracrine response of TGFs on the growth rate of a multicellular spheroid, and it examines the effects of the bifunctional behavior of TGF-β on cell proliferation. The concentrations, $C_i(r,t)$, of TGFs satisfy the following diffusion equations

$$\frac{\partial C_i}{\partial t} = D\nabla^2 C_i + \gamma f(r), \qquad 0 \leq r \leq R,$$

where C_1 denotes the concentration of TGF-α and C_2 denotes the concentration of TGF-β. The parameter γ represents the TGF production rate, R is the size of the tumor, and the function $f(r)$ is used to model the effects the autocrine mechanisms of TGFs. Diffusive equilibrium was assumed, and the following system was solved

$$-\frac{D}{r^2}\frac{d}{dr}\left[r^2\frac{dC_i}{dr}\right] = \begin{cases} -\gamma, & 0 \leq r \leq \hat{R}, \\ \gamma, & \hat{R} \leq r \leq R. \end{cases}$$

The model is based on the assumption that as the cell growth increases, so are the concentrations of TGFs, and their autocrine response begins when the concentrations C_i have reached some critical levels $\hat{C}_i$ at some distance $r = \hat{R}$ from the center of the tumor. Thus, $-\gamma$ represents a *sink* of TGFs in the region $[0, \hat{R}]$, and γ represents a source of TGFs in the region $[\hat{R}, R]$. The concentrations $C_i(r)$ and their fluxes $\frac{dC_i}{dr}$ are taken to be continuous at the interface $\hat{R}$, and it is assumed that, initially, there are TGFs present so that

$C_i(r) = (C_0)_i$ at $r = R$. A parameter λ was introduced to model the positive and/or negative effect of TGFs on cellular growth. Thus, positive λ denotes the stimulatory effect of TGF-α and β, while negative λ denotes the inhibitory effect of TGF-β. Since, as it was shown in [18], the tumor size plays a role in determining whether or not vascularization takes place, the growth rate of the multicellular spheroid, as a function of the TGFs and their diffusion into the intercellular space of the spheroid, was modelled by using the following integro-differential equation

$$\frac{4\pi}{3}\frac{dR^3}{dt} = 4\pi \left[\int_0^{\hat{R}} r^2 S(C_i) dr + \int_{\hat{R}}^R r^2 S(C_i) dr \right],$$

where

$$S(C_i) = \begin{cases} s, & C_i(r) \leq \hat{C}_i, \\ \dfrac{\lambda s C_i(r)}{\hat{C}_i}, & \hat{C}_i \leq C_i(r), \end{cases}$$

represents the cell proliferation rate (volume created per unit volume of viable cells) with s being the normal cell proliferation rate. When the tumor exceeds a certain size, the concentration of TAF reaches a critical level and is subsequently secreted into the surrounding tissue and triggers the angiogenesis process.

Self-activation and self-inhibition of TGF concentration due to spatially localized source were also studied in [3]. Time-independent and time-dependent models were examined, and the linear stability of the resulting steady states of the time-dependent model was discussed. This work was later supplemented by developing a nonlinear model [4] of growth factor production, which examined the uniqueness and stability criteria of low and high concentration steady states of TGF in a spatially homogeneous system. It was also shown that the uniqueness analysis carries over to the case of a localized TGF source in a spatially non-homogeneous system. Another one-dimensional model of growth control in a cell culture in which TGFs diffuse through intercellular spaces and act locally was constructed in [46]. The model examines the behavior of a cell culture subject to the presence of TGFs.

§3. Discussion

Angiogenesis is a highly complex process which must take place in order for circulation to develop during embryogenesis, for a wound to heal, and for a tumor to grow. In spite of the intense investigations that have been carried over in this field, many questions still remain unanswered. As it was mentioned in the introduction, the growth of a solid tumor proceeds through an avascular phase which soon turns into the rapidly growing vascular stage. It is during the vascularizaton phase that the tumor grows rapidly, and the process of invasion and metastasis can take place. The transition of the tumor from the avascular to vascular stage depends upon the process of angiogenesis and neovascularization, but tumors can remain dormant when vascularization is prevented. Thus, understanding the various patterns of vascularization is very important for the diagnosis, prognosis, and also therapy of cancer. It could be possible to inhibit tumor growth by preventing angiogenesis. To this end, a possible therapeutic approach in oncology, that of antiangiogenesis, i.e., the inhibition of growth of new vessels into the tumor, was proposed [28]. It was shown that laboratory animals could be cured of cancer by means of antiangiogenesis. Consequently, antiagiogenesis together with surgery and irradiation can become an important approach for tumor therapy. Clinicians, however, are skeptical about long-term antiangiogenesis treatment, because blood-vessel growth is critical to other processes such as wound healing.

Recently, it was reported in [12] that antiangiogenesis therapy is not the only means of inhibiting the blood supply of a tumor. An antivascular approach has been suggested in which the goal is to cause blood clots in the blood vessels through which tumors get oxygen and nutrients in order to live and grow. There are certain reservations about this approach when it comes to be used on humans. Researchers will have to make sure that this approach does not cause any clots in the non-tumor vessels. It is believed, however, that this problem can be solved based on the fact that blood vessels around tumors are much more disposed toward blood clotting than normal vessels are. It has also been suggested [4] that the angiopoietins Ang1 and Ang2, when they act alone and in combination with other agents, can act as positive and negative regulators of angiogenesis, and they can, therefore, be tested for their ability to manipulate the formation of blood vessels in a therapeutically beneficial way.

As can be easily expected, such highly complex processes as angiogenesis, tumor invasion, and metastasis leave many questions unanswered and stimulate the creation of new problems. The clinical observations, discussed in this paper, should prompt the development of mathematical models that will yield valuable insight into the dynamics of tissue growth and will discuss and formulate new approaches for designing therapies that target tumor blood vessels. Since there are no fundamental qualitative differences between the angiogenic capabilities of malignant and nonmalignant diseases [56], the results obtained from normal and malignant vascularization can be used to make comparisons and produce results that will aid in making progress independently of the system of investigation used. It is hoped that more mathematical models will be developed to aid in understanding this important process of tumor-related angiogensis and to provide insight on how to prevent it completely.

References

1. Aaronson, S. A., Growth factors and cancer, Science **254** (1991), 1146–1153.

2. Adam, J. A., Diffusion models of prevascular and vascular tumor growth. A Review, in *Lecture Notes in Pure and Applied Mathematics, Proceed-*

ings: Mathematical population dynamics, Marcel Dekker **131**, 1991, 625–652.

3. Adam, J. A., Self-activation and inhibition: A simple nonlinear model, Appl. Math. Lett. **4** (1991), 85–87.

4. Adam, J. A., Solution uniqueness and stability criteria for a model of growth factor prodcution, Appl. Math. Lett. **5** (1992), 89–92.

5. Adam, J. A. and C. Bellomo, Post-surgical passive response of local environment to primary tumor removal, Math. Comput. Modelling **25** (1997), 7–17.

6. Adam, J. A. and S. A. Maggelakis, Mathematical model of tumor growth: IV. Effects of a necrotic core, Math. Biosci. **97** (1989), 121–136.

7. Adam, J. A. and S. A. Maggelakis, Diffusion regulated growth characteristics of a spherical prevascular carcinoma, Bull. Math. Biol. **53** (1990), 549–582.

8. Assoian, R. K., A. Komoriya, C. A. Meyers, D. M. Miller and M. B. Sporn, Transforming growth factor-beta in human platelets, J. Biol. Chem. **258** (1983), 7155–7160.

9. Ausprunk, D. H., D. R. Knighton and J. Folkman, Vascularization of neoplastic tissues grafted to the chick chorioallantois, Am. J. Pathol. **79** (1975), 597–628.

10. Baird, A. and T. Durkin, Inhibition of endothelial cell proliferation by type beta transforming growth factor: Interactions with acidic and basic fibroblasts growth factors, Biochem. Biophys. Res. Commun. **138** (1986), 476–482.

11. Balding, D. and D. L. S. McElwain, A mathematical model of tumor-induced capillary growth, J. Theor. Biol. **114** (1985), 53–74.

12. Barinaga, M., Designing therapies that target tumor blood vessels, Science **275** (1997), 482–484.

13. Brown, M. T. and D. R. Clemmons, Platelets contain a peptide inhibitor of endothelial cell proliferation and growth, Proc. Natl. Acad. Sci. U.S.A. **83** (1986), 3321–3325.

14. Byrne, H. M. and M. A. J. Chaplain, Growth of necrotic tumors in the presence and absence of inhibitors, Math. Biosci. **135** (1996), 187–216.

15. Chaplain, M. A. J., The mathematical modeling of tumor angiogenesis and invasion, Acta Biotheoretica **43** (1995), 387–402.

16. Chaplain, M. A. J., D. L. Benson and P. K. Maini, Nonlinear diffusion of a growth inhibitory factor in multicell spheroids, Math. Biosci. **121** (1994), 1–13.

17. Chaplain, M. A. J. and N. F. Britton, On the concentration profile of a growth inhibitory factor in multicell spheroids, Math. Biosci. **115** (1993), 233–243.

18. Chaplain, M. A. J. and B. D. Sleeman, A mathematical model for the production and secretion of tumor angiogenesis factor in tumors, IMA J. Math. Appl. Med. Biol. **7** (1990), 93–108.

19. Chaplain, M. A. J. and A. M. Stuart, A mathematical model for the diffusion and of tumor angiogenesis factor into the surrounding host tissue, IMA J. Math. Appl. Med. Biol. **8** (1991), 191–220.

20. Chaplain, M. A. J. and A. M. Stuart, A model mechanism for the chemotactic response of endothelial cells to tumor angiogenesis factor, IMA J. Math. Appl. Med. Biol. **10** (1993), 149–168.

21. Cliff, W. J., Observations on healing tissue: A combined light and electron microscopic investigation, Philos. Trans. R. Soc. London B. **246** (1963), 305–325.

22. Denekamp, J., Vascular endothelium as the vulnerable element of tumors, Acta Radiol. Oncol. **23** (1984), 217–225.

23. Derynck, R., J. A. Jarrett, Y. C. Ellson, D. H. Eaton, J. R. Bell, R. K. Assoian, A. B. Roberts, M. B. Sporn and D. V. Goeddel, Human transforming growth factor-beta complementary DNA sequence and expression in normal and transformed cells, Nature **316** (1985), 701–705.

24. Derynck, R., A. B. Roberts, D. H. Eaton, M. E. Winkler and D. V. Goeddel, Human transforming growth factor-alpha: Precursor sequence, gene structure, and heterologous expression, growth factors and transformation, Feramisco, J., B. Ozanne and C. Stiles (eds.), Cold Spring Harbor Laboratory, Cold Spring Harbor, NY, 1985, 79–86.

25. Folkman, J., Tumor angiogenesis, in *Cancer 3, Biology of Tumors: Cellular Biology and Growth,* Becker, F. F., (ed.), Plenum Press, New York, 1975.

26. Folkman, J., Proceedings: Tumor angiogenesis factor, Cancer Research **34** (1974), 2109–2113.

27. J. Folkman, Tumor angiogenesis, Adv. Cancer Res. **43** (1985), 175–203.

28. Folkman, J., Antiangiogenesis: new concept for therapy of solid tumors, Ann. Surg. **175** (1972), 409–416.

29. Folkman, J. and R. Cotran, Relation of vascular proliferation to tumor growth, Int. Rev. Exp. Pathol. **16** (1976), 207–248.

30. Folkman, J. and H. P. Greenspan, Influence of geometry on control of cell growth, Biochem. Biophys. Acta. **417** (1975), 211–236.

31. Folkman, J. and M. Klagsburn, Angiogenic factors, Science **235** (1987), 442–447.

32. Folkman, J., R. Langer, R. J. Linhardt, C. Haudenschild and S. Taylor, Angiogenesis inhibition and tumor regression caused by heparin or a heparin fragment in the presence of cortisone, Science **221** (1983), 719–725.

33. Folkman, J., D. M. Long and F. F. Becker, Growth and metastasis of tumor in organ culture, Cancer **16** (1963), 453.

34. Form, D. M. and R. Auerbach, PGE_2 and angiogenesis, Proc. Soc. Exp. Biol. Med. **172** (1983), 214–218.

35. Frater-Schroeder, M., G. Mueller, W. Birchmeier and P. Boehlen, Transforming growth factor-beta inhibits endothelial cell proliferation, Biochem. Biophys. Res. Commun. **137** (1986), 295–302.

36. Gimbrone, M. A., R. H. Aster, R. S. Cotran, J. Corkery, J. H. Jandl and J. Folkman, Preservation of vascular integrity in organs perfused in vitro with a platelet rich medium, Nature **222** (1969), 33–36.

37. Goustin, A. S. E. B. Leof, G. D. Shipley and H. L. Moses, Growth factors and cancer, Cancer Research **46** (1986), 1015–1029.

38. Greenspan, H. P., Models for the growth of a solid tumor by diffusion, Stud. Appl. Math. **51** (1972), 317.

39. Greenspan, H. P., On the self inhibited growth of cell cultures, Growth **38** (1974), 81–95.

40. Heimark, R. L., D. R. Twardzik and S. M. Schwartz, Inhibition of endothelial regeneration by type-beta transforming growth factor from platelets, Science **233** (1986), 1078–1080.

41. Henry, N., Y. Eeckhout, A. L. van Lamsweerde and G. Vaes, Co-operation between metastatic tumor cells and macrophages in the degradation of basement membrane (type IV) collagen, FEBS Lett. **161** (1983), 243–246.

42. Holley, R. W., Control of growth of mammalian cells in cell culture, Nature **258** (1975), 487–490.

43. Lobb, R., J. Sasse, Y. Shing, P. A. D'Amore, R. Sullivan, J. Jacobs and M. Klagsburn, Purification and characterization of heparin-binding growth factors, J. Biol. Chem. **261** (1986), 1924–1928.

44. Maggelakis, S. A., The effects of tumor angiogenesis factor (TAF) and tumor inhibitor factors (TIFs) on tumor vascularization: A mathematical model, Math. Comput. Modelling **23** (1996), 121.

45. Maggelakis, S. A., Type α and type β transforming growth factors as regulators of cancer cellular growth: A mathematical model, Math. Comput. Modelling **18** (1993), 9.

46. Maggelakis, S. A., The effect of tumor growth factors on the growth rate of cell cultures, Appl. Math. Lett. **5** (1992), 53.

47. Maggelakis, S. A., Mathematical model of prevascular growth of a spherical carcinoma -Part II, Math. Comput. Modelling **17** (1993), 19.

48. Maggelakis, S. A., Effects of non-uniform inhibitor production on the growth of cancer cell cultures, Appl. Math. Lett. **5** (1992), 11.

49. Maggelakis, S. A. and J. A. Adam, Mathematical model of prevascular growth of a spherical carcinoma, Math. Comput. Modelling **13** (1990), 23–28.

50. Maisonpierre, P. C., C. Suri, P. F. Jones, S. Bartunkova, S. J. Wiegand, C. Radziejewski, D. Compton, J. McClain, T. H. Aldrich, N. Papadopoulos,

T. J. Daly, S. Davis, T. N. Sato and G. D. Yancopoulos, Angiopoietin-2, a natural antagonist for Tie2 that disrupts in vivo angiogenesis, Science **277** (1997), 55–60.

51. Marquardt, H., M. W. Hunkapiller, L. E. Hood and G. J. Todaro, Rat transforming growth factor type I: Structure and relation to epidermal growth factor, Science **223** (1984), 1079–1082.

52. Marx, J. L., Angiogenesis Research comes of age, Science **237** (1987), 23–24.

53. Michelson, S. and J. Leith, Autocrine and paracrine growth factors in tumor growth: A mathematical model, Bull. of Math. Biol. **53** (1991), 639.

54. Michelson, S. and J. Leith, Growth factors and growth control of heterogeneous cell populations, Bull. of Math. Biol. **55** (1993), 993–1011.

55. O'Reilly, M. S., L. Holmgren, Y. Shing, C. Chen, R. A. Rosenthal, M. Moses, W. S. Lane, Y. Cao, E. H. Sage and J. Folkman, Angiostatin: A novel angiogenesis inhibitor that mediates the suppression of metastases by a Lewis Lung carcinoma, Cell **79** (1994), 315–328.

56. Paweletz, N. and M. Knierim, Tumor-related angiogenesis, Critical Reviews in Oncology/Hematology **9** (1989), 197–242.

57. Pitot, H. C., *Fundamental of Oncology*, Marcel Dekker, New York, 1986.

58. Plate, K. H., G. Breier, H. A. Weich and W. Risau, Vascular endothelial growth factor is a potential tumor angiogenesis factor in human gliomas, (in vivo), Nature **359** (1992), 845–848.

59. Raju, K. S., G. Alessandri and P. Gullino, Characterization of a chemottractant for endothelium induced by angiogenesis effectors, Cancer Res. **44** (1984), 1579–1584.

60. Roberts, A. B., M. B. Sporn, R. K. Assoian, J. M. Smith, N. S. Roche, L. M. Wakefield and U. I. Heine, Transforming growth factor type beta: rapid induction of fibrosis and angiogenesis in vivo and stimulation of collagen formation in vitro, Proc. Natl. Acad. Sci. U.S.A. **83** (1986), 4167–4171.

61. Schoefl, G. I., Studies on inflammation. III. Growing capillaries: Their structure and permeability, Virchows Arch. Pathol. Anat. **337** (1963), 97.

62. Schoefl, G. I. And G. Majno, Regeneration of blood vessels in wound healing, Adv. Biol. Skin **5** (1964), 173.

63. Schreiber, A. B., M. E. Winkler and R. Derynck, Transforming growth factor-alpha: a more potent angiogenic mediator than epidermal growth factor, Science **232** (1986), 1250–1253.

64. Schweigerer, L., B. Malerstein and D. Gospodarowicz, Tumor necrosis factor inhibits the proliferation of cultured capillary endothelial cells, Biochem. Biophys. Res. Commun. **143** (1987), 997–1004.

65. Sholley, M. M., G. P. Ferguson, H. R. Seibel, J. L. Montour and J. D. Wilson, Mechanisms of neovascularization. Vascular sprouting can occur without proliferation of endothelial cells, Lab. Invest. **51** (1984), 624–634.

66. Shweiki, D., A. Itin, D. Soffer and E. Keshet, Vascular endothelial growth factor induced by hypoxia may mediate hypoxia-initiated angiogenesis, Nature **359** (1992), 843–845.

67. Shymko, R. M. and L. Glass, Cellular and geometric control of tissue growth and mitotic instability, J. Theor. Biol. **63** (1976), 355.

68. Sporn, M. B. and A. B. Roberts, Autocrine growth factors and cancer, Nature **313** (1985), 745–747.

69. Taylor S. and J. Folkman, Protamine is an inhibitor of angiogenesis, Nature **297** (1982), 307–312.

70. Thornton, S. C., S. N. Mueller and E. M. Levine, Human endothelial cells: Use of heparin in cloning and long term serial cultivation, Science **222** (1983), 623–625.

71. Warren, B. A., The ultrastructure of the microcirculation of the advancing edge of Walker 256 carcinoma, Microvasc. Res. **2** (1970), 443–453.

72. Warren, B. A., The vascular morphology of tumors, in *Tumor Blood Circulation*, Peterson, H. I., (ed.), CRC Press, Boca Raton, FL, 1979, Chapter 1.

Sophia A. Maggelakis
Department of Mathematics and Statistics
Rochester Institute of Technology
Rochester, NY 14623

Remarks on an Environmental Control Problem

Natalia Navarova and Horst R. Thieme

Abstract. The model by Thomas et al. [12] for zoo-plankton/pollu-
tant interaction in a fresh water environment is considered with a modified
pollutant input function. General conditions are presented under which a
relaxed feed-back control of the pollutant input drives the dynamics of the
model to a steady state where the environmental pollutant concentration
is below a prescribed threshold. Complementarily, a scenario is described
where the system converges towards a periodic orbit for almost all initial
conditions.

§1. Introduction

Thomas, Snell and Jaffar [12] present a feed-back control model for the interaction of a fresh-water population of zoo-plankton (e.g., rotifers) with a
toxic pollutant. The zoo-plankton population dynamics are described by a
standard logistic model where the Malthusian growth parameter $r(y)$ and the
carrying capacity $K(y)$ are monotone decreasing functions of the internal concentration y of the pollutant per unit zoo-plankton biomass. The model allows
for self-degradation of the pollutant and for degradation by the zoo-plankton.
The feed-back control is chosen in such a way that it forces the environmental
concentration of the pollutant to a limit, M (that is supposed to satisfy water
quality criteria). Thomas et al. [12] have analyzed the large-time behavior of
the controlled system for specific choices of the functions r and K, this note
will give conditions of a general form.

Our main result will be that the controlled system settles to a unique
equilibrium provided that $yr(y)$ and $yK(y)$ are strictly monotone increasing
functions of the internal pollutant concentration y. This condition is valid for
r and K considered in [12].

Conversely, if the derivative of $yK(y)$ is strictly negative for some $y > 0$,
a limit M can be chosen such that the system converges towards a periodic
orbit for almost all initial conditions.

We also look into the question whether the desired water quality limit can
be achieved by reducing the influx of the pollution alone, without an expensive

Mathematical Models in Medical and Health Sciences
Mary Ann Horn, Gieri Simonett, and Glenn Webb (eds.), pp. 267-279.

clean-up of the environment, and into the question what can be achieved by an open loop control. Finally we consider the problem in which the environmental concentration of the pollutant is not forced to a certain limit, but only below a certain threshold. We design a relaxed feed-back control that achieves this aim while granting some flexibility to adjust the input of pollutant to the internal needs of the polluting agent.

The paper is organized as follows. Section 2 describes the mathematical model. Section 3 gives a simple but general analysis of the system for a bounded influx of pollutant. In Section 4, the explicit formula for a feed-back controlled pollutant input is chosen, such that the environmental pollutant concentration converges to a prescribed limit, while Section 5 analyzes the resulting large-time behavior. In Section 6, we consider the relaxed feed-back control which forces the pollutant concentration below a prescribed threshold.

§2. The Model

The mathematical model by Thomas et al. [12] for the population-toxicant interaction consists of the following system of differential equations:

$$\frac{dx}{dt} = xr(y)\left(1 - \frac{x}{K(y)}\right),$$

$$\frac{dC_E}{dt} = -aC_Ex + bC_I - hC_E + u, \tag{2.1}$$

$$\frac{dC_I}{dt} = aC_Ex - \mu C_I,$$

where

$$y = \frac{C_I}{x},$$

with the initial conditions:

$$x(0) = x_0 > 0, \quad C_E(0) = C_E^0 \ge 0, \quad C_I(0) = C_I^0 \ge 0.$$

Here we have used the following notation:

$x(t)$, concentration of biomass of the population at time t,
$C_E(t)$, concentration of toxicant in the environment at time t,
$C_I(t)$, concentration of toxicant in the biomass at time t,
$y(t)$, concentration of toxicant per unit biomass at time t.
All parameters of the model, a, b, h, μ, are positive constants,

$$\mu = b + \beta, \quad \beta > 0.$$

The first equation in (2.1) represents the logistic model for the population of rotifers. Pollutant uptake by the zoo-plankton in the second and third equation are described by the law of mass action. hC_E describes the self-degradation of the pollutant in the environment. μC_I could be interpreted as the loss of internal pollutant due to zoo-plankton death where only part of the internal pollutant, bC_I (recall $b < \mu$), is recycled to the environment while the rest has been detoxicated by the zoo-plankton. The function u describes the input of toxicant into the environment.

From experimental data (see the references in [12]) it is known that the toxicant lowers both the growth rate r and the carrying capacity K. Therefore, we assume that $r = r(y), K = K(y)$ are continuously differentiable and non-increasing functions of $y \geq 0$. For convenience we further assume that r, K are bounded away from 0,

$$0 < \rho \leq r(y) \leq r(0),$$

$$0 < \delta \leq K(y) \leq K(0),$$

where $r(0)$ is the Malthusian growth parameter and $K(0)$ is the carrying capacity in the absence of toxicant.

The r, K notation obscures, however, that this may be a severe restriction of the model which becomes evident when one rewrites the first equation in (2.1) as

$$\frac{dx}{dt} = \beta(y)x - \mu_1(y)x - \mu_2(y)x^2,$$

with $\beta(y), \mu_1(y)$ being the per capita birth rate and the per capita mortality rate without crowding and $\mu_2(y)x$ the extra per capita mortality due to crowding. It is well conceivable that a high toxicant concentration makes the per capita death rate higher than the per capita birth rate which makes r, K strictly negative such that the model analysis both in [12] and in this paper no longer applies.

The input u can be governed by an open loop control that is independent of x, C_I, C_E, or by a feed-back control that, at any time instance $t \geq 0$, is adjusted according to the observable values of x, C_E, C_I.

Later the input u will be determined as a continuous function of t, x, C_E, C_I in such a way that it will force a convex combination of the environmental and internal pollutant concentrations

$$\zeta C_E + (1 - \zeta)C_I \longrightarrow M < \infty, \quad t \to \infty,$$

towards a prescribed limit M. Here $0 < \zeta \leq 1$ is some fixed arbitrary number, for example $\zeta = 1$ corresponds to the case considered in [12]. For $\zeta = 1/2$ we control the total pollutant concentration. As we will see later, this latter choice allows to take advantage of the self-cleaning properties of the system and to choose u always positive, i.e., an expensive clean-up of the environment can be avoided.

§3. Analysis of the Model with a Bounded Input

Let the pollutant input $u = u(t, x, C_E, C_I)$ be locally Lipschitz in $x, C_E, C_I \geq 0$ and

$$u(t, x, C_E, C_I) + bC_I \geq 0, \text{ whenever } C_E = 0, C_I \geq 0, x \geq 0, t \geq 0. \quad (3.1)$$

This assumption for the function u guarantees that, in the second equation in (2.1), $\frac{dC_E}{dt}$ is non-negative whenever $C_E = 0$; in other words, if there is no pollutant in the environment, there is nothing left one can remove.

Existence and uniqueness of a nonnegative solution.

In order to apply the standard theory of ordinary differential equations it is convenient to extend r, K, u to $\mathbb{R}$ by $r(y) = r(0), K(y) = K(0)$ for $y \leq 0$ and $u(t, x, C_E, C_I) = u(t, x_+, C_{E+}, C_{I+})$ with the subscript $+$ denoting the positive part of a number, e.g., $x_+ = \max\{x, 0\}$. This extension preserves Lipschitz continuity, and we obtain a unique solution of system (2.1) on a maximal interval $[0, c), c > 0$, with x being strictly positive. Furthermore, because of assumption (3.1), system (2.1) satisfies the conditions given in Proposition B.7 by Smith and Waltman [7]. Therefore, for any nonnegative data, there exists a unique solution which is nonnegative for all $t \geq 0$ for which it is defined. In particular, the above extension turns out to be redundant.

Since K is non-increasing, we readily see that

$$x(t) \leq \max\{x(0), K(0)\}.$$

Since we have assumed that r and K are bounded away from 0, we easily see that

$$x(t) \geq \min\{x(0), \inf K\} > 0.$$

Let $C = C_E + C_I$. Then it follows from (2.1) that C satisfies the differential equation

$$\frac{dC}{dt} = -\beta C_I - h C_E + u.$$

Let us introduce

$$\alpha = \min\{\beta, h\}, \quad \gamma = \max\{\beta, h\},$$

then

$$u - \gamma C \leq \frac{dC}{dt} \leq -\alpha C + u. \qquad (3.2)$$

Therefore, if u is bounded, C is bounded on $[0, c)$. However, $C = C_E + C_I$ and $C_E \geq 0, C_I \geq 0$, hence C_E and C_I are bounded on $[0, c)$. It follows that the local existence of a bounded nonnegative solution of (2.1) implies its global existence. In other words, for all $x(0) > 0$, $C_E(0), C_I(0) \geq 0$, there exists a unique nonnegative solution of (2.1), with x being globally bounded away from 0, which is defined on $[0, \infty)$.

We conclude this section by a simple, but universal result which applies to all bounded inputs u whether they are associated with an open loop control or a feed-back control. Let

$$u^\infty = \limsup_{t \to \infty} u(t),$$

and let analogous notation also hold for other functions.

Proposition 3.1. *Let the input u be bounded, $C = C_E + C_I$. Then*

$$C^\infty \leq \frac{u^\infty}{\alpha}, \qquad \alpha = \min\{\beta, h\}.$$

In particular $C_E(t) \longrightarrow 0$, $C_I(t) \longrightarrow 0$, as $t \to \infty$, when $u(t) \to 0$ as $t \to \infty$.

Proof: Apply the *method of fluctuation* that has been developed by Hirsch, Hanisch and Gabriel [4]. According to Proposition 2.1 given in Thieme [9] we can choose a sequence $t_n \to \infty$ $(n \to \infty)$ such that $C'(t_n) \to 0$, $C(t_n) \to C^\infty$, $n \to \infty$. By (3.2), $0 \leq -\alpha C^\infty + u^\infty$. $\square$

The practical meaning of this result is that the ecosystem cleans itself once pollution stops.

§4. Formula for the Feedback Input

Let us choose the input of toxicant into the environment as follows,

$$u(x, C_E, C_I) = \frac{1-\zeta}{\zeta}\Big[\mu C_I - aC_E x\Big] + aC_E x - bC_I + hC_E + \alpha(M - C_\zeta), \quad (4.1)$$

where

$$0 < \zeta \leq 1, \quad \alpha > 0,$$

and M is the desired limit of water quality in terms of

$$C_\zeta = \zeta C_E + (1 - \zeta)C_I. \tag{4.2}$$

Notice that $C_\zeta = C_E$ for $\zeta = 1$, the case studied in [12], while $C_\zeta = (1/2)(C_E + C_I)$ is proportional to the total pollutant concentration contained in the environment and the zoo-plankton biomass.

One easily checks that u has been chosen such that

$$\frac{dC_\zeta}{dt} = -\alpha\zeta(C_\zeta - M), \tag{4.3}$$

and so

$$\frac{d(C_\zeta - M)^2}{dt} = -2\alpha\zeta(C_\zeta - M)^2. \tag{4.4}$$

In order to satisfy the constraint

$$u(x, 0, C_I) + bC_I \geq 0 \quad \text{whenever } x, C_I \geq 0,$$

we notice that

$$u(x, 0, C_I) + bC_I \geq (1 - \zeta)\left[\frac{\mu}{\zeta} - \alpha\right]C_I.$$

So this constrained is satisfied if $\zeta = 1$ (the case considered in [12]) or if $\zeta\alpha \leq \mu$. Further observe that u is a locally Lipschitz continuous function.

A similar analysis as in the previous section establishes unique non-negative solutions x, C_E, C_I on a maximal interval $[0, c)$. It follows from (4.3) that

$$C_\zeta(t) \leq \max\{C_\zeta(0), M\}.$$

This implies that C_ζ is bounded on $[0, c)$, and so is $C_E \leq (1/\zeta)C_\zeta$. As before, x is bounded and bounded away from 0; it follows from the third equation in (2.1) that also C_I is bounded. Again, we can conclude that the solutions actually exist on $[0, \infty)$. The previous analysis shows that the solutions are globally bounded on $[0, \infty)$.

We summarize our consideration as follows.

Theorem 4.1. *Let u be chosen by (4.1) with $\zeta = 1$ or $\zeta\alpha \leq \mu$. Then, for $x(0) > 0, C_E(0) \geq 0, C_I(0) \geq 0$, there exist unique non-negative solutions x, C_E, C_I on $[0, \infty)$ of (2.1). These solutions are globally bounded on $[0, \infty)$. Moreover x is globally bounded away from 0. Finally*

$$C_\zeta(t) \to M, \quad t \to \infty.$$

Proof: Existence, uniqueness and boundedness on $[0, \infty)$ have been established before. As we already mentioned in the previous section, we have

$$x(t) \geq \min\{x(0), \inf K\} \quad \forall t \geq 0.$$

The convergence statement follows from (4.4). □

Notice, if $\zeta = 0.5$, the toxicant input u forces $C = C_E + C_I \to 2M$. At least in this case, u can be chosen nonnegative. Indeed, if $\zeta = 0.5$, and

$$\alpha \leq 2\min\{\beta, h\},$$

then

$$u = \beta C_I + h C_E + \alpha\left(M - \frac{1}{2}C\right) \geq \alpha M,$$

where $C = C_E + C_I$.

This means that for $\zeta = 0.5$ the suggested control strategy does not require to clean up the environment which would presumably be more expensive than reducing the input of pollutant.

We rewrite the third equation in (2.1) as

$$\frac{dC_I}{dt} = \frac{a}{\zeta}C_\zeta x + \left(a(1 - \frac{1}{\zeta})x - \mu\right)C_I.$$

As a result, the system (2.1) can be reduced to the following planar asymptotically autonomous system in terms of x and $y = C_I/x$:

$$\begin{aligned}
\frac{dx}{dt} &= xr(y)\left(1 - \frac{x}{K(y)}\right), \\
\frac{dy}{dt} &= \frac{aC_\zeta}{\zeta} - \left(\mu + a(\frac{1}{\zeta} - 1)x\right)y - yr(y)\left(1 - \frac{x}{K(y)}\right).
\end{aligned} \tag{4.5}$$

Since $C_\zeta(t) \to M$ as $t \to \infty$, this asymptotically autonomous system has the following limiting system:

$$
\begin{aligned}
\frac{dx}{dt} &= xr(y)\left(1 - \frac{x}{K(y)}\right) = f_1(x, y), \\
\frac{dy}{dt} &= \frac{aM}{\zeta} - \left(\mu + a(\frac{1}{\zeta} - 1)x\right)y - yr(y)\left(1 - \frac{x}{K(y)}\right) = f_2(x, y),
\end{aligned}
\tag{4.6}
$$

with initial conditions

$$
x(0) = x_0 > 0, \ y(0) = y_0 \geq 0.
$$

Since the system (4.5) is equivalent to (2.1) and (4.6) is equivalent to the limit system for (2.1), we have that all solutions to (4.5) and (4.6), with the appropriate initial data, are globally bounded, and x is globally bounded away from 0. Further direct analysis of the second equation in (4.5) or (4.6), respectively, shows that also y is globally bounded away from 0.

§5. The Long-Time Behavior of the Controlled System

While the solutions of an asymptotically autonomous differential equation do not always behave like the solutions of the associated limit system (see Thieme [10, Sections 2 and 3] for examples), they do so under quite general assumptions (see [5, 8, 13]). In particular there is a *Poincaré/Bendixson* type limit-set-trichotomy similar to the autonomous case if the system is planar [1,10,11]. This limit-set-trichotomy is identical to the autonomous case, if the system is rather quasi-autonomous than merely asymptotically autonomous [11, (1.2)], as is our system (4.5) because, by (4.4), C_ζ converges to M exponentially. The following result is stated somewhat loosely. The exact assumptions are the same as in [11, Theorem 1.5].

Theorem 5.1. *Consider a quasi-autonomous planar system (QA) with limit system (L). Let z be a forward bounded solution of (QA) that is defined for all forward times such that the closure of its forward orbit is contained in the domains of definition of (QA) and (L). Assume that there are at most finitely many equilibria of (L) in a sufficiently small neighborhood of ω, the ω-limit set of z. Then the following trichotomy holds:*
(i) ω consists of an equilibrium of (L).
(ii) ω is a periodic orbit of (L).
(iii) Every point in ω lies on an orbit cycle of (L) contained in ω.

An *orbit cycle* of (L) consists of equilibria $e_1, ..., e_m$ and of orbits $\gamma_1, ..., \gamma_m$ of (L) such that γ_j connects e_j to e_{j+1} for $j = 1, \ldots, m-1$ and γ_m connects e_m to e_1. If $m = 1$, an orbit cycle is a homoclinic orbit.

Proof: This theorem is almost identical to Theorem 1.5 in [11], except for the stronger statement (iii). In [2] and [5, Theorem 1.8], it is shown that ω is (internally) chain-recurrent. Option (iii) now follows from Theorem 1.1 in [1]. $\square$

Before we start applying this theorem, we observe from the first equation in (2.1), or (4.5), and the assumption that the carrying capacity K is globally bounded away from 0, that

$$\liminf_{t \to \infty} x(t) \geq \inf K > 0$$

for every non-negative solution with $x(0) > 0$. So every boundary equilibrium on the $x = 0$ axis is unstable, even a repeller. Moreover every ω-limit set of a non-negative solution of (4.6) with $x(0) > 0$ is bounded away from the $x = 0$ axis.

Let us first discuss the less interesting case that the target value M is 0. Then the limiting system (4.6) has three equilibria, which are all boundary equilibria, two on the $x = 0$ axis which, as we have seen, are repellers, and the equilibrium $y^* = 0, x^* = K(0)$ which is locally asymptotically stable, as seen by linearization. The system (4.6) has no periodic orbits, because they would need to surround an interior equilibrium. Both the repellers and the asymptotically stable equilibrium cannot be part of an orbit cycle of (4.6), so (4.6) has no orbit cycle. By Theorem 5.1, the ω-limit set of any non-negative solution of (4.5) with $x(0) > 0$ is an equilibrium. The nature of the three equilibria, as discussed above, implies that $y(t) \to 0, x(t) \to K(0)$ as $t \to \infty$.

In the following we **exclusively** consider the more interesting case $M > 0$. The steady states of the limiting system (4.6) then satisfy the algebraic equations:

$$x^* = 0, \quad \varphi(y^*) := \zeta\Big(\mu + r(y^*)\Big)y^* = aM, \tag{5.1}$$

$$x^* = K(y^*), \quad \psi(y^*) := \Big(\zeta\mu + a(1 - \zeta)K(y^*)\Big)y^* = aM. \tag{5.2}$$

Let us show that there exists at least one boundary equilibrium, i.e., a solution of (5.1). Obviously $\varphi(0) = 0$ and $\varphi(y) \to \infty$ as $y \to \infty$. Since $\varphi : [0, \infty) \to [0, \infty)$ is continuous, by the Intermediate Value Theorem there exists a solution $\varphi(y^*) = aM$. Thus, there exists at least one boundary equilibrium $(0, y^*)$. Since $r'(y) < 0, y > 0$, it is possible to have 3 or more boundary equilibria in the case when the function φ has one local maximum and one local minimum at least. On the other hand, if the function φ is strictly increasing, e. g., if $(yr(y))' > 0, \forall y > 0$, there is the only one boundary steady state $(0, y^*)$.

The solutions $(K(y^*), y^*)$ of (5.2) are interior equilibria of (4.6). The same analysis as before shows that there always exists an interior equilibrium and that it is unique if ψ is strictly increasing, e.g., if $yK(y)$ is strictly increasing. Again, in general, it is possible to have 3 or more interior equilibria.

Let $(K(y^*), y^*)$ be an interior equilibrium. Then

$$D(f_1, f_2)(K(y^*), y^*) =$$
$$\begin{pmatrix} -r(y^*) & r(y^*)K'(y^*) \\ -a\left(\frac{1}{\zeta} - 1\right)y^* + y^*\frac{r(y^*)}{K(y^*)} & -\left(\mu + a\left(\frac{1}{\zeta} - 1\right)K(y^*) + y^*\frac{r(y^*)}{K(y^*)}K'(y^*)\right) \end{pmatrix}$$

Since the sum of the eigenvalues is the trace of this matrix, we have that

$$\lambda_1 + \lambda_2 = -\left[\frac{r(y^*)}{K(y^*)}(y^*K(y^*))' + \mu + a\left(\frac{1}{\zeta} - 1\right)K(y^*)\right]$$

is negative if $(y^*K(y^*))' > 0$.

Since the determinant equals the product of the eigenvalues, we obtain that

$$\lambda_1\lambda_2 = \frac{r(y^*)}{\zeta}\psi'(y^*).$$

Proposition 5.2. *Let the function ψ in (5.2) be strictly monotone increasing (e.g., $\zeta = 1$). Then there exists a unique interior equilibrium of (4.6) which is either a sink or a source. Every solution x, y of (4.5) with $x(0) > 0, y(0) \geq 0$ converges towards the interior equilibrium of (4.6) or towards a periodic orbit of (4.6).*

We recall that a sink is an equilibrium with all the associated eigenvalues having strictly negative real part, while all the eigenvalues of a source have strictly positive real part.

Remark. If even the derivative of $yK(y)$ is strictly positive, the unique interior equilibrium is locally asymptotically stable.

We use the Bendixson-Dulac criterion to exclude periodic orbits of (4.6) and actually establish global stability of a (uniquely determined) interior equilibrium.

As the Dulac function to be we introduce

$$\chi(x, y) = \frac{1}{xyr(y)},$$

defined on $x > 0, y > 0$. Then

$$\frac{\partial(\chi f_1)}{\partial x}(x, y) + \frac{\partial(\chi f_2)}{\partial y}(x, y) = -\frac{(yK(y))'}{yK^2(y)} - \frac{aM(yr(y))'}{\zeta x(yr(y))^2}$$
$$+ \left(\mu + a(\frac{1}{\zeta} - 1)x\right)\frac{r'(y)}{xr^2(y)}$$
$$\leq -\frac{(yK(y))'}{yK^2(y)} - \frac{aM(yr(y))'}{\zeta x(yr(y))^2},$$

because $r = r(y)$ is non-increasing and $\mu + a(\frac{1}{\zeta} - 1)x > 0$.

Hence, if $(yK(y))', (yr(y))' > 0$ for all $y > 0$, the divergence

$$\frac{\partial(\chi f_1)}{\partial x}(x,y) + \frac{\partial(\chi f_2)}{\partial y}(x,y) < 0.$$

By the Bendixson-Dulac criterion, there are no periodic orbits in the interior of the positive quadrant. So we can conclude the following from Proposition 5.2 first for the solutions x, y of (4.5) and then the solutions of system (2.1).

Theorem 5.3. *Let the feed-back control u be given by (4.1) with the restrictions $\zeta = 1$ or $0 < \zeta < 1, \zeta \alpha \leq \mu$.*

If the functions $F_1(y) = yK(y), F_2(y) = yr(y)$ have strictly positive derivatives, there exists a unique interior equilibrium of (2.1) which attracts all solutions x, C_E, C_I of (2.1) with $x(0) > 0$, $C_E(0) \geq 0$, $C_I(0) \geq 0$.

The assumption for K is necessary in a certain way:

Theorem 5.4. *Let the feed-back control u be given by (4.1) and $\zeta = 1$. Assume that the derivative of $F_1(y) = yK(y)$ is strictly negative for some $y > 0$. Then there exist $M > 0, \mu > 0$ such that the solutions of (2.1) converge towards a periodic orbit for almost all initial data $x(0) > 0$, $C_E(0) \geq 0$, $C_I(0) \geq 0$.*

Proof: Choose $y^* > 0$ such that the derivative of $F_1(y) = yK(y)$ is strictly negative for $y = y^*$. Now choose $\mu > 0$ such that

$$\mu < -\frac{r(y^*)}{K(y^*)}(y^* K(y^*))'.$$

Set $M = (\mu/a)y^*$ and $(K(y^*), y^*)$ becomes an equilibrium of (4.6) which is a source. The associated interior equilibrium of (2.1) is a saddle with a one-dimensional stable and a two-dimensional unstable manifold. By Proposition 5.2, all solution of (4.5) and hence of (2.1) converge towards the interior equilibrium or a periodic orbit. But only the solutions starting on the stable manifold converge towards the interior equilibrium. Since the stable manifold of an unstable hyperbolic equilibrium has Lebesgue measure 0 (see [7, proof of Theorem F.1]), the assertion follows. $\square$

Alternatively to Theorem 5.4 we can try to employ the theory of competitive systems [3,6].

Let us introduce a time scale of the limit system (4.6):

$$\frac{d\tau}{dt} = r(y).$$

Then the scaled system (4.6) takes the form:

$$\frac{d\hat{x}}{d\tau} = \hat{x}\left(1 - \frac{\hat{x}}{K(\hat{y})}\right) = f_1(\hat{x}, \hat{y}),$$

$$\frac{d\hat{y}}{d\tau} = \frac{1}{r(\hat{y})} \left(\frac{aM}{\zeta} - \left(\mu + a(\frac{1}{\zeta} - 1)\hat{x} \right) \hat{y} \right) - \hat{y} \left(1 - \frac{\hat{x}}{K(\hat{y})} \right) = f_2(\hat{x}, \hat{y}).$$

Since

$$\frac{\partial f_1}{\partial \hat{y}} = \frac{\hat{x}^2 K'(\hat{y})}{K^2(\hat{y})} \le 0$$

and

$$\frac{\partial f_2}{\partial \hat{x}} = - \left(\frac{a(\frac{1}{\zeta} - 1)}{r(\hat{y})} - \frac{1}{K(\hat{y})} \right) \hat{y},$$

this system is competitive if the right hand side of the last equation is non-positive. Since planar competitive ODE systems have no periodic orbits (see, e.g., Theorem 2.2 in [6, Chapter 3], we obtain the following from Proposition 5.2.

Theorem 5.5. *Let the feed-back control u be given by (4.1) with the restrictions $0 < \zeta < 1, \zeta\alpha \le \mu$.*

Let the function ψ in (5.2) be strictly monotone increasing. Further let

$$a(\frac{1}{\zeta} - 1) \ge \frac{r(y)}{K(y)}, \quad \forall y \ge 0.$$

Then all solutions x, y of (4.5) with $x(0) > 0, y(0) \ge 0$ converge towards the uniquely determined interior equilibrium of (4.6).

This result does not apply to the case that is C_E controlled, $\zeta = 1$. In case that $C = C_E + C_I$ is controlled, $\zeta = 0.5$, the condition in Theorem 5.4 takes the form

$$a \ge \frac{r(y)}{K(y)} \quad \forall y \ge 0.$$

§6. A Relaxed Feedback Control

Actually, for restricting the pollution, it would be sufficient to achieve

$$\limsup_{t \to \infty} C_\zeta(t) \le M \tag{6.1}$$

rather than convergence of $C_\zeta(t)$ to $M > 0$. One wonders whether such a sufficient, but less precise target would allow to build some flexibility into the feed-back control to adjust the pollutant input to the internal needs of the polluting agent. This is the case, indeed. Consider the input

$$\bar{u}(t, x, C_E, C_I) = \frac{1-\zeta}{\zeta} \left[\mu C_I - aC_E x \right] + aC_E x - bC_I + hC_E$$

$$- \alpha[C_\zeta - M]_+ + \xi(t)[M - C_\zeta]_+ \tag{6.2}$$

with the restrictions $\zeta = 1$ or $0 < \zeta < 1, \zeta\alpha \leq \mu$.

Here $\xi : [0, \infty) \to [0, \infty)$ is an arbitrary non-negative function which the polluting agent can adjust as wished as long as it is piecewise continuous. Recall that $[\cdot]_+$ denotes taking the positive part.

We call $\bar{u}$ a relaxed feed-back control. We now obtain

$$\frac{dC_\zeta}{dt} = -\zeta\alpha[C_\zeta - M]_+ + \zeta\xi(t)[M - C_\zeta]_+.$$

Then

$$\frac{d}{dt}[C_\zeta - M]_+^2 = -2\zeta\alpha[C_\zeta - M]_+^2,$$

but also

$$\frac{d}{dt}[M - C_\zeta]_+^2 = -2\xi(t)\zeta[M - C_\zeta]_+^2.$$

Notice that $[C_\zeta - M]_+[M - C_\zeta]_+ = 0$. Hence, if $C_\zeta(0) \geq M$,

$$C_\zeta(t) = M + (C_\zeta(0) - M)e^{-\zeta\alpha t}$$

and $C_\zeta(t) \searrow M$ as $t \to \infty$. If $C_\zeta(0) < M$,

$$C_\zeta = M - (M - C_\zeta(0))\exp\left(-\zeta\int_0^t \xi(s)ds\right).$$

So there exists some number $\kappa \in [0, 1]$ such that

$$C_\zeta(t) \nearrow (1 - \kappa)M + \kappa C_\zeta(0), \quad t \to \infty, \qquad \text{if } C_\zeta(0) < M.$$

Depending on ξ the approach of C_ζ to its limit may or may not be exponentially fast. So the system (4.5) may be merely asymptotically autonomous, and not quasi-autonomous. Theorem 1.5 in [11] still allows us to draw the following conclusion from the local stability analysis of the interior equilibria in Section 5.

Proposition 6.1. *Let the function ψ in (5.2) be strictly monotone increasing. Then the following holds:*

There exists a uniquely determined interior equilibrium of (4.6) (with M being replaced by the limit of C_ζ) which is either a sink or a source.
Every solution x, y of (4.5) with $x(0) > 0, y(0) \geq 0$ either converges towards the unique equilibrium or has an ω-limit set that is the union of periodic orbits of (4.6).

It is sufficient to proceed as in Section 5 to draw the following conclusions from Proposition 6.1.

Theorem 6.2. *Let the relaxed feed-back control $u = \bar{u}$ be given by (6.2) with the restrictions $\zeta = 1$ or $0 < \zeta < 1, \zeta\alpha \leq \mu$. Then the Theorems 5.3 and 5.5 hold verbatim.*

Acknowledgments. This research has been partially supported by NSF grant DMS-9403884.

References

1. Benaïm, M. and M. W. Hirsch, Chain recurrence in surface flows, Disc. Cont. Dyn. Sys. **1** (1995), 1–16.

2. Benaïm, M. and M. W. Hirsch, Asymptotic pseudotrajectories and chain recurrent flows, J. Dyn. Diff. Eq. **8** (1996), 141–176.

3. Hirsch, M. W., Systems of differential equations which are competitive or cooperative I: Limit sets, SIAM J. Appl. Math. **13** (1982), 167–179.

4. Hirsch, W. M., H. Hanisch and J.P. Gabriel, Differential equation models for some parasitic infections; methods for the study of the asymptotic behavior, Comm. Pure Appl. Math. **38** (1985), 733–753.

5. Mischaikow, K., H. L. Smith and H. R. Thieme, Asymptotically autonomous semiflows, chain recurrence and Lyapunov functions, Trans. AMS **347** (1995), 1669–1685.

6. Smith, H. L., *Monotone Dynamical Systems: an Introduction to the Theory of Competitive and Cooperative Systems*, American Mathematical Society, Providence, RI, 1995.

7. Smith, H. L., and P. Waltman, *The Theory of the Chemostat*, Cambridge University Press, 1995.

8. Thieme, H. R., Convergence results and a Poincaré-Bendixson trichotomy for asymptotically autonomous differential equations, J. Math. Biol. **30** (1992), 755–763.

9. Thieme, H. R., Persistence under relaxed point-dissipativity (with applications to an endemic model), SIAM J. Math. Anal. **24** (1993), 407–435.

10. Thieme, H. R., Asymptotically autonomous differential equations in the plane, Rocky Mountain J. Math. **24** (1994), 351–380.

11. Thieme, H. R., Asymptotically autonomous differential equations in the plane II. Stricter Poincaré/Bendixson type results, Diff. Int. Eqs. **7** (1994), 1625–1640.

12. Thomas, D. M., T. W. Snell and S. M. Jaffar, A control problem in a polluted environment, Math. Biosci. **133** (1996), 139–163.

13. Zhao, X.-Q., Asymptotic behavior for asymptotically periodic semiflows with applications. Comm. Appl. Nonlin. Anal. **3**, 43–66.

Natalia Navarova and Horst R. Thieme
Department of Mathematics
Arizona State University
Tempe, AZ 85287-1804
asnxn@acvax.inre.asu.edu
thieme@math.la.asu.edu

The Mathematical Modelling of Cancer: A Review

John Carl Panetta, Mark A. J. Chaplain and John A. Adam

Abstract. Mathematical models have been used to describe almost every aspect of cancer, from its inception to treatment. This review will look into some of these models; discuss their results; determine how they relate to known medical information; and, speculate on some of the future avenues of research in cancer modelling. This review is not meant to be complete but rather touch on some areas of current research in cancer modelling.

§1. Introduction

When modelling cancer one of the first questions that comes to mind is, how will mathematics help in the quest to control cancer? At first, it might seem that there is little medical researchers can learn from mathematicians and their models. But with a closer look we can see that there can be much gained by mathematically modelling cancer. In general, the main areas that modelling can help are in gaining a better basic understanding of some of the different dynamics of cancer, the nonlinear interactions between cancer cells and their surroundings, and the treatment of cancer by various chemo- and radiotherapies. By developing nonlinear mathematical models to describe various aspects of cancer, we can demonstrate how non-intuitive dynamics might evolve from a given situation, thus giving us a better understanding of cancer.

Some of the areas of cancer growth that have been modeled mathematically include solid tumor growth (both prevascular and vascular), tumor progression, angiogenesis, metastases and tumor heterogeneity. Mathematical results arising from some of these models include: The prediction of the development of a necrotic core within a prevascular tumor; the prediction of the rate of growth of the necrotic core; the prediction of the ultimate thickness of the viable layer of proliferating cells in a multicell spheroid; the prediction of the stability of a cancer *vis-à-vis* cell-cell adhesion; the prediction of the

Mathematical Models in Medical and Health Sciences
Mary Ann Horn, Gieri Simonett, and Glenn Webb (eds.), pp. 281–309.

onset of invasion; the prediction of the rate of growth of a capillary network and how its development and morphology is influenced by various angiogenic cytokines and matrix macromolecules [12, 13, 14, 16, 63]. These models have helped in the understanding of the growth and progression of cancer.

Other areas of modelling have emphasized the treatment of cancer through methods such as chemotherapy and immunotherapy. Some approaches in these areas have been: to model the effects of the chemotherapeutic treatments to sensitive normal tissue, such as bone marrow, in an attempt to reduce the toxicity of the treatments; to utilize optimization methods to help determine optimal treatment regimens that can reduce the cancer while maintaining an acceptable level of bone marrow; to model the effects of cell-cycle-specific drugs on both the cancerous and normal tissue so the cell-cycle can be exploited to the advantage of the patient; and, to consider how the immune system interacts with the cancer and how that might be used to help control the cancer.

An example of an important modelling result that has come from the study of cell-cycle-specific chemotherapy is the concept that treatment regimens are not necessarily intuitive. For example, some of the models show that increasing just the dose strength of the drug does *not* relate to an increased cell kill. In fact, the various models have suggested that the treatment period, drug infusion time, and, in some cases, how each relates to the cell-cycle time have a much greater influence on the cell kill than merely increasing the drug strength. Furthermore, each of these model results have been shown the hold in various in vitro and in vivo studies.

In this review we will describe some of the areas mathematical researchers are helping in the fight against cancer. These topics range from the theoretical to the directly applicable. In this process, we hope to stimulate further research in these important areas of modelling.

§2. Immune-Tumor-Cytokine Interaction

One of the newer innovations in cancer treatment is the attempt to stimulate the immune system with cytokines such as interleukin-2 so that they can effectively destroy cancerous growth. This is known as immunotherapy. The basic premise is that cancer cells have unique markers on them called antigens which distinguish them as different from the antigens on normal cells. Immune system cells such as T-cells detect these cancer antigens as different from the normal tissue and thus mount an immune response against the cancer. Problems occur when the T-cells are unable to recognize the cancer's antigen or distinguish the antigen of the cancer as different from that of the normal tissue. When the T-cells do recognize a different antigen then they secrete an autocrine signal (similar to those described by Michelson and Leith—see section (4)) that stimulates a T-cell response to that antigen, and thus the cancer. Two common signals (or growth factors) that have been discovered are the cytokines interleukin-2 (IL-2) and interferon (IFN). In an attempt to use this signaling process to our advantage, scientist have isolated these two growth factors and have produced them artificially. These growth factors are then used in various ways to stimulate the immune response against cancer.

There are two forms of immunotherapy with IL-2 currently being investigated [72]. Either, IL-2 is given directly to the patient to boost the immune system, or it is given in the form of TIL therapy and LAK therapy. TIL (Tumor Infiltrating lymphocyte) Therapy are cells derived from lymphocytes recovered from patient tumors and are comprised of activated NK (natural killer) cells and CTL (cytotoxic T-Lymphocytes) cells. These lymphocytes are specifically adapted to killing the cancer cells from the region they are taken since they have been exposed to the specific antigen of that cancer. They are then incubated with high concentrations of IL-2 in vitro and injected back into the patient at the tumor site. LAK (lymphokine-activated killer cell) Therapy are cells derived from the in vitro culturing of peripheral blood leukocytes removed from patients, with high concentrations of IL-2. The LAK cells are then injected back at the cancer site.

In an attempt to better understand this process Kirschner and Panetta [45] have designed a mathematical model to describe the interactions between the immune system cells, the cancer, and the IL-2. Its form is

$$\frac{dE}{dt} = cT - \mu_2 E + \frac{p_1 E I_L}{g_1 + I_L} + s_1,$$

$$\frac{dT}{dt} = r_2(T)T - \frac{aET}{g_2 + T},$$

$$\frac{dI_L}{dt} = \frac{p_2 ET}{g_3 + T} - \mu_3 I_L + s_2,$$

where E are the effector (or immune system) cells, T are the tumor cells, and I_L is IL-2. This model is an extension of some previous models developed by Adam [3], DeLisi and Rescigno [22], and Kuznetsov et al. [46], with the addition of explicitly modelling the IL-2 concentration. This addition leads to some different and interesting (both mathematically and medically) dynamics.

The model is first used to show some interesting results without immunotherapy. For "low" antigenic cancers the immune system is not able to clear the cancer simply because it is unable to detect the cancer and therefore it cannot mount an immune response. But, the model shows that for cancers with "medium" antigenicity, stable limit cycles exist where the effector cell and tumor cell mass oscillates with periods in the range of 8 to 10 years. These oscillations are interesting in that during most of the period (all but about one month) the cancer is in a dormant state (undetectable). But, there is then a rapid growth where the cancer grows to very high levels. This effect can explain long term recurrence observed in cancers such as melanoma where the cancer is initially reduced to undetectable levels through various therapies then, in the range of 8 to 15 years later, there is a sudden recurrence of the disease. Finally, with a "highly" antigenic cancer the model predicts a dormant state where the cancer is not eradicated, but is undetectable (but not disease free). Thus any change in the environment, such as the cancer loosing its antigenicity, can lead to a recurrence of the cancer.

Next the model is used to investigate the use of IL-2, TIL, and LAK therapy to control the cancer. If TIL or LAK therapy is given at strong enough levels then the system predicts a cancer free state. But, even in this case if the antigenicity of the cancer is "small" then the model indicates a bistable situation where depending on the initial conditions either the cancer free or cancerous state is obtained. This indicates the need for starting treatment early, while the cancer is small, so that there is a better chance of obtaining the cancer free state.

Furthermore, the model indicates that the use of IL-2 alone to boost the immune system, thus eradicate the cancer, is not as successful as the TIL or LAK therapy. In fact this result is also seen clinically. What the model shows is that when IL-2 is administered at lower levels then the cancer will not be eradicated, but if it is given at the levels needed to remove the cancer then the immune system grows uncontrolled. This is an unsatisfactory result since this can lead to problems such as capillary leak syndrome. Therefore, the treatment must be reduced or stopped, thus preventing the destruction of the cancer. Thus, this model indicates that the best approach for immunotherapy is to give a combination of IL-2 and TIL or LAK therapy. Similar conclusions are also observed in the clinical studies of this therapy.

§3. Spatio-Temporal Dynamics of Immune Cell-Tumor Cell-Tumor Cell Interactions

In this section we continue to focus on the immune response to cancer but we add in an extra dimension to the modelling —that of space— and review a model which takes into account a possible spatio-temporal encounter between tumor cells and cells of the immune system.

The early stage of primary tumor formation often occurs in the absence of a vascular network. According to [27, 71], this stage may last up to several years. The tumor nodule grows to an approximate size of 1–3 mm in diameter, containing close to $(1-3) \times 10^6$ cells and then growth slows down and/or ceases. This limitation of growth is attributed by researchers to the competition between tumor cells for metabolites, the competition between tumor cells and cells of the immune system for metabolites and/or a direct cytostatic/cytotoxic effect produced by the tumor cells on each other. In addition, the early (avascular) stage and the subsequent stages of tumor growth are characterized by a chronic inflammatory infiltration of neutrophils, eosinophils, basophils, monocytes/macrophages, T-lymphocytes, B-lymphocytes and natural killer (NK) cells [53, 77, 86]. These cells penetrate the interior of the tumor and accumulate in it due to attractants secreted from the tumor tissue and the high locomotive ability of activated immune cells [70]. During the avascular stage, tumor development can be effectively eliminated by tumor-infiltrating cytotoxic lymphocytes (TICLs) [50]. The TICLs may be cytotoxic lymphocytes (CTLs), NK cells and/or lymphokine activated killer (LAK) cells [23, 35, 53, 86]. The cytostatic/cytotoxic activity of granulocytes and monocytes/macrophages located in the tumor is determined less frequently [23, 35, 80].

An important factor, which may influence the outcome of the interactions between tumor cells and TICLs in a solid tumor, is the distribution of the TICLs. A thick shell of lymphoid infiltration is often revealed around the tumor [8, 10] and even near the central hypoxic zone [51]. This would define an internal structure, whereby the regions of cell proliferation and cell death alternate, with the TICLs located near the groups of dying tumor cells [61]. In spite of some progress into the investigation of TICLs and their mechanisms of interaction with tumor cells, our understanding of the spatio-temporal dynamics of TICLs in small tumors and in micrometastases *in vivo* is still rather limited. It is perhaps not surprising therefore, that this complicated picture has not yet received an adequate explanation. Certainly, other components of the immune system (e.g. cytokines) are involved in modulating the local cellular immune response dynamics. Many cytokines are produced during cell-cell interactions, which can be focussed to perform their function over short ranges in space and over short intervals of time. Interestingly, strong local immune reactions are induced by the release of interleukin-1 (IL-1), IL-2, IL-3, IL-4, IL-5, IL-6, IL-7, IL-8, IL-10, IL-12, IL-13, IL-15, G-CSF, GM-CSF, INF-α, TNF-α, INF-γ etc. Each of these cytokines recruits and activates some distinct cell population, which could be tumor-infiltrating cells, or the tumor cells themselves [35, 69, 75]. Besides immune reactions, other processes (e.g. cell proliferation, development, locomotion and apoptosis) are governed in a feedback fashion by their own intensity. The experimental analysis of such *in vivo* functions requires gene transfer technology and adoptive cell transfer studies, among others. Such studies are, however, hampered by the availability of *in vitro* cloned TICLs and by the frustrating experience that these *in vitro* propagated killer cells perform relatively badly *in vivo*, due to, for example, the down-regulation of their homing receptors and up-regulation of many of the cytokines amongst other things.

The Mathematical Model

We consider a model of Chaplain et al. [17] which examines a simplified process of a small, growing, avascular tumor which produces signals (e.g. secretes chemicals) which attract a population of lymphocytes. These signals are recognized by TICLs and the tumor is directly attacked by TICLs [42, 43, 44]. The humoral immune response, the interactions between cells of the immune system and dynamics of cytokines in the tumor will be accounted for indirectly, because data related to these processes is often contradictory and many important mechanisms of cytokine dynamics in tumors are unknown.

Local interactions between TICLs and tumor cells *in vivo* may be described by the simplified kinetic scheme in Figure 1 (see [46] for full details), where E, T, C, E^* and T^* are the local concentrations of TICLs, tumor cells, TICL-tumor cell complexes, inactivated TICLs and 'lethally hit' or 'programmed-for-lysis' tumor cells, respectively. The parameters k_1, k_{-1} and k_2 are non-negative kinetic constants: k_1 and k_{-1} describe the rate of binding of TICL to tumor cells and detachment of TICL from tumor cells *without* damaging cells; k_2 is the rate of detachment of TICL from tumor cells, re-

$$E + T \underset{K_{-1}}{\overset{K_1}{\rightleftharpoons}} C \underset{k_2(1-p)}{\overset{k_2 p}{\underset{\searrow}{\nearrow}}} \begin{matrix} E + T^* \\ \\ E^* + T \end{matrix}$$

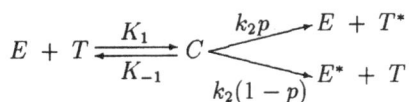

Fig. 1. TICL—Tumor kinetic scheme.

sulting in irreversibly programming tumor cells for lysis with probability p or inactivating TICLs with probability $(1 - p)$.

For the sake of simplicity we will consider the case of a one-dimensional tumor growth, (i.e. we shall assume that the cells lie on a straight line). This corresponds to the situation of the most malignant development of a primary neoplasm: that is, to invasive growth, when a cancer (e.g. malignant melanoma) grows not on the surface of the skin, but vertically downwards, growing directly into the tissue below. Invasive growth is extremely insidious and dangerous, giving rise to metastases or secondary tumors [18, 19].

The influence of other tissue cells on TICLs and tumor cells will be taken into account by specifying precise values for the model parameters, together with appropriate initial and boundary conditions. For a simplified description of the spatio-temporal growth of a solid tumor in the very early stages of its development, we will use a simple reaction-diffusion equation and we suppose that when the front of invading tumor cells moves into the tissue to a certain depth, they encounter TICLs which are migrating towards them. The dynamics of the interaction between TICLs and tumor cells may be presented in the following form:

$$\frac{\partial E}{\partial t} = \frac{\partial}{\partial x}\left[D_1 \frac{\partial E}{\partial x}\right] + F_1(E, T, C), \tag{1}$$

$$\frac{\partial T}{\partial t} = \frac{\partial}{\partial x}\left[D_2 \frac{\partial T}{\partial x}\right] + F_2(E, T, C), \tag{2}$$

$$\frac{\partial C}{\partial t} = F_3(E, T, C), \tag{3}$$

$$\frac{\partial E^*}{\partial t} = F_4(E^*, C), \tag{4}$$

$$\frac{\partial T^*}{\partial t} = F_5(T^*, C), \tag{5}$$

where E, T, C, E^*, and T^* are the population densities of: unbound TICLs, unbound tumor cells, TICL-tumor cell complexes, inactivated TICLs and 'lethally hit' tumor cells, respectively; $D_i (i = 1, 2)$ are the cell diffusion (random motility) coefficients.

We assume that inactivated and 'lethally hit' cells are quickly eliminated from the tissue (for example, by macrophages) and do not substantially influence the immune processes being analyzed. Also, we shall confine ourselves to consider the situation in which the cell diffusion (random motility) coefficients are independent of the spatio-temporal disposition of the cells (i.e. they are constant).

As suggested in the ordinary differential equation model [46] of the CTL response to the growth of an immunogenic tumor, the functions of local changes in the population density $F_i (i = 1 \ldots 5)$ are defined as follows:

$$F_1(E, T, C) = sh(x - l) + \frac{fET}{g + T} - d_1 E - k_1 ET + (k_{-1} + k_2 p)C,$$

$$F_2(E, T, C) = a(1 - bT)T - k_1 ET + (k_{-1} + k_2(1 - p))C,$$

$$F_3(E, T, C) = k_1 ET - (k_{-1} + k_2)C,$$

$$F_4(E^*, C) = k_2(1 - p)C - d_2 E^*,$$

$$F_5(T^*, C) = k_2 pC - d_3 T^*,$$

where s is the 'normal' (non-enhanced by the presence of tumor cells) rate of flow of mature TICLs into the tumor; and d_1, d_2 and d_3 are positive constants representing the rates of elimination of E, E^* and T^*, respectively, resulting from spontaneous death and/or migration from the region of tissue being considered. We assume that the tumor does not metastasize and that there is no migration of TICL-tumor cell complexes. The maximal growth rate of the tumor cells population is a, which incorporates both cell multiplication (mitosis) and death. Owing, for example, to competition for resources, mutual inhibition of growth and limited tissue space, the maximum density of the tumor cells is defined, and is represented by the parameter b^{-1}. In the region of tumor cell localization, the maximum rate of accumulation of the TICL population, due to the presence of the tumor, is f. Both TICL multiplication due to stimulation by the tumor cells, and enhanced TICL migration induced by TICL-tumor cell interactions, after which there is the production of many attractor factors for lymphocytes (e.g. IL-1, IL-2, IL-8, INF-γ etc.) may contribute to this process [11, 25]. It is important to note that a maximum rate of stimulated accumulation of TICLs is consistent with limitations in the rate of transport of TICLs to the tumor. These rate limitations could occur in the circulation, in the rate of exit from the circulation or in the rate of movement through the tissue to the tumor. The density of tumor cells, at which the maximum rate of accumulation of TICLs diminishes by a factor of two, is g.

It is easy to see that equations (4) and (5) are only coupled to the full system through the complexes C i.e. T^* and E^* have no effect on each other or the variables T and E. Thus, for the remainder of this paper, it is sufficient to analyze equations (1), (2) and (3) which essentially dictate the behavior of the complete system. With a suitable non-dimensionalization, equations (1),

(2) and (3) can be written in the form:

$$\frac{\partial E}{\partial t} = \frac{\partial^2 E}{\partial x^2} + \sigma h(x - l) + \frac{\rho ET}{\eta + T} - \sigma E - \mu ET + \epsilon C,$$

$$\frac{\partial T}{\partial t} = \omega \frac{\partial^2 T}{\partial x^2} + \alpha(1 - \beta T)T - \phi ET + \lambda C,$$

$$\frac{\partial C}{\partial t} = \mu ET - \chi C.$$

Values for the ten non-dimensional parameters are obtained from the estimated dimensional parameters [46]. Both diffusion coefficients were taken to be $10^{-6} cm^2 day^{-1}$, since these are close to the estimates obtained in [46]. Numerical simulations of the above system yields solutions which exhibit a rich spatio-temporal behavior (see Figures 2, 3, and 4).

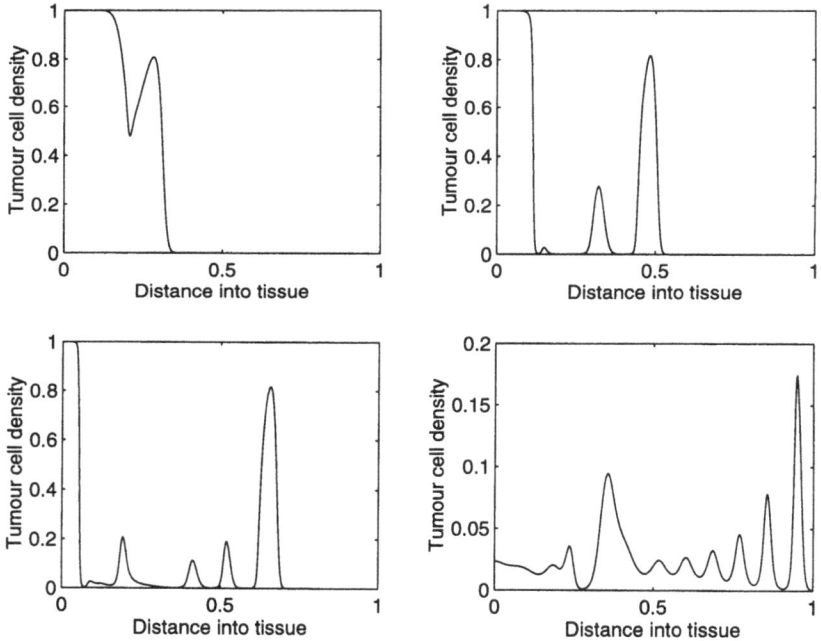

Fig. 2. Spatial distribution of tumor cell density within the tissue at times corresponding to 100, 300, 500 and 1000 days respectively.

The numerical predictions of the model make it possible to comprehend the mechanisms involved in the appearance of spatio-temporal heterogeneities detected in solid tumors infiltrated by cytotoxic lymphocytes. These are described in numerous immunomorphological investigations [8, 61]. However,

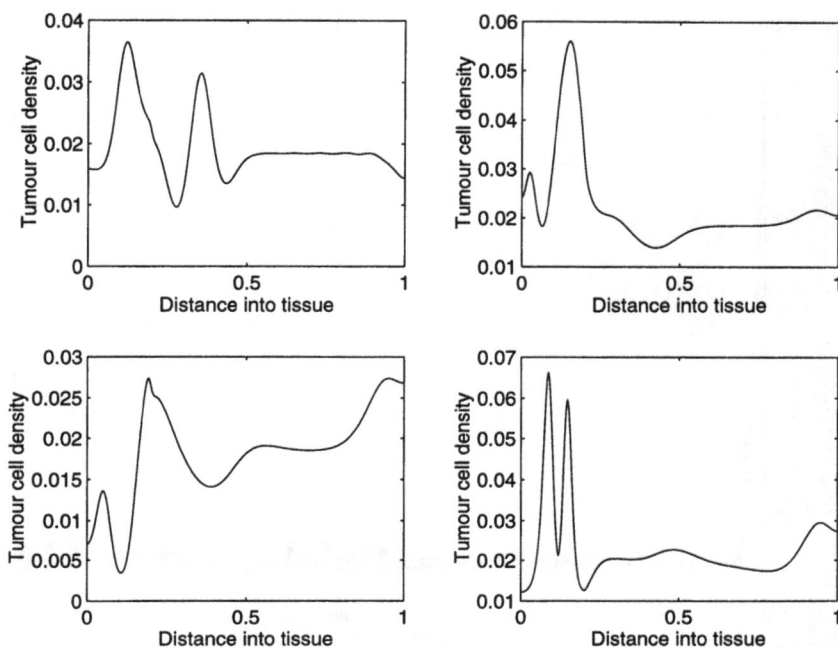

Fig. 3. Spatial distribution of tumor cell density within the tissue at times corresponding to 2000, 4000, 6000 and 10000 days respectively.

in the material discussed above, only some general problems associated with the mathematical theory, of the interaction of TICLs with TCs have been examined. Other issues to be further investigated include stability, the specific character of the dynamic behavior of the system (both spatial and temporal), and the role of parameters, especially those of diffusion, on the cells in the tissue. The investigation and solution of these 'formal' problems are not only of theoretical importance, but of practical importance as well.

§4. Growth Control and Growth Factors

Lack of growth control in cancer is one of the main reasons for its spread. Michelson and Leith have developed a series of models which attempt to explain the various pathways of tumor growth control [55, 56, 57, 58]. These pathways include: the autocrine, where cells stimulate themselves; the paracrine, where cells stimulate other cells in the local environment; and, the endocrine, where the cells are stimulated by some remote signal. Examples of some of these signals include growth factors such as Transforming Growth Factor (TGF), Epidermal Growth Factor (EGF), and Fibroblast Growth Factor (FGF).

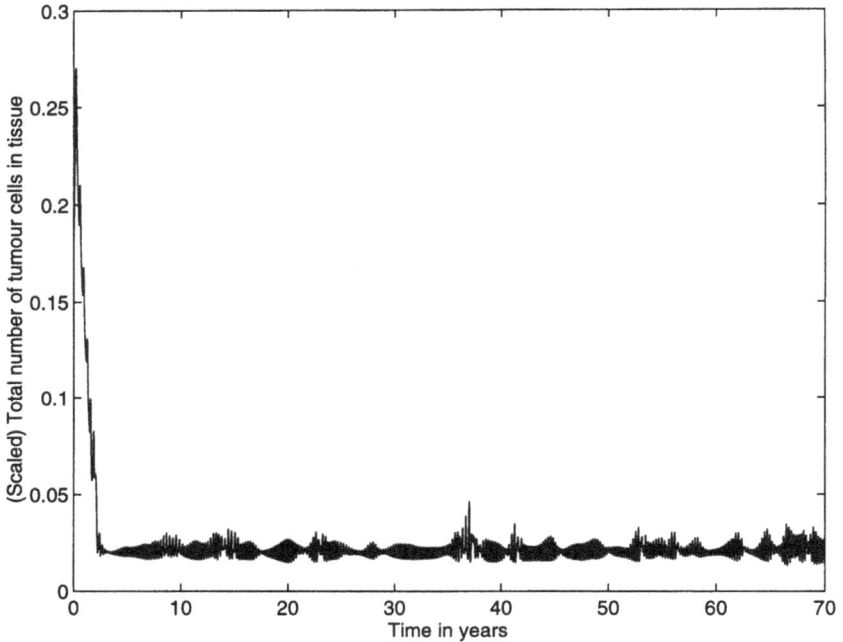

Fig. 4. Total number of tumor cells within tissue over a period of 70 years.

The basic model they use is a variation on the competition model from population dynamics describing two distinct and interacting tumor cell populations (one proliferating and one quiescent). The model also takes into account that cells from the proliferating population are allowed to differentiate to a quiescent population. The form of their model is

$$\frac{dX}{dt} = rX \left(1 - \frac{X}{K} - cY \right) - mX,$$
$$\frac{dY}{dt} = mX,$$

where X are the proliferating cells, Y are the quiescent cells, r is the growth rate, K is the carrying capacity of the proliferating cells, c is the competitive effects of Y on X (or a negative signal from the quiescent cells), and m is the differentiation rate. Some of the various signaling pathways are modeled by assuming that the carrying capacity (K) and/or the differentiation rate (m) are non-constant.

One common method that tumors have to manipulate their environment is by producing growth factors that induce angiogenesis (also see section 5). This is termed a paracrine signal and can be modeled by an increase in the carrying capacity (since more blood vessels mean more nutrients for the tumor). One possible form suggested for the carrying capacity to model this paracrine signal is

$$K = A + BX^{\alpha},$$

where A is the baseline carrying capacity. In this case the carrying capacity increases proportional to the number of proliferating cells, thus suggesting that the angiogenesis signal is originating from the proliferating compartment. They suggest that if the angiogenic response is proportional to the surface area of the tumor, then $\alpha = 2/3$ is a reasonable approximation for the growth of a sphere. If the signal is strong enough then the tumor will be able to grow uncontrolled eventually leading to the death of the patient. This type of uncontrolled growth due to vascularization is seen experimentally with the "tumor-with-a mouse" syndrome. That is, the tumor is able to grow as large or larger than the mouse. But, if the signal is not strong enough and the carrying capacity (K) is increasing at a rate slower than the growth rate of the proliferating compartment (r) then the ability of the host to support the tumor is eventually overtaken by X and the tumor will eventually stop growing.

Switches in the size of the carrying capacity K can also be explained by the protein angiostatin—a angiogenesis inhibitor (see section (5)). In its presence K is "small"—blood vessels are not growing towards the tumor bringing it nutrients. Folkman [33] notes that in some cases angiostatin is released by large tumors which can keep small metastases from growing (therefore small K at the metastasis site). But, if the large tumor is removed then so is the angiostatin signal, therefore K switches to a value large enough to allow growth of the metastases.

The parameter m relates to a differentiation signal. Depending on the form of m (a constant or a function of other variables or parameters), the cancer can grow uncontrolled or not. If $m > 0$ (and other parameters are considered constant) then the cancer will eventually reach a state where it is totally quiescent. This is considered the normal state of the system. But, if some signal exists that can "switch" it such that $m < 0$ then the quiescent cells can begin to proliferate again. This is observed, for example, when your skin is cut. A growth signal is given that switches $m < 0$ thus the cells start to proliferate and heal the wound. But, when the wound is healed the signal is turned off ($m > 0$). One explanation for the uncontrolled cell growth in cancer is that this signal is never turned off. For example, there are several oncogenes that signal cells to grow even when no growth factor is present. One example is the oncogene Erb-B2 in breast and ovarian cancer. (see Weinberg [85]). An example of uncontrolled growth related to cancer has been observed after a partial hepatectomy (used to remove a primary liver tumor). In this case dormant secondary tumors (previously undetected) start to grow uncontrolled. A possible explanation for this is that the primary tumor emitted a growth inhibitory signal (therefore $m > 0$) that causes the cells in the secondary tumor to differentiate, but when the primary tumor is removed so is the signal, (therefore $m < 0$) and the secondary tumor starts to grow again.

There are many other possible growth factor signals that could possibly be explained by this model or variations to it. For example section (2) discusses the growth factor interleukin-2 which stimulates the immune system in response to "foreign" cells such as cancer cells. In this case the growth factor signals are between the immune system and the cancer as opposed to two difference types of cancer cells. Also, the next section discusses various growth factors related to angiogenesis.

§5. Tumor Angiogenesis

It has been know for a long time that solid tumors cannot grow beyond a size of approximately 10^6 cells or about 1–2 mm in diameter in the absence of a blood supply [30, 34]. This initial pre-vascular or avascular growth phase is followed by a vascular growth phase, in which tumor-induced angiogenesis [28, 30, 34] is the rate limiting step for further tumor growth and also provides tumor cells direct access to the circulation. Over the last few years several mathematical models have been developed to describe some of the important features of tumor-induced angiogenesis [7, 15, 64, 79]. In this section we review a mathematical model of Chaplain and Anderson [16] which focuses on three particularly important variables involved in tumor angiogenesis; namely, endothelial cells, tumor angiogenic factors (e.g. vascular endothelial growth factor, VEGF) and matrix macromolecules (e.g. fibronectin, laminin). Each of these variables has a crucial role to play in orchestrating the sequence of events which constitutes angiogenesis beginning with the rearrangement and migration of endothelial cells from pre-existing vasculature and culminating in the formation of an extensive capillary network [54]. The first event of tumor-induced angiogenesis involves the tumor cells secreting chemicals, collectively known as tumor angiogenic factors [29] which, in turn, induce any neighboring endothelial cells to secrete matrix-degrading enzymes (proteases, collagenases) which degrade the vascular basement-membrane. The cells then migrate through the disrupted membrane towards the tumor. The cells of the capillary sprout-tip region subsequently proliferate, leading to further extension of the sprouts [6, 20, 73, 76, 83] and this process of sprout-tip migration and proliferation of sprout-wall cells forms solid strands of endothelial cells amongst the extracellular matrix. At first, the sprouts arising from the parent vessel grow essentially parallel to each other and later, at a certain distance from the parent vessel, they tend to incline toward each other [67] leading to numerous tip-to-tip and tip-to-sprout fusions and the formation of loops. Following this, the first signs of circulation can be recognized and from the primary loops, new buds and sprouts emerge repeating the angiogenic sequence of events and providing for the further extension of the new capillary network. As the sprouts approach the tumor their branching dramatically increases, and the tumor is eventually penetrated, resulting in vascularization [60]. In making their way to the tumor, the cells must penetrate the extracellular matrix of the surrounding tissue which consists of various components including collagen fibre and fibronectin [49], an important matrix macromolecule which is known to enhance cell adhesion to collagen [74] and is also produced by endothelial cells [59]. The mathematical model of Chaplain and Anderson consists of three coupled partial differential equations describing the response of endothelial cells to angiogenic factors via chemotaxis and to matrix macromolecules (fibronectin) via haptotaxis. Simple kinetic terms modelling TAF uptake, fibronectin production and uptake are also included.

$$\frac{\partial n}{\partial t} = D\nabla^2 n - \nabla \cdot (\chi(c)n\nabla c) - \nabla \cdot (\rho(f)n\nabla f),$$
$$\frac{\partial c}{\partial t} = -anc,$$
$$\frac{\partial f}{\partial t} = bn - dnf.$$

The above equations were scaled with appropriate variables and solved numerically with parameter values based on experimental data. By treating the discretezed form of these equations as a biased random walk in two dimensions, Chaplain and Anderson were able to generate realistic capillary network structures. In addition to the rules for cell movement it was also possible to incorporate rules for sprout branching, anastomosis and cell proliferation.

Figure 5 shows the results of simulated endothelial cell movement towards a small circular tumor (e.g. carcinoma). We see that by a time of 4.5 days, four of the loops have already achieved anastomosis. The network continues to grow and branch until connection with the tumor and vascularization are achieved at around 15 days.

§6. Cell-Cycle-Specific Chemotherapy

One of the more common types of chemotherapeutic drugs currently used to treat cancers are cell-cycle-specific drugs. These are drugs that only affect cells in a specific phase or phases of the cell-cycle. For example: antimetabolites such as methotrexate and fluorouracil; alkylating agents such as cyclophosphamide; and platinum agents such as cisplatin all affect the cell's DNA in various ways. Therefore, each of these drugs are designated as S-phase (DNA synthesis phase) drugs since they block the replication of the DNA thus prevent cell reproduction. Another common type of chemotherapeutic drugs are Alkaloids such as paclitaxel and vinblastine. These drugs disrupt mitosis and are referred to as M-phase drugs. Cells that are not in the active phase of the cell-cycle are in the resting or quiescent phase (referred to as the G_0-phase) and are resistant to the drugs. This is sometimes referred to as kinetic resistance. One of the advantages of cell-cycle-specific drugs is that many of the normal cells of the body are not actively reproducing thus are not in any of the active phases (G_1, S, G_2, M) of the cell-cycle, therefore, they are not susceptible to the cell-cycle-specific treatment. But, some normal tissue such as the bone marrow and cells of the gastrointestinal track are actively reproducing thus they are affected by cell-cycle-specific treatments. Thus, treatment

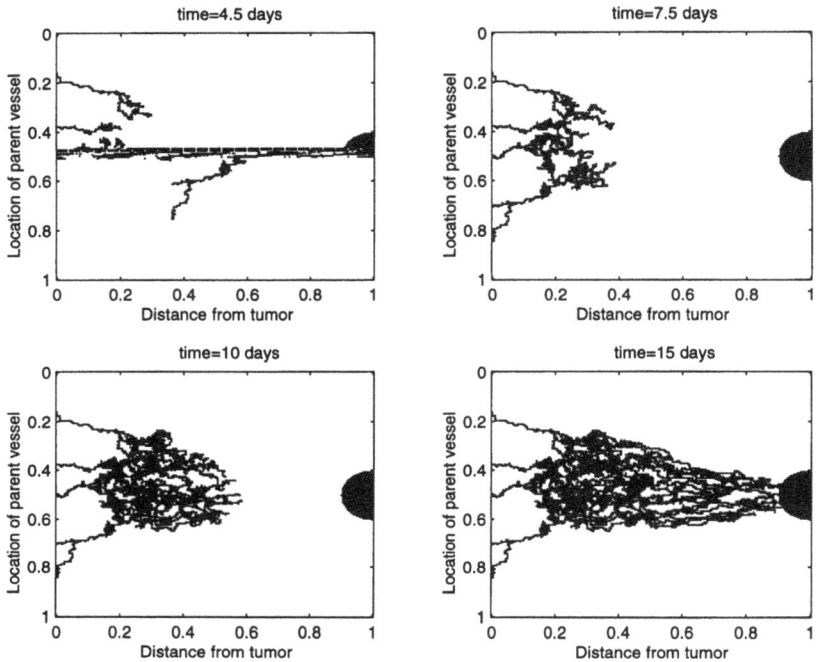

Fig. 5. Computer simulation of the evolution of a capillary network in response to a solid tumor over a 15 day period. The figures show the migration, branching and anastomosis of the capillary sprouts as they make their way from the parent vessel through the tissue to the tumor.

regimens need to be designed to take advantage of these cell-cycle kinetics and maximize the damage to the cancer while minimizing the damage to the sensitive normal tissue.

In the process of modelling cell-cycle-specific chemotherapy we first need to describe the important aspects of the cell-cycle. These include the proliferating cells (P) which are susceptible (in various degrees) to the cell-cycle-specific treatment and the resting or quiescent cells (Q) which are resistant to the treatment. Figure 6 shows diagrammatically what this model looks like. The arrows indicate rates of cell flow between compartments. Eisen and Schiller [25], Webb [84], Adam and Panetta [5], Panetta and Adam [65], and Panetta [66] have used this general scheme in various ways to model the cell-cycle of cancer and also the effects of cell-cycle-specific treatments.

To help better understand how to deliver cell-cycle-specific treatments it is useful to be able to compare the model to a specific cancer and drug. Usually this is very difficult since often drugs are given in combination and their kinetics and interactions are not known (see conclusions). But, in the case of the chemotherapeutic drug paclitaxel, which is often used alone to treat breast and ovarian cancer, its mechanics are fairly well known. For example

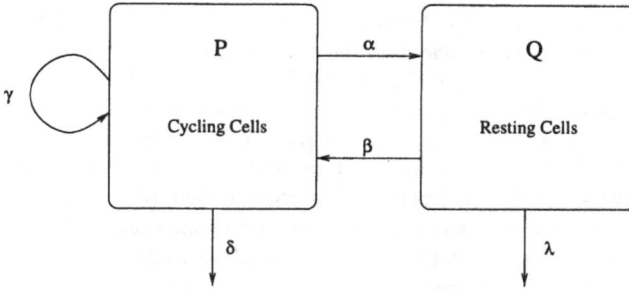

Fig. 6. Cell-Cycle Model.

it is known to be M-phase specific, that is it disrupts mitosis, and also its 1/2-life in the body is estimated to be between 3 and 8 hours [78]. Thus, it is an appropriate drug to study with this model. The main question to ask is: what is the most effective method of delivering this treatment so that we get increased cancer cell kill?

The typical drug regimen of paclitaxel for treating either breast or ovarian cancer has a treatment period of 21 days, a drug infusion time of 24 hours, and a dose around 135 mg/m^3 [78]. The model in Panetta [66] attempts to use the cell-cycle-specific model (diagrammatically described in Figure 6) to determine if the above regimen is the "best" or if the model suggests other regimens that lead to larger cell kills. In each of the following cases the same total dose is used. 1.) Shorter periods are better since they can reduce the cancer mass while longer periods cannot. This is analytically shown in Webb [84] and also observed numerically in Panetta [66]. 2.) Shorter drug infusion times kill fewer cancer cells (and bone marrow cells). This is also observed in a variety of clinical studies [9, 38]. Conversely, longer infusion times not only kill more cancer cells but also normal tissue such as bone marrow. Therefore, there must be some intermediate infusion time such that the cancer is reduced without overly destroying the bone marrow. 3.) The cell kill is directly related to the proliferating fraction—the percentage of cells in the proliferating compartment. 4.) Finally, it is observed that changes in dose has less effect on the reduction of the cancer than changes in the infusion time and period. This is also observed clinically. One conclusion of Panetta [66] along with some clinical studies suggest that treatment periods between 7 to 14 days might be more effective than the more common 21 day period.

There are many other questions to be asked or considered with variations of these models. These include: what is the optimal treatment regimen (see section (7)); and, what is the best method of delivering a combination of different cell-cycle-specific drugs (see section (9)).

§7. Optimization Methods

Section (6) indicates some interesting and yet unanswered questions in cell-cycle-specific chemotherapy such as: should the drug infusion time be shortened to reduce toxicity to the bone marrow or should it be increased to destroy more cancer cells? One possible way to answer this and other questions about how treatment regimens should be given is with the use of optimal control theory. The idea is that researchers attempt to develop optimal control problems that try to maximize cancer cell kill while minimizing the ill effects of the drugs. Much mathematical work has been done in this area with non-cell-cycle-specific treatment and a good review of this is given in Swan [81]. Swan's review also has some material on optimal control with cell-cycle-specific chemotherapy, but this area has not been studied nearly as much. An early attempt to use optimal control theory on cell-cycle-specific treatments is given in Eisen [26]. He designed a model similar to that of Figure 6. The control he used was to reduce the cancer to a fixed level over a given interval while minimizing the total drug used. This optimal control problem turns out to be singular and does not have a unique solution. Swierniak et al. [82] has also developed a similar model. They attempt to minimize the total cancer mass at the end of some specified time interval using the least amount of drug possible. Like the control problem in Eisen, this is also a singular problem and also does not have a unique solution. These problems are known as bang-bang type and they can be solved numerically by solving a resulting two-point-boundary-value-problem (TPBVP). Since there are not unique solutions to these problems it turns out that there exist solutions that optimize the mathematical problem but are clinically unrealistic. An example of this, given in Swierniak et al. [82], is that one solution exist where the cancer mass is allowed to grow to nearly twice its original mass before treatment is given to reduce it to the given end value.

Since this area of modelling can have direct and fairly fast implications on how chemotherapeutic treatment regimens are designed, much effort should be made to improve these models and design new ones to help clinicians determine optimal or near optimal methods of treatment. Improved models should be designed to eliminate mathematically acceptable but clinically unacceptable results. Also, the models need to be designed so that the parameters are obtainable through measurements made by clinicians. Furthermore, from a clinical standpoint, the "solution" does not necessarily have to be optimal, just "close" (better than current treatment methods). If designed well, it is perceived that a computer could directly aid the clinician in the proper administration of the treatment so that the patients' cancer is reduced with minimal adverse effects.

§8. Catastrophe Theory

Models of tumor growth historically have fallen into several broad categories: "demographic" (i.e. exponential, logistic, Gompertz); diffusion (ranging from "generic" to deterministic and time evolutionary); reaction-diffusion (describing angiogenesis, vascularization and invasion); elasticity (invasion and tumor classification). Details of these have been mentioned earlier in this paper, and can also be found in the chapters by Chaplain and Adam in [4].

Although the results so far have been encouraging in many ways, the question should still be asked: can we think usefully about cancer in different, perhaps non-traditional terms? Such "models", being more speculative than usual are perhaps better termed metaphors or similes. The distinction is made clearer using the cartoon in Figure 7.

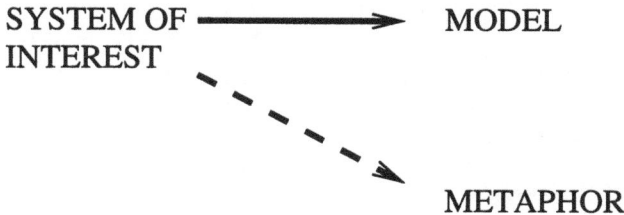

SYSTEM OF ⟶ MODEL
INTEREST

METAPHOR

Fig. 7. Speculative Models.

For a traditional mathematical model there exists a direct connection (kinetic, thermodynamic, mechanistic, etc.) between the system of interest and its mathematical representation. For a mathematical metaphor, no such direct connection may be known as yet, though the system behavior may well indicate its existence. This is probably typical of many biological systems! Perhaps no intermediate levels of description are in existence, to fill in the gaps, so to speak, between the system and the metaphor. This might be referred to as mathematical "lateral thinking" in the spirit of Edward DeBono's famous book [21]!

Catastrophe theory, (à la René Thom and Christopher Zeeman; see references in Adam and Bellomo [4]), a profound and beautiful system of ideas, has in many respects played the (sometimes controversial) role of a mathematical metaphor in the sense described above. Briefly, as is well known, the phenomenon of interest is assumed to be governed by a potential function V of some kind, the minima of which are regarded as defining stable states of the system. Thus, more than one such state may be accessible to the system; in Figure 8, several levels of description of the "cancer problem" are shown, each exhibiting bistability.

Under such circumstances the cusp catastrophe may be an appropriate descriptor of the system (at whatever level) in terms of the double-well potential function $V(a, b; X)$, defined by

$$V = \frac{1}{4}X^4 + \frac{1}{2}aX^2 + bX. \tag{6}$$

In this expression, X is the "behavior" variable, and a and b are "control" parameters; changing these may alter the form of V so as to change the positions, relative height or total number of local minima. Thus the observed state of a system may change discontinuously (or "catastrophically") as the control parameters are changed smoothly. Such a metaphor exhibits (under appropriate circumstances) behavior characteristic of many biological systems,

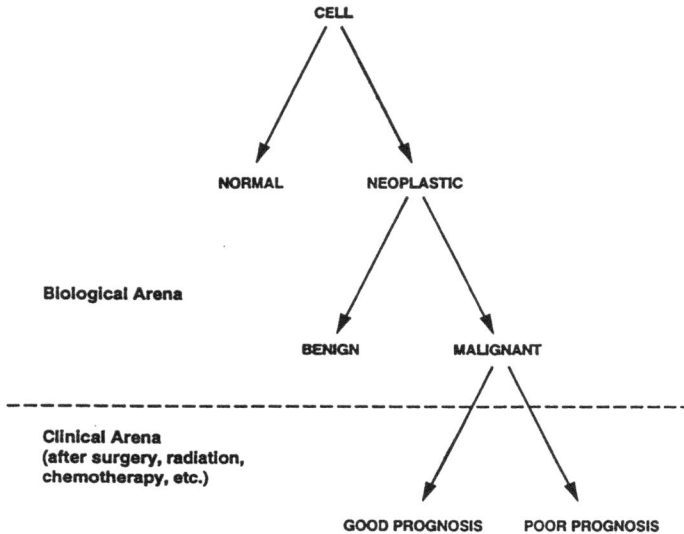

Fig. 8. Cancer States Exhibiting Bistability.

including bimodality, discontinuity, hysteresis, and divergence of initially close steady states. The cusp catastrophe surface defined by equation (6) is shown in Figure 9.

If we focus on the different levels of bistability in Figure 9, we need to ask questions like:

(i) What physiological/genetic/environmental factors, or what combinations of them, determine the control parameters for each level?

(ii) How do we find them? (Lots of raw data?)

If we can answer these questions to our satisfaction, then in "solving" this "inverse problem" (i.e. given the exhibited behavior, what is the nature of the control parameters?) we have a potentially valuable prognostic and possibly diagnostic tool. It may be, however, that the control parameters are unique to each individual, and a "personalized" catastrophe surface is called for.

There is an interesting catastrophe-theoretic description of the local interaction between cancer cells and the cell-mediated immune response mechanisms, based on work of Garay and Lefever [37]. This description is closer to being a model than a metaphor because a potential function $V(a, b; X)$

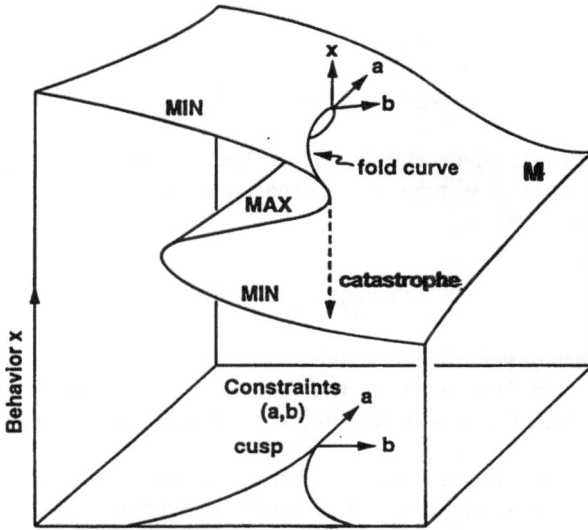

Fig. 9. Cusp Catastrophe Surface.

arises naturally out of the governing nonlinear differential equation for the behavior variable x (tumor cell population). The description is still partially "metaphorical" because the quartic potential function is associated with the zeros of the numerator of a rational function, rather than the rational function itself. (Bistability still occurs for complete potential function, but it is no longer a pure polynomial function, and it is not possible to describe the overall qualitative behavior in simple terms). Details may be found in Adam and Bellomo [4].

The dimensionless form of the governing differential equation is

$$\frac{dx}{dt} = \alpha + x(1 - \theta x)x - \frac{\beta x}{1 + x},$$

where α, β and θ^{-1} are respectively measures of the mutation rate of normal cells to neoplastic cells, the efficiency of the cell-mediated immune response to the presence of tumor cells (x), and the local saturation limit for cancer cells. Steady states of the system are defined by

$$-\theta x^3 + (1 - \theta)x^2 + (1 + \alpha - \beta)x + \alpha = 0$$

or in canonical form

$$X^3 + aX + b = 0,$$

where

$$X = x - x_c, \qquad x_c = \frac{1 - \theta}{3\theta},$$

$$a = -3x_c^2 - \left(\frac{1 + \alpha - \beta}{\theta}\right),$$

$$b = -2x_c^3 - x_c\left(\frac{1 + \alpha - \beta}{\theta}\right) - \frac{\alpha}{\theta}.$$

The cusp catastrophe surface is defined by $X = X(a, b)$. The projection of this surface on the (b, a) plane defines the catastrophe set: A cusped region on the boundary of which

$$b = \pm\left(-\frac{4}{27}a^3\right)^{\frac{1}{2}}, \quad a \leq 0.$$

For appropriate variations in a and b (and hence in the biological parameters α, β and θ) it may be shown that both high $X \to$ low X (remission) and low $X \to$ high X (metastic growth) rapid transitions (catastrophes) are possible.

One important deficiency of this and all the deterministic models is that in real biological systems, environmental fluctuations may cause significant modifications in the steady state properties. Interestingly, this was investigated in depth by Lefever and Horsthemke [48] shortly after the above-mentioned paper by Garay and Lefever [37] was published (1978). Earlier work by Horsthemke and Malek-Mansour [39] had shown that distinct classes of steady state solutions can exchange stability at bifurcation points which do not show up in the stability diagrams associated with the deterministic equations. Furthermore, environmental fluctuations may stabilize macroscopic states which do not even appear as steady state solutions in deterministic treatments (Horsthemke and Lefever [40]).

As pointed out by Lefever and Horsthemke [48], in vivo, the cytotoxic parameters and replication constants of the cells are influenced by many environmental factors (e.g. the supply of oxygen, nutrients, degree of vascularization of tissues, immunological state of the host, temperature, etc.). This will cause the systemic parameters to undergo random variations superimposed upon their average behavior, giving them a stochastic character. To this end, the authors examine in turn the effect of externally induced fluctuations of β and of the normal cellular replication rate. In each case the idealized assumption of gaussian white noise is made, the corresponding stochastic differential equation stated, and the stationary solution of the associated Fokker-Planck equation is derived. While the deterministic phenomenological model predicts that the immune response is generally insufficient to always ensure tumor rejection (i.e. high $X \to$ low X), the stochastic analysis shows that in each of the above cases, the effect of external "noise" consistently acts, it appears, in favor of tumor cell rejection, i.e. noise appears to enhance the efficiency of immune defense mechanisms, and this has been shown without requiring the average value of the fluctuating parameters to vary.

Again, though, hard questions must be asked. Clearly, the administration of cytotoxic drugs and/or radiation corresponds at some level to the imposition of external fluctuations on the tumor cell environment. Are the therapeutic implications of the stochastic analysis observed in practice? The answer would appear to be "no" in general, and so we must ask further, what is missing from the model? Or is it the wrong model?

There is a related phenomenon that may be worth pursuing in the cancer-metaphor/model arena: that of stochastic resonance (SR). To quote Bulsara and Gammaitoni [11], "Stochastic resonance has become widely recognized as a paradigm for noise-induced effects in driven nonlinear dynamic systems." The necessary requirements for SR are (i) a bistable system; (ii) a periodic driving signal, and (iii) a noise signal (Lanzara et al. [47]). The periodic component may be associated for our purposes either normal daily variations of the system, or with the periodicity of chemotherapeutic or other regimens. In the absence of noise, a low amplitude periodic signal may be insufficient to cause transitions from one minimum to the other of the bistable potential. When low or moderate amplitude additive noise is introduced, random transitions over the central potential barrier occur. Eventually, with increasing noise amplitude, synchronized noise-induced transitions may occur between the wells. If the noise amplitude is too great, this synchrony is destroyed. A stochastic resonance condition can be derived in terms of the escape time for a bistable system, the height of the well, and other parameters of the system, based in part on the curvature of the potential at the top of the barrier and the bottom of the well (details are supplied along with many references in the paper by Lanzara et al. [47]). It might well be worth pursuing these ideas in the context of the system bistability mentioned above.

There is another metaphor — this time a more extreme one — that should be mentioned in passing. It concerns the application of quantum scattering ideas to bistable potentials. Very little appears in the literature on general asymmetric quartic potentials, though some progress can be made on double asymmetric rectangular wells (Adam, in preparation). It is debatable whether or not quantum mechanical (QM) ideas have any relevance to macroscopic (i.e. at the cellular and inter-cellular scale) biological systems. Nevertheless, it is possible that the eigenfunctions and eigenvalues associated with these potentials do have some useful interpretation in the context of a system passing from non-cancerous to cancerous (or vice versa) steady states. The eigenvalues ("energy levels") might be associated with some type of metastatic potential, or propensity of a cell to become neoplastic, while the square of the eigenfunction (or, if complex, the square of its modulus) might indicate the probability of a cell being found in one state or the other (as in keeping with the standard interpretation in quantum mechanics).

The concept of transmission amplitude from one well to the other might be related to the likelihood or not of "tunneling" taking place between the two states. And resonances, "leaky" bound states with long but finite lifetimes, related to the tunneling concept, might well serve as a metaphor for a normal cell eventually becoming neoplastic.

At the present time, these latter two topics (SR and QM) are speculations without substance. Perhaps they are not worth pursuing because of that, but perhaps they are sufficiently outrageous, even offensive, to the cancer modelers, that they will stimulate new and better ideas and models to describe what has to be one of the most multifaceted of modern problems — the scourge of cancer.

§9. Conclusions

By considering what is currently being done in cancer modelling along with the direction of current clinical research one can speculate on some directions of future mathematical research. Some are discussed directly in the previous sections, but we would like to emphasize a few here.

For example, in the works by Michelson and Leith (see section 4) they discuss some possible signal pathways between various cancerous cells. Currently medical researchers are discovering new oncogenes that have various effects on the growth control of cancer. Variations on Michelson and Leith's models relating to these discoveries in genetics and how they related to growth control can play an important role in understanding how researchers can control cancer.

The models of sections 3 and 5 illustrate two important, complementary areas of mathematical modelling of cancer growth and development - qualitative and quantitative modelling. The model of section 3 concerning a possible spatio-temporal immune response to a cancer is slightly more speculative in that less facts are known about an *in vivo* immune response to a cancer at a very early stage of its development. Nonetheless the model uses as much *in vitro* data as possible in order to provide a quantitative framework in which to work. The results of the model are interesting in both mathematical (spatio-temporal complexity) and biological (tumor dormancy) terms. The model of section 5 concerning the development of a tumor-induced capillary network strongly demonstrates the potential of mathematical models for quantitative prediction. The parameters of this model are based, as far as possible, on available experimental data, thus rendering the model quantitative as well as qualitative. Once this basic model is developed and perhaps subsequently refined, it may be possible to use the theoretical networks generated by the model as test-beds for any anti-angiogenic strategies being developed clinically. In this way an "optimal" anti-angiogenic strategy may be developed more quickly than would be possible with drug trials alone. If mathematical models of cancer are to have a real clinical impact in the future then they must, in addition to replicating known results and providing qualitative solutions (which they must at least do to be a good model), possess the capacity to be predictive in their own right and provide quantitative information to clinicians. Only by working closely with experimentalists and clincians will this come about.

Another area that mathematics can lend much insight to is in the delivery of combination chemotherapy. Various clinical studies have shown that for many combinations of drugs (expecially cell-cycle-specific ones) the sequencing of the drugs becomes very important. In some cases the clinical evidence shows that if combinations of drugs are given in an inappropriate sequence the treatment can have more adverse effects on the patient than treating with any one of the drugs of the combination seperately. For example, it is well documented that when treating with the combination of chemotherapeutic drugs cisplatin and paclitaxel, paclitaxel should always preceed cisplatin. Among other things the reverse order is more mylosuppressive. The clinical evidence suggests that there are possibly many cell-kinetic and pharmacokinetic interactions that may affect the outcome of this and other treatments—many of which are currently not understood. This suggest that some mathematical method for determing the effects of various combinations of drugs could be instrumental in understanding what some of the interactions are and how to better design combination chemotherapy. Furthermore, this is another excellent area to consider optimal control theory since it could automate the process of combination chemotherapy and determine the "best" regimen of treatment that will reduce the cancer while minimizing normal tissue damage.

There are many other possibilities for mathematical modelling in cancer and they are only limited by the imagination and creativity of the researcher. The hope is that each of these efforts will help researchers understand the growth and control of cancer a little better with each new model.

Acknowledgments.
John A. Adam: I would particularly like to thank the following mathematical scientists for (a) listening to some of my wild speculations without ridiculing me, (b) actually encouraging me to pursue these thoughts, however tortuous the path to enlightenment may be! I am very grateful you all: Zeljco Bajzer, David Cameron, Larry Greller, Seth Michelson, Frank Tobin, and, of course, my co-authors, Mark Chaplain and Carl Panetta.
Mark Chaplain: I would like to thank Carl for organizing the cancer modelling session and getting together such an interesting and diverse group of people.
J. Carl Panetta: I would like to thank all the speakers in the sessions on cancer modelling at the International Conference on Mathematical Models in Medical and Health Sciences.

References

1. Adam, J. A., The dynamics of growth-factor-modified immune response to cancer growth: One dimensional models, Math. Comp. Modell. **17** (1993), 83–106.

2. Adam, J. A., Mathematical models of prevascular spheroid development and catastrophe-theoretic description of rapid metastatic growth/tumor remission, Invasion and Metastasis **16** (1996), 247–267.

3. Adam, J. A., Effects of vascularization on lymphocyte/tumor cell dynamics: qualitative features, Math. Comput. Model. **23** (1996), 1–10.

4. Adam, J. A. and N. Bellomo, *A Survey of Models for Tumor-Immune System Dynamics*, Birkhäuser, Boston, 1997.

5. Adam, J. A. and J. C. Panetta, A simple mathematical model and alternative paradigm for certain chemotherapeutic regimens, Math. Comput. Model. **22** (1995), 49–60.

6. Ausprunk, D. H. and J. Folkman, Migration and proliferation of endothelial cells in preformed and newly formed blood vessels during tumour angiogenesis, Microvasc. Res. **14** (1977), 53–65.

7. Balding, D. and D. L. S. McElwain, A mathematical model of tumour-induced capillary growth, J. Theor. Biol. **114** (1985), 53–73.

8. Berezhnaya, N. M., L. V. Yakimovich, R. A. Semenova-Kobzar, V. D. Lyulkin and A. Yu. Papivets. The effect of interleukin-2 on proliferation of explants of malignant soft-tissue tumours in diffusion chambers, Experimental Oncology **8** (1986), 39–42.

9. Bokkel Huinink, W. W. ten, E. Eisenhauser and K. Swenerton, Preliminary evaluation of a multcenter randomized comparative study of TAXOL (paclitaxel) dose and infusion length in platinum-treated ovarian cancer, Cancer Treat. Rev. **19** Suppl. C (1993), 79–86.

10. Brocker, E. B., G. Zwaldo, B. Holzmann, E. Macher and C. Sorg, Inflammatory cell infiltrates in human melanoma at different stages of tumour progression, Int. J. Cancer **41** (1988), 562–567.

11. Bulsara, A. R. and L. Gammaitoni, Tuning in to noise, Physics Today (March issue) (1996), 39–45.

12. Byrne, H. M. and M. A. J. Chaplain, Growth of necrotic tumours in the presence and absence of inhibitors, Math. Biosci. **135** (1996), 187–216.

13. Byrne, H. M. and M. A. J. Chaplain, On the role of cell-cell adhesion in models for solid tumour growth, Math. Comp. Modell. **24** (1996), 1–17.

14. Chaplain, M. A. J., S. M. Giles, B. D. Sleeman and R. J. Jarvis, A mathematical analysis of a model for tumour angiogenesis, J. Math. Biol. **33** (1995), 744–770.

15. Chaplain, M. A. J., Avascular growth, angiogenesis and vascular growth in solid tumors: the mathematical modelling of the stages of tumor development, Math. Comput. Modell. **23** (1996), 47–87.

16. Chaplain, M. A. J. and A. R. A. Anderson, Mathematical modelling, simulation and prediction of tumour-induced angiogenesis, Invasion Metastasis **16** (1997), 222–234.

17. Chaplain, M. A. J., V. A. Kuznetsov, Z. H. James and L. A. Stepanova, Spatio-temporal dynamics of the immune system response to cancer, in *Mathematical Models in Medical and Health Sciences*, Vanderbilt University Press, Nashville, 1998, to appear.

18. Clark, W. H., Tumour progression and the nature of cancer, Brit. J. Cancer **64** (1991), 631–644.

19. Clark, W. H., D. E. Elder and M. Vanhorn, The biologic forms of malignant melanoma, Human Pathology **17** (1986), 443–450.

20. Cliff, W. J., Observations on healing tissue: A combined light and electron microscopic investigation, Trans. Roy. Soc. London **B246** (1963), 305–325.

21. De Bono, E., *Lateral Thinking: Creativity Step by Step*, Harper & Row, New York, 1970.

22. DeLisi, C. and A. Rescigno, Immune surveillance and neoplasia–I a minimal mathematical model, Bull. Math. Biol. **39** (1977), 201–221.

23. Deweger, R. A., B. Wilbrink, R. M. P. Moberts, D. Mans, R. Oskam and W. den Otten. Immune reactivity in SL2 lymphoma-bearing mice compared with SL2-immunized mice, Cancer Immun. Immunotherapy **24** (1987), 1191–1192.

24. Durand, R. E. and R. M. Sutherland, Growth and cellular characteristics of multicell spheroids, Recent Results in Cancer Research **95** (1984), 24–49.

25. Eisen, M. and J. Schiller, Stability analysis of normal and neoplastic growth, Bull. Math. Biol. **39** (1977), 597–605.

26. Eisen, M., *Mathematical Models in Cell Biology and Cancer Chemotherapy*, Volume 30 of Lecture Notes in Biomathematics, Springer-Verlag, New York, 1979.

27. Folkman, J., How is blood-vessel growth regulated in normal and neoplastic tissue, Proc. Amer. Assoc. Cancer Res. **26** (1985), 384–385.

28. Folkman J. Tumor angiogenesis, Adv. Cancer Res. **43** (1985), 175–203.

29. Folkman, J. and M. Klagsbrun, Angiogenic factors, Science **235** (1987), 442–447.

30. Folkman J. What is the evidence that tumors are angiogenesis dependent? J. Natn. Cancer Inst. **82** (1990), 4–6.

31. Folkman, J., Angiogenesis in cancer, vascular, rheumatoid and other disease, Nature Medicine **1** (1995), 21–31.

32. Folkman, J. New Prospectives in Angiogenesis Research, European Journal of Cancer **32A** (1996), 2534–2539.

33. Folkman, J., Fighting cancer by attacking its blood supply, Scientific American **275**(3), (1996), 150–156.

34. Folkman, J., K. Watson, D. Ingber and D. Hanahan, Induction of angiogenesis during the transition from hyperplasia to neoplasia, Nature **339** (1989), 58–61.

35. Forni, G., G. Parmiani, A. Guarini and R. Foa, Gene Transfer in tumour therapy, Annals Oncol. **5** (1994), 789–794.

36. Friedl, P., P. B. Noble and K. S. Zanker, T-Lymphocyte Locomotion in a 3-Dimensional Collagen Matrix – Expression and Function of Cell-Adhesion Molecules, J. Immunol. **154** (1995), 4973–4985.

37. Garay, R. P. and R. Lefever, A kinetic approach to the immunology of cancer: Stationary state properties of effector-target cell reactions, J. Theor. Biol. **73** (1978), 417–438.

38. Hainsworth, J. D. and F. A. Greco, Paclitaxel administered by 1-hour infusion, Cancer **74** (1994), 1377–1382.

39. Horsthemke, W. and M. Malek-Mansour, The influence of external noise on non-equilibrium phase transitions, Z. Physik B **24** (1976), 307–313.

40. Horsthemke, W. and R. Lefever, Phase transition induced by external noise, Phys. Lett. **64A** (1977), 19–21.

41. Hynes, R. O., *Fibronectins*, Springer-Verlag, New York, 1990.

42. Ioannides, C. G. and T. L. Whiteside, T-cell recognition of human – Implications for molecular immunotherapy of cancer, Clin. Immunol. Immunopath. **66** (1993), 91–106.

43. Jaaskelainen, J., A. Maenpaa, M. Patarroyo, C. G. Gahmberg, K. Somersalo, J. Tarkkanen, M. Kallio and T. Timonen. Migration of recombinant Il-2-activated T-cells and natural killer cells in the intercellular space of human H-2 glioma spheroids in vitro – A study on adhesion molecules involved, J. Immunol. **149** (1992), 260–268.

44. Kawakami, Y., M. I. Nishimura, N. P. Restifo, S. L. Topalian, B. H. O'Neil, J. Shilyansky, J. R. Yannelli and S. A. Rosenberg. T-cell recognition of human-melanoma antigens, J. Immunotherapy **14** (1993), 88–93.

45. Kirschner, D. and J. C. Panetta, Modeling immunotherapy of the tumor–immune interaction, J. Math. Biol., to appear.

46. Kuznetsov, V. A., I. A. Makalkin, M. A. Taylor and A. S. Perelson, Nonlinear dynamics of immunogenic tumors: parameter estimation and global bifurcation analysis, Bull. Math. Biol. **56** (1994), 295–321.

47. Lanzara, E., R. N. Mantegna, B. Spagnolo and R. Zangara, Experimental study of a nonlinear system in the presence of noise; the stochastic resonance, Am. J. Phys. **65** (1977), 341–349.

48. Lefever, R. and W. Horsthemke, Bistability in fluctuating environments. Implications in tumor immunology, Bull. Math. Biol. **41** (1979), 469–490.

49. Liotta, L. A., C. N. Rao and S. H. Barsky, Tumour invasion and the extracellular matrix, Lab. Invest. **49** (1983), 636–649.

50. Loeffler, D. and S. Ratner. In vivo localization of lymphocytes labeled with low concentrations of HOECHST-33342, J. Immunol. Meth. **119** (1989), 95–101.

51. Loeffler, D., G. Heppner and E. Lord, Influence of hypoxia on T-lymphocytes in solid tumours, Proc. Amer. Assoc. Cancer Res. **29** (1988), 378.

52. Lord, E. M. and G. Burkhardt, Assessment of in situ host immunity to syngeneic tumours utilizing the multicellular spheroid model, Cell. Immunol. **85** (1984), 340–350.

53. Lord, E. M. and G. Nardella, The multicellular tumour spheroid model. 2. Characterization of the preliminary allograft response in unsensitized mice, Transplantation **29** (1980), 119–124.

54. Madri, J. A. and B. M. Pratt, Endothelial cell-matrix interactions: in vitro models of angiogenesis, J. Histochem. Cytochem. **34** (1986), 85–91.

55. Michelson, S. and J. T. Leith, Growth factors and growth control of heterogeneous cell populations, Bull. Math. Biol. **55** (1993), 993–1011.

56. Michelson, S. and J. T. Leith, Dormancy, regression and recurrence: towards a unifying theory of tumor growth control, J. Theoret. Biol. **169** (1994), 327–338.

57. Michelson, S. and J. T. Leith, Interlocking triads of growth control in tumors. Bull. Math. Biol. **57** (1995), 733–747.

58. Michelson, S. and J. T. Leith, Positive feedback and angiogenesis in tumor growth control. Bull. Math. Biol. **59** (1997), 233–254.

59. Monaghan, P., M. J. Warburton, N. Perusinghe and P. S. Rutland, Topographical arrangement of basement membrane proteins in lactating rat mammary gland: comparison of the distribution of Type IV collagen, laminin, fibronectin and Thy-1 at the ultrasructural level, Proc. Natn. Acad. Sci. **80** (1983), 3344–3348.

60. Muthukkaruppan, V. R., L. Kubai and R. Auerbach, Tumor-induced neovascularization in the mouse eye. J. Natn. Cancer Inst. **69** (1982), 699–705.

61. Nesvetov, A. M. and A. S. Zhdanov, Relationship of the morphology of the immune response and the histological structure of tumours in stomach cancer patients. Voprosy Onkologii **27** (1981), 25–31.

62. O'Reilly M. S., L. Holmgren, Y. Shing, C. Chen, R. A. Rosenthal, M. Moses et al. Angiostatin: A novel angiogenesis inhibitor that mediates the suppression of metastases by a Lewis lung carcinoma, Cell **79** (1994), 315–328.

63. Orme, M. E. and M. A. J. Chaplain, A mathematical model of vascular tumour growth and invasion, Math. Comp. Modell. **23**(10) (1996), 43–60.

64. Orme, M. E. and M. A. J. Chaplain, Two-dimensional models of tumor angiogenesis and anti-angiogenesis strategies, IMA J. Math. App. Med. and Biol. **14** (1997), 189–205.

65. Panetta, J. C. and J. A. Adam, A Mathematical Model of Cycle-Specific Chemotherapy, Math. Comput. Model. **22** (1995), 67–82.

66. Panetta, J. C., A mathematical model of breast and ovarian cancer treated with paclitaxel, Math. Biosci. **146**(2) (1997), 89–113.

67. Paweletz, N. and M. Knierim, Tumor-related angiogenesis, Crit. Rev. Oncol. Hematol. **9** (1989), 197–242.

68. Pleass, R. and R. Camp, Cytokines induce lymphocyte migration in vitro by direct, receptor-specific mechanisms, Euro. J. Immunol. **24** (1994), 273–276.

69. Puri, R. K. and J. P. Siegel, Interleukin-4 and cancer therapy, Cancer Invest. **11** (1993), 473–486.

70. Ratner, S. and G. H. Heppner, Mechanisms of lymphocyte traffic in neoplasia, Anticancer Res. **6** (1986), 475–482.

71. Retsky, M. W., R. H. Wardwell, D. E. Swartzendruber and D. L. Headley, Prospective computerized simulation of breast-cancer – Comparison of computer-predictions with 9 sets of biological and clinical data, Cancer Res. **47** (1987), 4982–4987.

72. Rosenberg, S. A., M. T. Lotze, Cancer immunotherapy using interleukin-2 and interleukin-2-activated lymphocytes, Annual Review of Immunology **4** (1986), 681–709.

73. Schoefl, G. I., Studies on inflammation III. Growing capillaries: Their structure and permeability, Virchows Arch. Pathol. Anat. **337** (1963), 97–141.

74. Schor, S. L., A. M. Schor and G. W. Brazill, The effects of fibronectin on the migration of human foreskin fibroblasts and syrian hamster melanoma cells into three-dimensional gels of lattice collagen fibres, J. Cell Sci. **48** (1981), 301–314.

75. Schwartzentruber, D. J., S. L.Topalian, M. Mancini and S. A. Rosenberg, Specific release of granulocyte-macrophage colony-stimulating factor, tumour necrosis factor-α and IFN–γ by human tumour-infiltrating lymphocytes after autologous tumour stimulation, J. Immunol. **146** (1991), 3674–3681.

76. Sholley, M. M., G. P. Ferguson, H. R. Seibel, J. L. Montour and J. D. Wilson, Mechanisms of neovascularization. Vascular sprouting can occur without proliferation of cells, Lab. Invest. **51** (1984), 624–634.

77. Sordat, B., H. R. MacDonald and R. K. Lees, The multicellular spheroid as a model tumour allograft. 3. Morphological and kinetic analysis of spheroid infiltration and destruction, Transplantation **29** (1980), 103–112.

78. Spencer, C. M. and D. Faulds, Paclitaxel. A Review of its Pharmacodynamic and Pharmacokinetics Properties and Therapeutic Potential in the Treatment of Cancer, Drugs **48** (1994), 794–847.

79. Stokes, C. L. and D. A. Lauffenburger, Analysis of the roles of microvessel endothelial cell random motility and chemotaxis in angiogenesis, J. Theor. Biol. **152** (1991), 377–403.

80. Suzuki, Y., C. M. Liu, L. P. Chen, D. Bennathan and E. F. Wheelock, Immune regulation of the L5178Y murine tumour dormant state. 2. Interferon-gamma requires tumour necrosis factor to restrain tumour cell growth in peritoneal cell cultures from tumour dormant mice, J. Immunol. **139** (1987), 3146–3152.

81. Swan, G. W., Role of optimal contro theory in cancer chemotherapy, Math. Biosci. **101** (1990), 237–284.

82. Swierniak, A., A. Polanski and M. Kimmel, Optimal control problems arising in cell-cycle-specific cancer chemotherapy, Cell Prolif. **29** (1996), 117–139.

83. Warren, B. A., The growth of the blood supply to melanoma transplants in the hamster cheek pouch, Lab. Invest. **15** (1966), 464–473.

84. Webb G. F., A Cell Population Model of Periodic Chemotherapy Treatment, Biomedical Modeling and Simulation, Elsevier Science Publishers, 1992, 83–92.

85. Weinberg R. A., How cancer arises, Scientific American **275** (1996), 62–70.

86. Wilson, K. M. and E. M. Lord, Specific (EMT6) and non-specific (WEHI-164) cytolytic activity by host cells infiltrating tumour spheroids, Brit. J. Cancer **55** (1987), 141–146.

John Carl Panetta
Mathematics Program
Penn State Erie, The Behrend College
Station Road
Erie, PA 16563–0203
panetta@wagner.bd.psu.edu

Mark A. J. Chaplain
Department of Mathematics
University of Dundee
Dundee DD1 4HN
United Kingdom
chaplain@mcs.dundee.ac.uk

John A. Adam
Department of Mathematics and Statistics
Old Dominion University
Norfolk, VA 23529–0077
adam@math.odu.edu

The Hodgkin-Huxley Equations of Nerve Impulse Propagation

Mary E. Parrott

§1. Introduction

Hodgkin and Huxley, in their celebrated work done in the late 1940s and early 1950s, [21–25], for which they received the Nobel prize, obtained a quantitative explanation of the process of nerve impulse propagation. A measure of the power and influence of their accomplishments is the fact that since their work, most experimental and theoretical studies of electrically excitable cells have been based on the techniques they developed. In the present paper, we will look at the work of Hodgkin and Huxley and also at some recent work which is based on their fundamental contribution.

§2. Physiological Background

We begin by giving a brief description of the physiological process of nerve impulse conduction. For a thorough treatment of this background we refer the reader, for example, to the book of Cronin [6]. (Some of the description below is taken from [6].)

When a signal carries a command from the brain to a muscle, for example, it travels along a series of neurons having roughly the shape indicated in [6, page 7].

When an input signal arrives at the dendrites on the left-hand side of the neuron, the stimuli given the dendrites are integrated at the cell body to form a nerve impulse having roughly the shape of a sawtooth wave. This impulse travels along the axon to the branches (dendrites) on the right-hand side of the neuron. Various voltage-gated ion channels now open and a neurotransmitter chemical is released; this chemical diffuses across a gap (the synapse) to the dendrites of another neuron where chemically-gated ion channels open, and the process continues.

It was known by the end of the eighteenth century that nerves could be stimulated by an electric shock, so the basic problem of nerve conduction was known to be electrical in nature. One might have conjectured that nerve

Mathematical Models in Medical and Health Sciences
Mary Ann Horn, Gieri Simonett, and Glenn Webb (eds.), pp. 311–326.
Copyright © 1998 by Vanderbilt University Press, Nashville, TN.
ISBN 0-8265-1310-7.

conduction consists of an electric current, but Helmholtz showed in 1850, in his experiments on the sciatic nerve of a frog, that the signal velocity is fairly slow (about 27m/s) compared to the speed of electric current in a wire (i.e., the speed of light). This suggested that nerve impulse is not carried by an electric current, but is in some way reinforced as it travels along the nerve fiber. The main objective of the work of Hodgkin and Huxley was to explain not only this reinforcing process, but also the many phenomena observed in experiments conducted by physiologists over a long period of time.

Hodgkin and Huxley performed their experiments on the "giant" axon of the squid. The term giant axon is relative; its diameter of roughly .5mm is unusually large compared to those of other axons known in the animal kingdom. This large size makes experimental work possible.

For the Hodgkin-Huxley work, the axon can be regarded as a cylinder of radius a, containing a homogeneous aqueous gel called axoplasm, enclosed by a thin membrane consisting of protein and lipid fat. The axon is surrounded by an interstitial fluid containing sodium (Na^+), potassium (K^+), chloride (Cl^-) and other ions.

The propagation of nerve impulses is a combination of transmission down the core and continuous excitation of voltage impulses across the surrounding membrane. This excitation is due to the selective permeabilities of the membrane to potassium and sodium ions that, by the work of Hodgkin and Huxley, are known to depend on the voltage. Letting E denote the potential difference across the axon membrane at a particular point and time, what can be observed is as follows: If the amplitude of a stimulus at the point (provided, for example, by the insertion of an electrode) is large enough so that E is greater than a certain critical ("threshold") value, then E increases rapidly to form a roughly triangular solitary wave, called the "action potential," which splits immediately into two separate waves that travel away from the stimulating electrode in opposite directions along the fiber at a constant conduction velocity. The so-called all-or-nothing law in physiology refers to the fact that only the presence or absence of the travelling wave can be recorded. After a stimulus which produces an action potential there is a time interval of about 1ms (called the absolute refractory period) during which no stimulus, however strong, can produce an action potential.

The axon of the squid, as described above, is an example of a so-called unmyelinated axon. In most vertebrates the structure is more complicated; the axon is surrounded by a sheath of fatty material called myelin. The sheath is interrupted at intervals of about 1mm by short gaps (or nodes); in the gaps the axon consists of axoplasm surrounded by a thin membrane. We will see that the speed of propagation of the action potential in the unmyelinated squid axon studied by Hodgkin and Huxley is proportional to the square root of the radius of the axon (cylinder). In myelinated nerves, the action potential seems to skip from one node to another. This method of conduction is about 100 times faster than that of an action potential in an unmyelinated neuron. (See, for example, [34].)

In the absence of an external stimulus, the nerve axon is at a certain "resting potential," E_r, of about -70mV. A new variable $v = E - E_r$ is usually used to measure the (relative) potential difference across the axon membrane at a certain point and time; at the resting potential then, $v = 0$. This resting potential is a non-equilibrium, steady-state phenomenon common to all living cells. It is now known that the resting potential is maintained by two competing processes; one passive, involving leakage diffusion of K^+ from inside to outside the axon membrane (leaving behind Na^+ and other large organic ions to which the membrane is impermeable), and the other active (and energy requiring), involving the action of so-called molecular $Na - K$ pumps. These pumps repeatedly push three Na^+ ions out of the cell, against a concentration gradient, while pushing two K^+ ions into the cell, also against a concentration gradient. The resting potential can be changed by either changing the membrane permeability to any ion, or changing the external concentration of various ions. The current understanding of the process by which the action potential is propagated after the introduction of a stimulus involves the opening and closing of various voltage and chemically-gated Na^+ and K^+ channels along the axon membrane, as well as the restoring action of the $Na - K$ pumps. We refer the reader to the description of the process in [36], and the recent review article [1].

§3. Work of Hodgkin and Huxley

As mentioned, Hodgkin and Huxley sought to obtain a physical explanation of the processes that produced the experimentally observed phenomena that have been described. Through a series of carefully thought out and executed experiments, they achieved a substantial part of their goal.

As Cronin points out in [6], when the physiologists Hodgkin and Huxley initiated their work, they were not looking for a set of differential equations. They were concerned with studying the flow of electric current through the membrane surface, and finding an explanation for how these currents occur. There were no first principles of quantitative physiology to guide them, as there are, for example, in problems of mathematical physics.

It was observed that, in addition to its role as a variable conductor of electrically-charged particles, the axon membrane also functions as the dielectric of an electrical capacitor (in that charged particles accumulate on either side of it). Denoting the total membrane current density by I, the current density due to the capacitor effect by I_c, the membrane capacitance by C_m, the current density due to ion flow by I_{ion}, and the membrane potential difference by $v (= E - E_r)$, Hodgkin and Huxley considered the equation

$$I = I_c + I_{ion} = C_m \frac{dv}{dt} + I_{Na} + I_K + I_\ell, \qquad (3.1)$$

where I_{Na}, I_K and I_ℓ denote the current densitites due to ion flows of sodium, potassium, and other (leakage) ions respectively.

Using Ohm's law and the Nernst equation, one obtains

$$I_{Na} = g_{Na} \left(E - E_{Na} \right),\tag{3.2}$$

where g_{Na} is the conductance of sodium, and

$$E_{Na} = \frac{\overline{R}T}{F} \ln \frac{[Na]_0}{[Na]_i},$$

with $\overline{R}$ = the gas constant, T = absolute temperature, F = Faraday's constant and $[Na]$ = concentration of sodium (outside or inside). In terms of $v = E - E_r$, (3.2) takes the form

$$I_{Na} = g_{Na} \left(v - v_{Na} \right),\tag{3.3a}$$

with similar expressions for I_K and I_ℓ:

$$I_K = g_K \left(v - v_K \right),\tag{3.3b}$$
$$I_\ell = g_\ell \left(v - v_\ell \right).\tag{3.3c}$$

One of the landmark discoveries of the Hodgkin-Huxley study was that membrane permeability to Na and K ions varies with voltage and with time as an action potential occurs. They postulated that

$$\frac{dv}{dt} = F \left(t, v, g_{Na}, g_K \right),$$
$$\frac{dg_{Na}}{dt} = G \left(t, v, g_{Na}, g_K \right),$$
$$\frac{dg_K}{dt} = H \left(t, v, g_{Na}, g_K \right),$$

and were able to determine explicit forms for these functional relationships by means of their "voltage-clamped" and "space-clamped" experiments.

In the voltage-clamped experiments, the interior axon was "clamped" at -45mV; the fixed voltage in these conductance experiments was maintained by controlling the current fed to an implanted electrode. The entire axon membrane acts in unison in this situation; there are no spatial effects, and the ionic conductances depend only on time.

In order to capture the features of the observed behavior of g_K, g_{Na} and g_ℓ from the voltage-clamped experiments (see, for example, [36, Chap. 8]), Hodgkin and Huxley described the conductances g_K, g_{Na} and g_ℓ by:

$$g_K = \overline{g}_K n^4,\tag{3.4a}$$
$$g_{Na} = \overline{g}_{Na} m^3 h,\tag{3.4b}$$
$$g_\ell = \overline{g}_\ell.\tag{3.4c}$$

Here $\bar{g}_K$, $\bar{g}_{Na}$, and $\bar{g}_\ell$ are the (measurable) maximum conductances of K, Na, and leakage ions respectively, which are attained over all depolarizing voltages (that is, voltages whose magnitudes are less than that of the resting potential). The new variables n, m, and h are dimensionless variables of exponential type with values in $[0, 1]$; they can be considered as proportions of ions in a specific location, or as probabilities. The variables n, m, and h can be cast as the solutions, respectively, of the differential equations

$$\frac{dn}{dt} = \alpha_n(1 - n) - \beta_n n, \tag{3.5a}$$

$$\frac{dm}{dt} = \alpha_m(1 - m) - \beta_m m, \tag{3.5b}$$

$$\frac{dh}{dt} = \alpha_h(1 - h) - \beta_h h, \tag{3.5c}$$

where, experimentally, the coefficients were found to vary with the voltage. Hodgkin and Huxley fit the experimental relations by:

$$\alpha_n = \frac{0.01(v + 10)}{e^{.1(v+10)} - 1}, \quad \beta_n = 0.125 e^{v/80}, \tag{3.6a}$$

$$\alpha_m = \frac{0.1(v + 25)}{e^{.1(v+25)} - 1}, \quad \beta_m = 4 e^{v/18}, \tag{3.6b}$$

$$\alpha_h = 0.07 e^{0.05v}, \quad \beta_h = \frac{1}{e^{.1(v+30)} + 1}. \tag{3.6c}$$

From (3.3a–c) and (3.4a–c), the expressions for the ionic currents are

$$I_k = \bar{g}_K n^4 (v - v_K), \tag{3.7a}$$

$$I_{Na} = \bar{g}_{Na} m^3 h (v - v_{Na}), \tag{3.7b}$$

$$I_\ell = \bar{g}_\ell (v - v_\ell). \tag{3.7c}$$

Not surprisingly, Hodgkin and Huxley obtained the correct prediction of total current during the voltage-clamped experiments using these expressions. What is surprising (given the somewhat arbitrary nature of the derivation of the expressions (3.4a–c)) is how well theoretical and experimental results of the full Hodgkin-Huxley equations using (3.7a–c) (as described in the next section) agree.

In the space-clamped experiments (still an artificial situation), electrodes are fixed along the entire length of the axon as before, but now the electrodes are used to measure the voltage as it is varied during a depolarizing event. As a shock is applied, the entire axon undergoes an action potential at the same time. The so-called space-clamped equations which emerge can be regarded as describing the variations of membrane potential and ion conductances that occur at a fixed point on the axon. From (3.1),

$$I_c = C_m \frac{dv}{dt} = I - I_{Na} - I_K - I_\ell.$$

Using (3.7a–c) with the above and (3.5a–c), and specifying initial conditions, yields the space-clamped equations (SC):

$$\frac{dv}{dt} = \frac{1}{C_m} \left[I - \bar{g}_K n^4 \left(v - v_K\right) - \bar{g}_{Na} m^3 h \left(v - v_{Na}\right) - \bar{g}_\ell \left(v - v_\ell\right) \right],$$

$$\frac{dn}{dt} = \alpha_n(1 - n) - \beta_n n, \qquad\qquad\qquad\qquad\qquad \text{(SC)}$$

$$\frac{dm}{dt} = \alpha_m(1 - m) - \beta_m m,$$

$$\frac{dh}{dt} = \alpha_h(1 - h) - \beta_h h,$$

$$v(0) = v_0, \quad n(0) = n_0, \quad m(0) = m_0, \quad h(0) = h_0.$$

Here α_i, b_i, $i = n, m, h$, are given by (3.6a–c).

Numerical analysis of (SC) gives good agreement between the predicted and experimental observations of the duration of the refractory period, and changes in $v(t)$ as the membrane returns to the normal resting condition. There is not, however, entirely satisfactory agreement between the theoretical and experimental results for v. (See the discussion, for example, in [6].)

§4. The Hodgkin-Huxley Equations

In reality, with the normal physiological functioning of the nerve axon, the potential varies with the position on the axon as well as time; the action potential is propagated along the axon in time. The extended model is usually obtained by combining the models of the voltage and space-clamped experiments of Hodgkin and Huxley with a few facts from standard electrical theory. In what follows, t = time, x = distance along the axon from the cut end, a = axon radius, v = potential difference across membrane ($= E - E_r$), i = membrane current/unit length, I = membrane current density $= i/2\pi a$, i_a = axon current/unit length, r = axon resistance/unit length, R = specific resistance of axon $= \left(\pi a^2\right) r$, L = axon specific self-inductance, C_m = membrane capacitance, C_a = axon self-capacitance/unit area/unit length, $C = \frac{a}{2} C_a + C_m$.

The cable equations (which relate current and voltage on a transmission line with allowance for a current lost to the line) are used to relate the axon current, voltage, and membrane current:

$$\frac{-\partial i_a}{\partial x} = i + \pi a^2 C_a \frac{\partial v}{\partial t}, \qquad\qquad\qquad\qquad \text{(4.1a)}$$

$$\frac{-\partial v}{\partial x} = r i_a + \frac{L}{\pi a^2} \frac{\partial i_a}{\partial t}. \qquad\qquad\qquad\qquad \text{(4.1b)}$$

Applying $\left(r + \dfrac{L}{\pi a^2}\dfrac{\partial}{\partial t}\right)$ to (4.1a) and using (4.1b), (3.1), (3.7a–c) and (3.5a–c), one obtains the Hodgkin-Huxley system of equations which we call $(HH)_L$:

$$\frac{\partial^2 v}{\partial x^2} - \frac{2}{a}LC\frac{\partial^2 v}{\partial t^2} = \frac{2}{a}RC\frac{\partial v}{\partial t} + \frac{2}{a}L\left(\bar{g}_K n^4 + \bar{g}_{Na}m^3 h + \bar{g}_\ell\right)\frac{\partial v}{\partial t}$$

$$+ \bar{g}_K\left(\frac{2}{a}Rn^4 + 4\left(\frac{2L}{a}\right)n^3\frac{\partial n}{\partial t}\right)(v - v_K)$$

$$+ \bar{g}_{Na}\left[\frac{2}{a}Rm^3 h + \frac{2}{a}L\left(3m^2 h\frac{\partial m}{\partial t} + m^3\frac{\partial h}{\partial t}\right)\right](v - v_{Na})$$

$$+ \bar{g}_\ell\left(\frac{2}{a}R\right)(v - v_\ell), \tag{HH$_L$}$$

$$\frac{\partial n}{\partial t} = \alpha_n(1 - n) - \beta_n n,$$

$$\frac{\partial m}{\partial t} = \alpha_m(1 - m) - \beta_m m,$$

$$\frac{\partial h}{\partial t} = \alpha_h(1 - h) - \beta_h h.$$

Recognizing that the axon self-capacitance, C_a, and the specific self-inductance, L, are small quantities, and that the partial differential equations which result from using (4.1a–b) (i.e., $(HH)_L$ above) are a complicated system, Hodgkin and Huxley dropped the terms involving C_a and L in (4.1a–b). We denote the equations which result from letting $L = 0$ and $C_a = 0$ in (4.1a–b) by (HH); these equations are

$$\frac{\partial^2 v}{\partial x^2} = \frac{2}{a}RC_m\frac{\partial v}{\partial t} + \bar{g}_K\left(\frac{2}{a}Rn^4\right)(v - v_K)$$

$$+ \bar{g}_{Na}\left(\frac{2}{a}Rm^3 h\right)(v - v_{Na}) + \bar{g}_\ell\left(\frac{2}{a}R\right)(v - v_\ell),$$

$$\frac{\partial n}{\partial t} = \alpha_n(1 - n) - \beta_n n, \tag{HH}$$

$$\frac{\partial m}{\partial t} = \alpha_m(1 - m) - \beta_m m,$$

$$\frac{\partial h}{\partial t} = \alpha_h(1 - h) - \beta_h h.$$

In the spirit of Hodgkin and Huxley, most of the mathematical work on nerve impulse transmission which has subsequently appeared deals either with the space-clamped equations (SC) or the extended system (HH) (under various initial and boundary conditions). We mention here again the work of Cronin [6] and references therein, and the work of Carpenter [5], Evans [7–10], Evans and Shenk [11], Hastings [20], Mascagni [30], McKean and Moll [31], and Meves [32]. An early exception, which deals with the system $(HH)_L$, is the 1967 work of Lieberstein [26, 27]. Lieberstein noted that if one lets

$\Theta = \left(\dfrac{a}{2LC}\right)^{1/2}$, then the left-hand side of the first equation of (HH)$_L$ becomes

$$\frac{\partial^2 v}{\partial x^2} - \frac{1}{\Theta^2}\frac{\partial^2 v}{\partial t^2},$$

which points clearly to the hyperbolic character of this equation for v. This is expected when one notes the type of observable wave propagation behavior, and allows the finite wave propagation speed Θ to be defined in a natural fashion in terms of physical parameters. We note that the equation for v given in (HH) is a parabolic equation.

It is interesting to note here the ad-hoc procedure which Hodgkin and Huxley used to determine the wave propagation speed. From the equations (HH), Hodgkin and Huxley looked for a travelling wave solution (with hypothetical speed Θ) of the form $(v(x - \Theta t), n(x - \Theta t), m(x - \Theta t), h(x - \Theta t))$. Letting $z = x - \Theta t$, (HH) yields

$$\frac{\partial^2 v}{\partial z^2} = \frac{2}{a}RC(-\Theta)\frac{\partial v}{\partial z} + \bar{g}_K\left(\frac{2}{a}Rn^4\right)(v - v_K)$$
$$+ \bar{g}_{Na}\left(\frac{2}{a}Rm^3h\right)(v - v_{Na}) + \bar{g}_\ell\left(\frac{2}{a}R\right)(v - v_\ell),$$

$$\frac{\partial n}{\partial z} = -\frac{1}{\Theta}\left[\alpha_n(1 - n) - \beta_n n\right],$$

$$\frac{\partial m}{\partial z} = -\frac{1}{\Theta}\left[\alpha_m(1 - m) - \beta_m m\right],$$

$$\frac{\partial h}{\partial z} = -\frac{1}{\Theta}\left[\alpha_h(1 - h) - \beta_h h\right].$$

Hodgkin and Huxley numerically looked for a value of Θ for which solutions of the above system are such that $\lim\limits_{z\to\infty} v(z) = 0$. They showed that, for a particular axon, $\Theta = 18.8\text{m/s}$, close to the experimentally-observed velocity for the same axon of 21.2m/s. This prediction of the wave propagation speed is considered the most spectacular prediction of Hodgkin-Huxley theory.

Lieberstein used a modified method of characteristics/finite-difference method to obtain numerical results for (HH)$_L$ which show the transient development of the action potential, and are generally in good agreement with the experimental results of Hodgkin and Huxley (cf. [26]). Lieberstein's work is not widely known, probably because the spirit of that time leaned toward simplification of the Hodgkin-Huxley equations. For example, one of these simplified models, proposed by Fitzhugh [16] and later developed by Nagumo et al. [33], consists of a diffusion equation for the potential difference v and one equation for the "recovery" variable w (in place of n, m or h),

$$\frac{\partial v}{\partial t} = \frac{\partial^2 v}{\partial x^2} + f(v) - w, \qquad\qquad\qquad \text{(FN)}$$

$$\frac{\partial w}{\partial t} = c(v + a - bw),$$

where a, b, c are nonnegative constants, and $f \in C^2(R)$ is a curve with a prescribed shape (for example, $f(v) = v - v^3$). Several analytical and numerical results were obtained for the (FN) model which fit qualitatively with the expected nerve fiber behavior. More recently, València [35] put together the simplification of Fitzhugh and Nagumo and the modification of Lieberstein to obtain a model of the form

$$\epsilon \frac{\partial^2 v}{\partial t^2} + (1 - \epsilon f'(v)) \frac{\partial v}{\partial t} = \frac{\partial^2 v}{\partial x^2} + f(v) - w,$$

$$\frac{\partial w}{\partial t} = \delta \frac{\partial^2 w}{\partial x^2} + c(v + a - bw), \quad (x,t) \in R \times R^+, \tag{V}$$

where $\epsilon > 0$, $\delta \geq 0$, and a, b, c and f are as above. In this work, information on the asymptotic behavior of solutions of (V) was obtained by considering positively-invariant regions for the solutions of (V) containing its constant steady-state solutions.

§5. Relationship of Solutions of $(HH)_L$ and (HH)

In a series of recent papers, Fitzgibbon, Martin and Parrott [12], Fitzgibbon and Parrott [13], and Fitzgibbon, Parrott and You [14, 15], have examined the relationship of solutions of the system $(HH)_L$ to solutions of the system (HH). Since L is small, $(HH)_L$ was viewed as a singular perturbation of (HH). The reduced systems considered (for simplicity) in these papers, corresponding to $(HH)_L$ and (HH), respectively, have the form:

$$\epsilon \frac{\partial^2 v}{\partial t^2} + (\epsilon f_3(w) + 1) \frac{\partial v}{\partial t} = \frac{\partial^2 v}{\partial x^2} - f_1(w)v + f_2(w), \quad x \in (0,1), \quad t > 0, \tag{5.1a}$$

$$\frac{\partial w}{\partial t} = -h_1(v)w + h_2(v), \quad x \in (0,1), \quad t > 0, \tag{5.1b}$$

$$\frac{\partial v}{\partial x}(0,t) = \frac{\partial v}{\partial x}(1,t) = 0, \quad t > 0, \tag{5.1c}$$

$$v(x,0) = v_0(x), \quad w(x,0) = w_0(x), \quad x \in (0,1), \tag{5.1d}$$

$$\frac{\partial v}{\partial t}(x,0) = v_1(x), \quad x \in (0,1), \tag{5.1e}$$

and

$$\frac{\partial v}{\partial t} = \frac{\partial^2 v}{\partial x^2} - f_1(w)v + f_2(w), \quad x \in (0,1), \quad t > 0, \tag{5.2a}$$

$$\frac{\partial w}{\partial t} = -h_1(v)w + h_2(v), \quad x \in (0,1), \quad t > 0, \tag{5.2b}$$

$$\frac{\partial v}{\partial x}(0,t) = \frac{\partial v}{\partial x}(1,t) = 0, \quad t > 0, \tag{5.2c}$$

$$v(x,0) = v_0(x), \quad w(x,0) = w_0(x), \quad x \in (0,1). \tag{5.2d}$$

It is assumed in the above equations that ϵ is a small positive constant; f_i, $i = 1, 2, 3$, and their derivatives are continuous, polynomially-bounded functions;

h_i, $i = 1, 2$, are uniformly bounded functions and their derivatives are locally bounded; v_0, w_0, $v_1 \in C^\infty(0, 1)$. In [13], the uniform convergence of solutions of (5.1a–e) to solutions of (5.2a–d) as $\epsilon \to 0$ is shown; the following theorem gives this result. In the theorem, $\| \cdot \|_\infty$ denotes the supremum norm on the space of continuous functions on $[0, 1]$.

Theorem 1. *([13, Thm. 6.4]) Let (v_ϵ, w_ϵ) be the solution of (5.1a–e) and let (v, w) be the solution of (5.2a–d). Under the given conditions (and a compatibility condition on the initial data),*

$$\lim_{\epsilon \to 0^+} \|v_\epsilon(\cdot, t) - v(\cdot, t)\|_\infty = 0$$

and

$$\lim_{\epsilon \to 0^+} \|w_\epsilon(\cdot, t) - w(\cdot, t)\|_\infty = 0$$

for all $t \in [0, T]$ and any $T > 0$.

The relationship between the dynamics of solutions of (5.1a–e) and (5.2a–d) was considered in [14] and [15]. In these papers, besides the hypotheses stated above, it is assumed that $f_1(w) \geq a$ with $a > 0$ a small constant, $h_1(v) \geq b$ with $b > 0$ a small constant, $h_2(v) \geq 0$, and $w^* \geq w_0(x) \geq 0$ for $x \in [0, 1]$, where w^* is a fixed constant. In [14], the existence of global attractors A_ϵ for (5.1a–e), for each $\epsilon > 0$ sufficiently small, is established. The solutions of (5.1a–e) are shown to define a semiflow $\sigma(t, \cdot)$ with associated semigroup $\{S(t) : t \geq 0\}$ in the Banach space $X = H^1(0, 1) \times L^2(0, 1) \times L^2(0, 1)$. (Here $H^1(0, 1)$ is the usual Sobolev space of $L^2(0, 1)$ functions whose first derivatives (in the distribution sense) are in $L^2(0, 1)$.) A set $A \subset X$ is called a "global attractor" for a semiflow σ if it is compact, functional invariant (i.e. $S(t)A = A$ for any $t \geq 0$), and dist$(S(t)B, A) \to 0$ as $t \to \infty$ for any bounded set B in X. The existence of a global attractor A for (5.2a–d) follows from results of Marion [29]. In [15], the authors show that the global attractors A_ϵ have finite Hausdorff and fractal dimensions. (This property was established for the attractor A in [29].) They also show in [15] that the attractors A_ϵ converge to the attractor A, as $\epsilon \to 0^+$, in the sense that

$$\lim_{\epsilon \to 0^+} \text{dist}_X(A_\epsilon, A_0) = \lim_{\epsilon \to 0^+} \sup_{a \in A_\epsilon} \inf_{b \in A_\epsilon} \|a - b\|_X = 0,$$

where A_0 is an embedding of the global attractor A in X.

The estimated bound of the fractal dimension of A_ϵ found in [15] depends on ϵ, and goes to infinity when ϵ goes to zero. In a recent paper [18], Galusinski shows the existence of so-called exponential attractors for (5.1a–e); these sets attract trajectories of solutions with a uniform (with ϵ) rate and have a bounded (uniformly in ϵ) fractal dimension.

The above discussion seems to justify the assumption of Hodgkin and Huxley that, since the line inductance L of the system is small, the terms containing L can be ignored, and suggests that one can continue to use the model (HH) with confidence. The discussion also suggests that the long-term ("steady-state") behavior of the two models should be the same. However, we have already noted that $(HH)_L$ preserves the correct hyperbolic form expected for the equation for v, and allows for a natural description of the wave propagation speed Θ. Another reason which supports the use of the model $(HH)_L$ instead of (HH) involves the further consideration of steady-state behavior.

§6. Steady-State Equations

As previously noted, it can be observed that fully-developed impulses form rapidly and travel with a constant velocity of propagation and without appreciable alteration of wave form. This suggests (though a mathematical theorem to prove the result is needed) that the potential difference v eventually (i.e., in the "steady-state") obeys the wave equation

$$\frac{\partial^2 v}{\partial x^2} - \frac{1}{\Theta^2}\frac{\partial^2 v}{\partial t^2} = 0, \tag{6.1}$$

where Θ is the rate of propagation.

From the equation for v in (HH), if we replace $\dfrac{\partial^2 v}{\partial x^2}$ by $\dfrac{1}{\Theta^2}\dfrac{\partial^2 v}{\partial t^2}$ we obtain the second-order ordinary differential equation:

$$\left(\frac{a}{2C_m\Theta^2}\right)\frac{d^2v}{dt^2} = R\frac{dv}{dt} + \frac{R}{C_m}\left(I_{Na} + I_K + I_\ell\right). \tag{6.2}$$

Using (6.2) in the steady-state formulation for (HH) has led to much confusion in obtaining numerical solutions, mainly due to the need to specify $\dfrac{dv}{dt}(0)$ (an artificial side condition) as well as $v(0)$, and there was extreme sensitivity of solutions to Θ (cf. [26]). This approach has mostly been abandoned. We remark that (6.2) was used by Hodgkin and Huxley to predict that $\Theta \sim \sqrt{a}$. They noted that since only the term on the left-hand side of (6.2) depends on a, this implies that the coefficient $\dfrac{a}{2C_m\Theta^2}$ must be constant with respect to a, which further implies that $\Theta = (\text{const.})\sqrt{\dfrac{a}{2C_m}}$. (This can be compared with Lieberstein's observation of $\Theta = \sqrt{\dfrac{a}{2LC}}$.)

Using the Hodgkin-Huxley observation that the total current becomes negligible after a brief interval following the application of a shock to an axon, the space-clamped equations (SC) with $I = 0$ are sometimes used as a system of ordinary differential equations to predict steady-state behavior. One drawback of this approach is that, except for a narrow range of values of I, there is a periodic solution of (SC). This has been shown by Fitzhugh [16], and more recently by Golubitsky and Schaeffer [19]. But, in laboratory experiments on the squid giant axon, for sawtooth inputs of current above a threshold value, only one action potential occurs; for stimulation by a step current, only a train of up to four impulses is observed.

An attempt has been made (cf. [2]) to modify the equations (SC) by taking into account the phenomenon of "accomodation," so that closer agreement between theory and experiments can be obtained. This phenomenon is a physiological process that produces a slow decay in a train of nerve impulses that result from a constant subthreshhold stimulation.

We believe, however, that the space-clamped equations represent an artificial situation which cannot be expected to accurately model steady-state behavior, and that the approach described below, using the equations $(HH)_L$, leads to the correct formulation of steady-state equations.

Following Lieberstein [27], we let $\dfrac{\partial^2 v}{\partial x^2} - \dfrac{1}{\Theta^2}\dfrac{\partial^2 v}{\partial t^2} = 0$, where $\Theta^2 = \dfrac{a}{2LC}$, in the first equation of $(HH)_L$, and add a term $r(t)$ to provide an initial voltage impulse, where

$$r(t) = \begin{cases} r_0, & 0 \le t < 1 \text{ ms}, \\ -\tfrac{1}{2}r_0, & 1 \le t < 3 \text{ ms}, \\ 0, & t \ge 3 \text{ ms}. \end{cases}$$

Here r_0 is a constant which indicates the amplitude of an initiating impulse. We obtain the following system of ordinary differential equations which we call the steady-state equations (SS):

$$\begin{aligned}
\frac{dv}{dt} = &-\left\{\left[\frac{2}{a}RC + \left(\frac{1}{\Theta^2 C}\right)(\bar{g}_K n^4 + \bar{g}_{Na}m^3 h + \bar{g}_\ell)\right]^{-1}\right\} \\
&\times \left\{\bar{g}_K\left[\frac{2}{a}Rn^4 + \left(\frac{4}{\Theta^2 C}\right)n^3\frac{dn}{dt}\right](v - v_K)\right. \\
&+ \bar{g}_{Na}\left[\frac{2}{a}Rm^3 h + \left(\frac{1}{\Theta^2 C}\right)\left(3m^2 h\frac{dm}{dt} + m^3\frac{dh}{dt}\right)\right](v - v_{Na}) \\
&\left. + \bar{g}_\ell\left(\frac{2}{a}R\right)(v - v_\ell)\right\} + r(t),
\end{aligned}$$ (SS)

$$\frac{dn}{dt} = \alpha_n(1 - n) - \beta_n n,$$

$$\frac{dm}{dt} = \alpha_m(1 - m) - \beta_m m,$$

$$\frac{dh}{dt} = \alpha_h(1 - h) - \beta_h h,$$

$$v(0) = 0, \quad n(0) = \frac{\alpha_n(0)}{\alpha_n(0) + \beta_n(0)},$$

$$m(0) = \frac{\alpha_m(0)}{\alpha_m(0) + \beta_m(0)}, \quad h(0) = \frac{\alpha_h(0)}{\alpha_h(0) + \beta_h(0)}.$$

Lieberstein [27] noted that for fixed L and C, the equations (SS) are invariant with respect to changes in either the propagation rate Θ or the axon radius a. (This can be seen from the equation for v in (SS); since

$$\Theta^2 = \frac{a}{2LC}, \quad \text{then} \quad \frac{1}{\Theta^2 C} = \frac{2}{a}L,$$

and the factor $2/a$ divides out of the equation.) Thus, for fixed electrical properties, the sensitivity of the equations (SS) to Θ is eliminated altogether. Although $\Theta \sim \sqrt{a}$, at any given position on the axon, the steady-state voltage as a function of time is independent of a, a fact which has been discovered empirically [4].

Recently, a further numerical study of (SS) has been begun by Parrott and a graduate student, Bill Reynolds. Using, for example, MAPLE, the numerical solution of (SS) is no more difficult than that of (SC). Good agreement with Lieberstein's work has been obtained for the comparison of numerical integration of (SS) (using Hodgkin-Huxley parameter values and $r_0 = -15$mV/ms, which initiates the occurrence of a -15mV sawtoothed impulse) , and an empirical curve obtained by Hodgkin and Huxley (cf. [26, Fig. 5 I, II]).

To see the close comparison of the numerical integration of the equations (SS) with the wave developed by $(HH)_L$ from an initial sawtoothed wave of amplitude -15mV applied to a cut end (where a shift in the time scale allows for the development of the initiating impulse), see [27, Fig. 1].

Using again the parameter values of Hodgkin and Huxley, we have also verified Lieberstein's calculation of the threshold value of $r_0 = -7.94$mV from (SS); that is, no action potential is fired for $r_0 = -7.94$mV; one, and only one, is fired for $|r_0| > 7.94$mV.

As suggested by Lieberstein in [27], adaptation of the model (SS) may be possible to provide a model for electrical activity of other membrane cells such as receptors, pacemaker cells and heart cells (see also [3]). In this endeavor, the previous viewpoint that the electrical activity of a nerve axon is a consequence of an initiating sawtooth voltage impulse is now altered to account instead for a sustained membrane current input. The addition of a sustained constant membrane current density I_0 applied at an active point of the membrane can be accounted for in (SS) by the addition of the term (replacing $r(t)$):

$$\frac{-\frac{2}{a} R I_0}{\frac{2}{a} RC + \left(\frac{1}{\Theta^2 C}\right)\left(\overline{g}_K n^4 + \overline{g}_{Na} m^3 h + \overline{g}_\ell\right)}.$$

By considering various values of I_0 and allowing the maximum sodium or potassium conductances, $\overline{g}_{Na}$ or $\overline{g}_K$, to vary, we have obtained early numerical results which verify and extend those of [27]. These results show promise for yielding information on certain types of cell behavior including the so-called repetitive firing phenomenon of receptors and pacemaker cells (where a finite or infinite train of action potentials is produced), and the plateau behavior shown by certain heart cells (where the membrane voltage eventually levels off to a sustained plateau). This project is ongoing; the results will be the subject of a future paper.

§7. Conclusions and Directions for Further Mathematical Research

We have seen that the work of Hodgkin and Huxley has provided a fundamental basis for the understanding of the process of nerve impulse propagation, and has had a profound influence on the subsequent research in this area which continues today.

We mention several topics related to the Hodgkin-Huxley equations where further mathematical research is needed. First of all, in order to prove that the equations (SS) correctly model the steady-state behavior of the Hodgkin-Huxley equations, the following mathematical results should be established:

1) As $t, x \to \infty$, the solution of the equation for v in $(HH)_L$ obeys the wave equation $\dfrac{\partial^2 v}{\partial x^2} - \dfrac{1}{\Theta^2}\dfrac{\partial^2 v}{\partial t^2} = 0$.

2) The attractor of (SS) contains only the physically-observed equilibrium point; i.e.

$$\lim_{t \to \infty} (v(t), m(t), n(t), h(t)) = (0, m_\infty, n_\infty, h_\infty).$$

We mention here a recent paper of Manganaro and Migliardo [28], which might prove useful in helping to answer item 1 above. In [28], the authors consider a hyperbolic system consisting basically of the cable equations defined in (4.1a-b) plus one equation for the recovery variable w,

$$\frac{\partial w}{\partial t} + \phi(v, w)\frac{\partial v}{\partial t} = \psi(v, w).$$

Under certain conditions on ϕ and ψ, the authors use a reduction method established in [17] for quasilinear hyperbolic systems of PDEs to determine the exact solutions to their nerve impulse propagation model. Their approach works, for example, for the Fitzhugh-Nagumo model (FN).

Even with the above results, we still don't know mathematically whether the solutions of $(HH)_L$ or (SS) describe such phenomena as the refractory period and threshold behavior. As Cronin points out [6], we need other mathematical concepts that correspond to these physiological notions, and we need to show that the Hodgkin-Huxley equations behave in accordance with these concepts.

References

1. Ackerman, M. and D. Clapham, Ion channels – basic science and clinical disease, The New England J. of Medicine **336** (1997), 1575–1586.

2. Adelman, W. and R. Fitzhugh, Solutions of the Hodgkin-Huxley equation modified for potassium accumulation in a periaxonal space, Fed. Amer. Soc. Exp. Biol. Proc. **34** (1975), 1322–1329.

3. Awiszus, F., J. Dehnhardt and T. Funke, The singular perturbed Hodgkin-Huxley equations as a tool for the analysis of repetitive nerve activity, J. Math. Biol. **28** (1990), 177–195.

4. Baker, P., A. Hodgkin and T. Shaw, Replacement of the axoplasm of giant nerve fibers with artificial solutions, J. Physiol. **164** (1962), 330–354.

5. Carpenter, G., A geometric approach to singular perturbation problems with applications to nerve impulse equations, J. Differential Equations **23** (1977), 335–367.

6. Cronin, J., *Mathematical Aspects of Hodgkin-Huxley Neural Theory*, Cambridge University Press, Cambridge, 1987.

7. Evans, J., Nerve axon equations I: linear approximations, Indiana Univ. Math. J. **21** (1972), 877–885.

8. Evans, J., Nerve axon equations II: stability at rest, Indiana Univ. Math. J. **22** (1972), 75–90.

9. Evans, J., Nerve axon equations III: stability of the nerve impulse, Indiana Univ. Math. J. **22** (1972), 577–593.

10. Evans, J., Nerve axon equations IV: the stable and the unstable impulse, Indiana Univ. Math. J. **24** (1975), 1160–1190.

11. Evans, J. and N. Shenk, Solutions to axon equations, Biophy. J. **10** (1970), 1090–1101.

12. Fitzgibbon, W., C. Martin and M. Parrott, Hodgkin-Huxley models of neural conduction, Seminar Notes in Functional Analysis and PDEs, LSU Dept. of Math. (1991–1992), 96–107.

13. Fitzgibbon, W. and M. Parrott, Convergence of singularly perturbed Hodgkin-Huxley systems, Nonlinear Anal. TMA **22** (1994), 363–379.

14. Fitzgibbon, W., M. Parrott and Y. You, Global dynamics of singularly perturbed Hodgkin-Huxley equations, *Semigroups of Linear and Nonlinear Operations and Applications*, G. Goldstein and J. Goldstein (eds.), Kluwer Acad. Publ., 1993, 159–176.

15. Fitzgibbon, W., M. Parrott and Y. You, Finite dimensionality and upper semicontinuity of the global attractor of singularly perturbed Hodgkin-Huxley systems, J. Differential Equations **129** (1996), 193–237.

16. Fitzhugh, R., Impulses and physiological states in theoretical models of nerve membrane, Biophys. J. **1** (1961), 445–466.

17. Fusco, D. and N. Manganaro, A method for finding exact solutions to hyperbolic systems of first-order PDEs, IMA J. Appl. Math. **57** (1996), 223–242.

18. Galusinski, C., Existence and continuity of uniform exponential attractors of singularly perturbed Hodgkin-Huxley systems, preprint.

19. Golubitsky, M. and D. Schaeffer, *Singularities and Groups in Bifurcation Theory*, Vol. 1, Appl. Math. Sci. **51**, Springer-Verlag, Berlin, 1985.

20. Hastings, S., On travelling wave solutions of the Hodgkin-Huxley equations, Arch. Rat. Mech. Anal. **60** (1975/76), 229–257.

21. Hodgkin, A. and A. Huxley, Currents carried by sodium and potassium ions through the membrane of the giant axon of Logio, J. Physio. **116** (1952), 449–472.

22. Hodgkin, A. and A. Huxley, Components of membrane conductance in the giant axon of Logio, J. Physio. **116** (1952), 473–496.

23. Hodgkin, A. and A. Huxley, The dual effect of membrane potential on sodium conductance in the giant axon of Logio, J. Physio. **116** (1952), 497–506.

24. Hodgkin, A. and A. Huxley, A quantitative description of membrane current and its application to conduction and excitation in nerve, J. Physio. **117** (1952), 500–544.

25. Hodgkin, A., A. Huxley and B. Katz, Measurement of current-voltage relations in the membrane of the giant axon of Logio, J. Physio. **116** (1952), 424–448.

26. Lieberstein, H., On the Hodgkin-Huxley partial differential equation, Math. Biosci. **1** (1967), 45–69.

27. Lieberstein, H., Numerical studies of the steady-state equations for a Hodgkin-Huxley model, Math. Biosci. **1** (1967), 181–211.

28. Manganaro, N. and M. Migliardo, Reduction procedure for a model describing nerve pulse propagation, IMA J. Appl. Math., to appear.

29. Marion, M., Finite dimensional attractors associated with partially dissipative reaction diffusion systems, SIAM J. Math. Anal. **20** (1989), 815–844.

30. Mascagni, M., An initial-boundary value problem of physiological significance for equations of nerve conduction, Comm. Pure and Appl. Math. XLII (1989), 213–227.

31. McKean, H. and V. Moll, Stabilization to the standing wave in a simple caricature of the nerve equation, Comm. Pure and Appl. Math. XXXIX (1986), 485–529.

32. Meves, H., Hodgkin-Huxley: Thirty years after, Current Topics in Membranes and Transport **22** (1984), 279–329.

33. Nagumo, J., S. Arimoto and S. Yoshizawa, An active pulse transmission line simulating nerve axon, Proc. IRE **50** (1962), 2061–2070.

34. Scott, A., The electrophysics of a nerve fiber, Rev. Med. Phys. **47** (1975), 487–533.

35. València, M., Invariant regions and asymptotic bounds for a hyperbolic version of the nerve equation, Nonlinear Anal., TMA **16** (1991), 1035–1052.

36. Yeargers, E., R. Shonkwiler and J. Herod, *An Introduction to the Mathematics of Biology: With Computer Algebra Models*, Birkhäser, Boston, 1996.

Mary E. Parrott
Department of Mathematics
University of South Florida
Tampa, FL 33620-5700
parrott@math.usf.edu

The Effect of Anisotropy on the Meandering of Spiral Waves in Cardiac Tissue

Bradley J. Roth

Abstract. Spiral waves of electrical activity underlie many cardiac arrhythmias. The tip of a spiral wave can trace out a complicated path as it meanders through cardiac tissue. In previous research, the tip meandering was studied for isotropic tissue. However, anisotropy has an important impact on the electrical behavior of the heart. In this paper, I explain how the anisotropy of cardiac tissue influences the meandering of spiral waves.

§1. Introduction

Heart disease is the leading cause of death in the United States. Mathematical modeling provides important insights into the causes of cardiac arrhythmias, and therefore plays an essential role in the battle against heart disease. *Spiral waves* underlie many cardiac arrhythmias [11]. What are spiral waves? Figure 1 shows a simulation of a spiral wave propagating through cardiac tissue. A wave front of electrical activity (white) propagates outward in a spiral pattern. At the center of the spiral (called the "tip" of the wave front) the dynamics are quite complex. Often the tip is stationary, but under some conditions it may meander throughout the heart. My goal is to understand the behavior of the tip of the spiral wave. In particular, I am interested in the effect of anisotropy on the tip path. I use the bidomain model to analyze spiral waves in cardiac tissue, and I show that anisotropy plays an important role in determining how the tip meanders.

My discussion of the mathematics of spiral waves consists of three parts (Figure 2). First, I review a simple model for cardiac excitability. Second, I represent cardiac tissue as a spatial distribution of excitable elements and develop a reaction-diffusion model. Third, I extend the reaction-diffusion model to account for the anisotropy of both the intracellular and extracellular spaces, and derive a bidomain model.

Mathematical Models in Medical and Health Sciences
Mary Ann Horn, Gieri Simonett, and Glenn Webb (eds.), pp. 327–336.
Copyright © 1998 by Vanderbilt University Press, Nashville, TN.
ISBN 0-8265-1310-7.

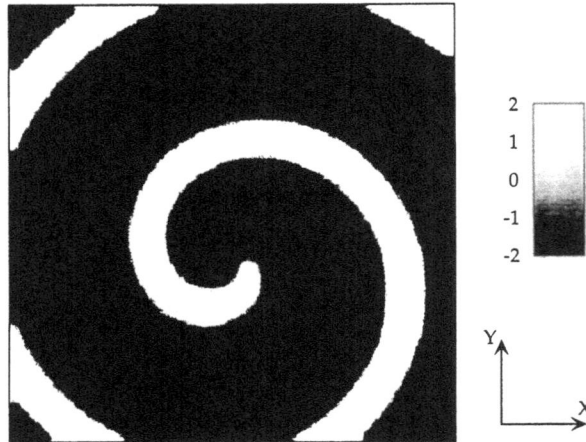

Fig. 1. The transmembrane potential, $\Phi_m(X, Y)$, of a fully developed spiral wave, for $\varepsilon = 0.2$, $\beta = 0.8$, $e = 0$. A gray scale indicates the value of Φ_m, where white is $+2$ and black is -2 (dimensionless units). The plot is 60 by 60 space units.

The Mathematics of Spiral Waves

Excitability $\longrightarrow$ Reaction-Diffusion $\longrightarrow$ Bidomain

Fig. 2. Mathematical models describing the electrical behavior of tissue.

§2. Excitability

I am not going to study a detailed model of cardiac excitability. That task would be long and complicated (see, for example, [4]). Instead, I analyze an extremely simple model that is a caricature for *excitability*: The *FitzHugh-Nagumo (FN) model* [1,5]. This model consists of two ordinary differential equations governing two variables: The electrical potential across the cell membrane (the transmembrane potential), Φ_m, and a recovery variable, v,

$$\frac{\partial \Phi_m}{\partial T} = \frac{1}{\varepsilon}\left(\Phi_m - \frac{\Phi_m^3}{3} - v\right), \tag{1}$$

$$\frac{\partial v}{\partial T} = \varepsilon(\Phi_m + \beta - \gamma v), \tag{2}$$

a)

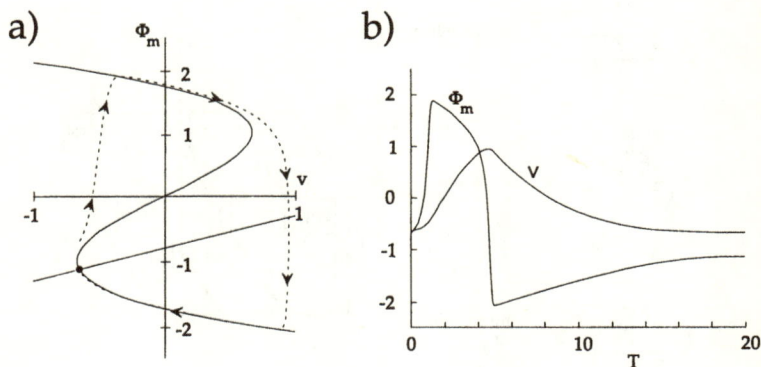

b)

Fig. 3. a) A phase space plot of the nullclines of Φ_m and v. The dot represents the steady state ($\Phi_m = -1.13$, $v = -0.65$). The dashed curve shows the phase portrait of an action potential, with the arrows indicating the direction in time. b) A plot of Φ_m and v as functions of time during an action potential. In both cases, $\varepsilon = 0.2$, $\beta = 0.8$ and $\gamma = 0.5$; and the initial values ($T = 0$) are $\Phi_m = -0.70$, $v = -0.65$.

where T is time and ε, β, and γ are parameters. When ε is small, Φ_m changes more rapidly than v. Thus, Φ_m is the "fast" variable and v is the "slow" variable. The FN model is *nonlinear* because of the cubic term in (1). One way to analyze a nonlinear dynamical system such as the FN model is to plot the *nullclines* of the system in *phase space*. The nullclines are curves relating Φ_m and v when the time derivatives on the left-hand-side of (1) and (2) are zero. Equation (1) yields a cubic ("z"-shaped) curve when plotted in phase space (Φ_m versus v), and (2) yields a straight line (Figure 3a). The point where the two nullclines intersect (dot) is the steady state solution of the FN model. It corresponds the resting state for cardiac tissue. The upper and lower branches of the cubic curve are stable; if the transmembrane potential is perturbed away from the curve, it returns. The middle branch of the cubic curve is unstable; if Φ_m is perturbed away from that section of the curve, it moves further away. The point on the middle branch of the cubic curve directly above the resting state is the *threshold* for electrical activity. If Φ_m increases to above threshold, the membrane fires an *action potential* shown by the dashed curve in Figure 3a. Figure 3b shows the behavior of Φ_m and v as functions of time.

The FN model has three parameters: ε, β, and γ. As discussed before, ε governs the relative rate of change of Φ_m and v; if ε is small, Φ_m rises and falls abruptly. The parameter β determines the location where the linear nullcline in Figure 3a intersects the Φ_m axis. If the line is lower, the steady-state point is farther vertically from the middle branch of the cubic curve, so a greater displacement of Φ_m is required to trigger an action potential. Thus β corresponds to a measure of the threshold for an action potential,

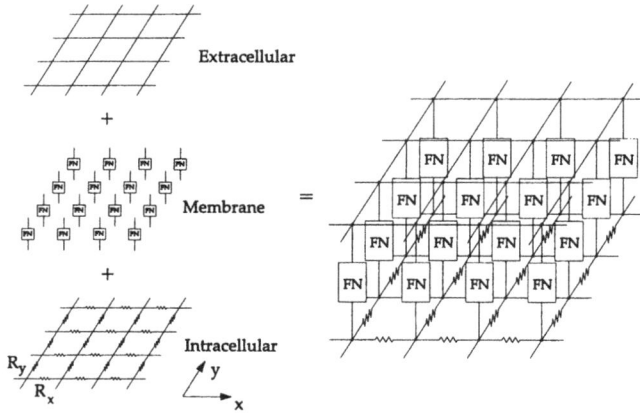

Fig. 4. A schematic representation of the two-dimensional reaction-diffusion model. This is a monodomain model, because the resistance of the extracellular space is neglected.

or the excitability (increasing β corresponds to decreasing excitability). The parameter γ determines the slope of the linear nullcline. Like β, γ affects the excitability. For my calculations, I consider γ a constant ($\gamma = 1/2$).

§3. Reaction-Diffusion Model

The FitzHugh-Nagumo model provides a simple picture of the electrical behavior of a patch of excitable membrane (a single cell). However, cardiac tissue does not consist of isolated single cells. Instead, cardiac tissue is a *syncytium*: Each cell is connected to its neighbors through intercellular channels. Thus, electrical current can pass from one cell to the next without ever crossing the cell membrane. Consider a two-dimensional syncytium, as shown in Figure 4. The intracellular space is represented by a two-dimensional grid of resistors, which accounts for the electrical resistance of the intercellular channels and the intracellular fluid. For the moment consider the extracellular space to be grounded (later I will relax this assumption). The intracellular and extracellular spaces are connected at each point by a patch of membrane represented by the FN model. The result is a two-dimensional cable model of cardiac tissue, sometimes called a *monodomain* model.

If you analyze the circuit in Figure 4 mathematically (assuming that the grid spacing between discrete resistors is small enough that the tissue acts like a continuum), you obtain two differential equations [9]:

$$\frac{\partial \Phi_m}{\partial T} = \frac{1}{\varepsilon}\left(\Phi_m - \frac{\Phi_m^3}{3} - v\right) + \frac{\partial^2 \Phi_m}{\partial X^2} + \frac{\partial^2 \Phi_m}{\partial Y^2}, \tag{3}$$

$$\frac{\partial v}{\partial T} = \varepsilon(\Phi_m + \beta - \gamma v), \tag{4}$$

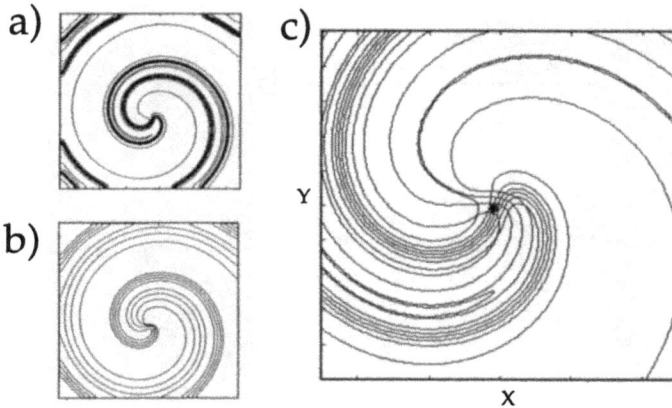

Fig. 5. Contour plots of a) Φ_m and b) v for a fully developed spiral wave ($\varepsilon = 0.2$, $\beta = 0.8$ and $\gamma = 0.5$). c) A magnified view of the tip of the spiral wave, with Φ_m and v contours superimposed. The dot indicates the location of the tip, defined as the maximum of the magnitude of $\nabla\Phi_m \times \nabla v$.

The box encloses the FN model (identical to (1) and (2)). The terms outside the box represent the coupling of FN patches by current through the resistor grid. Equations (3) and (4) are called a *reaction-diffusion* model. The "reaction" is the excitability of the FN model: The transmembrane potential reacts to a threshold increase in Φ_m by triggering an action potential. However, if in (3) you ignore the terms in parentheses, you are left with a first temporal derivative on the left and second spatial derivatives on the right: The "diffusion" equation. Thus, both excitability and diffusion play a role in determining the action potential. In fact, it is the interplay between excitability and diffusion that underlies propagation of *wave fronts* through the tissue. If one region of tissue has a positive transmembrane potential because of an action potential, this positive Φ_m diffuses into adjacent tissue, where it triggers an action potential, which results in more positive Φ_m, which diffuses into other nearby tissue, and so on.

Wave fronts can have several geometries. They can be plane waves, target patterns (circular wave fronts propagating outward from a central site), or spiral waves. Winfree has performed extensive simulations of spiral waves using a two-dimensional reaction-diffusion model with FN kinetics [10]. He was interested primarily in calculating the path of the tip of the spiral wave. In order to determine the path quantitatively, I need to define precisely what I mean by the spiral wave tip. (Note: The following definition was used by Winfree and his colleagues in another study [3]. It is also used in my own calculations described below. However, it is slightly different from the definition Winfree used in reference [10].)

Figures 5a and 5b show contour plots of Φ_m and v at one instance in time for a spiral wave. Figure 5c shows a magnified view of the spiral wave tip with

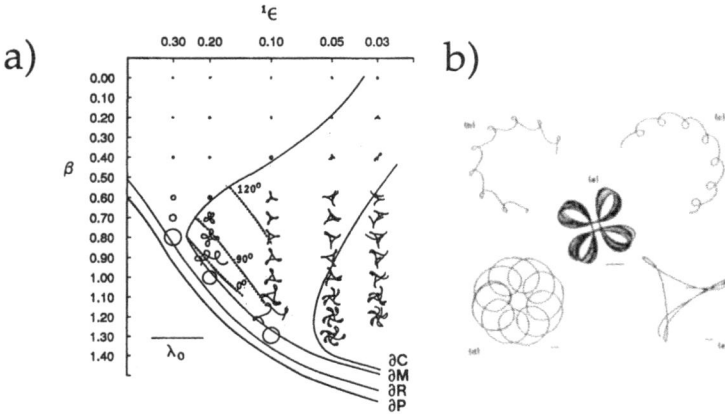

Fig. 6. a) The path of the tip of a spiral wave, as a function of ε and β.
b) Some tip paths in more detail. Reprinted with permission from A. T.
Winfree, Varieties of spiral wave behavior: An experimentalist's approach
to the theory of excitable media, Chaos **1** (1991), 303–334. Copyright 1991
American Institute of Physics.

the Φ_m and v contours superimposed. Contour lines are close together where
Φ_m and v are changing most rapidly in space. Throughout most of the wave
front, contours of Φ_m and v are nearly parallel. However, near the tip the two
sets of contours are almost perpendicular. This behavior suggests a definition
of the tip: The point where the magnitude of the cross product of the gradient
of Φ_m and the gradient of v is largest. The use of the gradient ensures that
the tip lies on the wave front, where Φ_m and v are changing rapidly in space.
The cross-product is large where the gradients are large and perpendicular
to each other, which selects a point on the wave front at the tip. With this
definition of the wave front tip, I can calculate the path that the tip travels
in time. The dot indicates the position of the tip in Figure 5c.

As Winfree varied the parameters in his calculations (ε and β), the tip
of his spiral wave traced out a variety of paths, from a circle to a regular
isogon to a chaotic-appearing contour (Figure 6a) [10]. When the tip path
is more complicated than a circle, the spiral wave tip is said to *meander*.
Many of these meander paths resemble curves produced by the children's toy
Spirograph® (Figure 6b). In general, meandering becomes more pronounced
when the difference between the time constants for Φ_m and v is large (small
ε) and when the excitability is low (large β).

§4. The Bidomain Model

Winfree's calculations using the reaction-diffusion model provide valuable in-

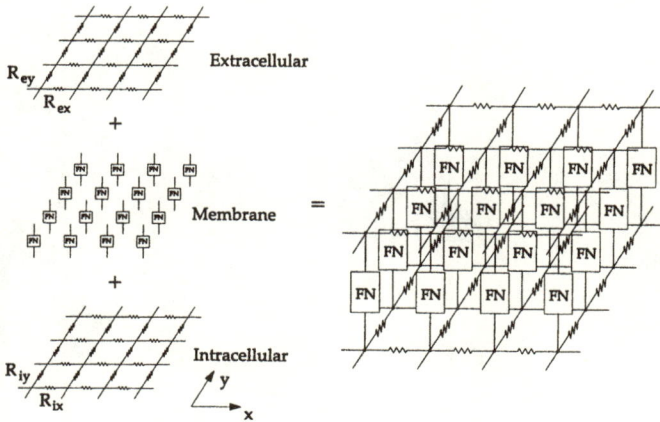

Fig. 7. A schematic representation of the two-dimensional bidomain model.

sight into the behavior of spiral waves in cardiac tissue. The heart, however, has unique electrical properties that cause behavior not predicted by generic reaction-diffusion models. These properties arise from the *anisotropy* of cardiac tissue: The electrical properties of the tissue depend on the direction. In particular, the different degree of anisotropy in the intracellular and extracellular spaces (*unequal anisotropy ratios*) plays a central role in the behavior of cardiac tissue [6]. Winfree's model was a monodomain, implying that it did not take into account unequal anisotropy ratios. I extend his calculations to include the effect of the *bidomain* model, which does account for the different anisotropies of the intra- and extracellular spaces.

The bidomain model is a two- or three-dimensional cable model often used to represent the electrical properties of cardiac tissue [2,6]. Figure 7 shows a circuit representation of a two-dimensional bidomain. The difference between the monodomain model in Figure 4 and the bidomain model in Figure 7 is that the bidomain model takes into account the resistance of the extracellular space.

In the bidomain model, both the intracellular and the extracellular spaces are anisotropic: The resistors parallel to the fibers (x-direction) are smaller than the resistors perpendicular to the fibers (y-direction). Moreover, the ratio of resistances in the x- and y-directions is different in the two domains. I define a dimensionless parameter e [7] that measures how different the anisotropy ratios are in the intracellular (i) and extracellular (e) domains:

$$e = 1 - \frac{\left(\frac{R_{ey}}{R_{ex}}\right)}{\left(\frac{R_{iy}}{R_{ix}}\right)}. \tag{5}$$

If the tissue has equal anisotropy ratios, then $e = 0$. If the intracellular space is much more anisotropic than the extracellular space, then $e = 1$. For ventricular muscle, e is about 0.75 [8].

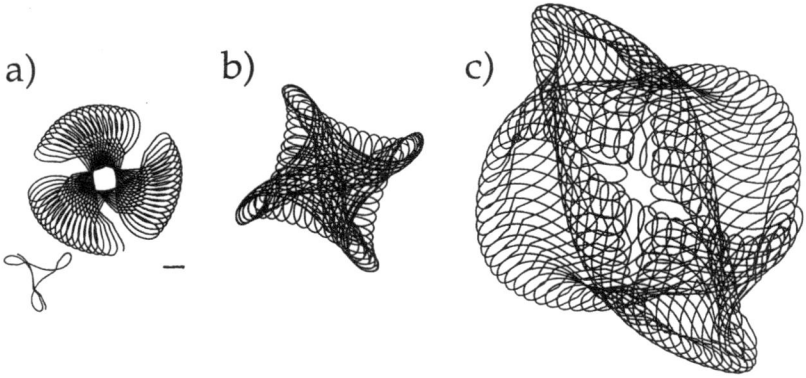

Fig. 8. Path of the tip of the spiral wave, for $\varepsilon = 0.1$, $\beta = 1.0$ and a) $e = 0$, b) $e = 0.75$ and c) $e = 0.9$. The inset shows the $e = 0$ case for a shorter time.

The bidomain model consists of two coupled partial differential equations [7] and one ordinary differential equation,

$$\frac{\partial \Phi_m}{\partial T} = \frac{1}{\varepsilon}\left(\Phi_m - \frac{\Phi_m^3}{3} - v\right) + \frac{\partial^2 \Phi_m}{\partial X^2} + \frac{\partial^2 \Phi_m}{\partial Y^2} + \frac{\alpha e}{1 + \alpha(1 - e)}\frac{\partial^2 \Psi}{\partial X^2}, \quad (6)$$

$$\frac{\partial v}{\partial T} = \varepsilon(\Phi_m + \beta - \gamma v), \quad (7)$$

$$\left(2 + \alpha + \frac{1}{\alpha}\right)\frac{\partial^2 \Psi}{\partial X^2} + \left(2 + \alpha(1 - e) + \frac{1}{\alpha(1 - e)}\right)\frac{\partial^2 \Psi}{\partial Y^2}$$
$$= e\left(1 + \frac{1}{\alpha(1 - e)}\right)\frac{\partial^2 \Phi_m}{\partial Y^2} \quad (8)$$

Inside the box is the reaction-diffusion model, identical to that given in (3) and (4). The term outside the box in (6) is unique to the bidomain model and represents the influence of the unequal anisotropy ratios. When $e = 0$, the bidomain model reduces to the reaction-diffusion model. Equation (8) governs the auxiliary potential, Ψ, which is a linear combination of the intracellular and extracellular potentials [7]. The parameter α is equal to the ratio of conductivities parallel to the myocardial fibers in the intracellular and extracellular spaces [7]. In my simulations, $\alpha = 1$ [8].

Figure 8 shows the meander path of the spiral wave tip for $\varepsilon = 0.1$ and $\beta = 1$. For equal anisotropy ratios ($e = 0$), the path of the wave front tip is nearly a trefoil (Figure 8a, inset), but does not quite close, resulting in a slow, Spirograph-like precession of the flower orientation (Figure 8a). Figure 8b shows the tip path for $e = 0.75$. This complex pattern arises as the three-petal flower makes an intricate dance, with the net result of forcing a four-fold symmetry onto the meander path. The spiral wave tip meanders through a tortuous path for $e = 0.9$ (Figure 8c). It roams over a large area, sometimes drifting nearly linearly and other times making hairpin turns.

§5. Conclusion

The heart can be described by a reaction-diffusion model. In particular, spiral waves are characteristic of a reaction-diffusion system, and exist in the heart. But in order to quantitatively predict the path of the tip of a spiral wave, one must go further than the "standard" reaction-diffusion model. One must take into account the bidomain structure of cardiac tissue. Of special importance is the unequal anisotropy ratios in the intracellular and extracellular domains. This feature influences the meandering of spiral waves, and has important implications for the path of the spiral wave tip.

Acknowledgments. This research is supported by the Whitaker Foundation and the College of Arts & Sciences, Vanderbilt University. I thank Art Winfree for supplying me with copies of Figs. 6a and 6b, and Jon Bennett for his valuable suggestions about the manuscript.

References

1. FitzHugh, R., Impulses and physiological states in theoretical models of nerve membrane, Biophys. J. **1** (1961), 445–465.
2. Henriquez, C. S., Simulating the electrical behavior of cardiac tissue using the bidomain model, Crit. Rev. Biomed. Eng. **21** (1993), 1–77.
3. Jahnke, W., W. E. Skaggs and A. T. Winfree, Chemical vortex dynamics in the Belousov-Zhabotinsky reaction and in the 2-variable Oregonator model, J. Phys. Chem. **93** (1989), 740–749.
4. Luo, C.-H. and Y. Rudy, A dynamic model of the cardiac ventricular action potential, Circ. Res. **74** (1994), 1071–1096.
5. Nagumo, J. S., S. Arimoto and S. Yoshizawa, An active pulse transmission line simulating nerve axon, Proc. IRE **50** (1962), 2061–2071.
6. Roth, B. J., How the anisotropy of the intracellular and extracellular conductivities influences stimulation of cardiac muscle, J. Math. Biol. **30** (1992), 633–646.
7. Roth, B. J., Approximate analytical solutions to the bidomain equations with unequal anisotropy ratios, Phys. Rev. E **55** (1997), 1819–1826.
8. Roth, B. J., Electrical conductivity values used with the bidomain model of cardiac tissue, IEEE Trans. Biomed. Eng. **44** (1997), 326–328.
9. Winfree, A. T., Stable particle-like solutions to the nonlinear wave equations of three-dimensional excitable media, SIAM Rev. **32** (1990), 1–53.
10. Winfree, A. T., Varieties of spiral wave behavior: An experimentalist's approach to the theory of excitable media, Chaos **1** (1991), 303–334.
11. Winfree, A. T., *Theory of spirals, in Cardiac Electrophysiology, From Cell to Bedside*, 2nd ed., D. P. Zipes and J. Jalife (eds.), Saunders, Philadelphia, 1995, 379–389.

Bradley J. Roth
Department of Physics and Astronomy
Vanderbilt University
Nashville, TN 37235
roth@compsci.cas.vanderbilt.edu

Sister, Mother-Daughter and Cousin Cell Generation Time Correlations and Cell Cycle Progression

Roland Sennerstam and Jan-Olof Strömberg

Abstract. In this work we linked recent knowledge concerning regulation of cell cycle progression to classical problems still under discussion regarding the correlation of cell generation times of intraclonally closely related cells, in particular from tissue cultures of growing murine embryonal carcinoma cells. Pedigrees of intermitotic times recorded over several generations were compared with results in published studies. As the correlation of cousin-cell generation times has not previously been considered in depth, it was regarded in the present investigation as an informative complement to elucidate the mother-daughter intermitotic time correlation and cell cycle progression in general. Data obtained from the murine embryonal cell line were inserted into a computer program in a unifying cell cycle model, recently published. The mother-daughter intermitotic time correlation in the cell line analysed was found to be close to zero, whereas a strong positive sister-sister and a positive cousin-cell pair intermitotic time correlation were found, both experimentally and by simulation. Comparison with data reported in the literature spanning several decades revealed a similar phenomenon. How it might be possible for a near zero mother-daughter generation time correlation to accord with epigenetic and genetic inheritance transferred from mother to daughters is discussed and a solution to the problem is proposed.

Abbreviations: IDT: Intermitotic time; TSCM: Two-subcycle cell cycle model; DDC: DNA-division cycle; CGC: Cell-growth cycle; Rb: Retinoblastoma protein; PGRR: Point of growth rate regulation.

§1. Introduction

Studies on intermitotic time (IDT) correlations obtained by means of TV-video time-lapse filming experiments that generate pedigrees of growing cell populations, can reveal the type of IDT correlation existing between closely related cells. However, such a macro-cell level type of investigation may do no more than hint at how the cell's own surveillance mechanism regulates

Mathematical Models in Medical and Health Sciences
Mary Ann Horn, Gieri Simonett, and Glenn Webb (eds.), pp. 337–350.

the progression of the cell cycle, whereas micromolecular regulation of various checkpoints in the cell cycle offers another approach by which to gain knowledge, in a field of cell cycle research that has expanded vastly in the last decade [9,19,20,21]. Various avenues of study can, however, prove mutually complementary to ovecome for example, misinterpretation of how the cell monitors growth in size in relation to DNA content leading to erroneous interpretations of micromolecular results, and vice-versa. In this report, we show how information regarding correlations between IDTs of related cells can clarify our understanding of cell cycle progression in general. The data obtained have been inserted into a structured model, published elsewhere called the Two- subcycle cell cycle model (TSCM). In the model various Gaussian distributed parameters are selected randomly at certain points in time and the program runs like Markov processes [33].

1.1. Intermitotic time correlations

It is well known from numerous studies that the coefficient of correlation between sister cell IDTs (r_{ss}) is positive, whereas the mother-daughter cell IDT correlation (r_{md}) has been reported to be both positive [4,6,37] and negative [26] and even zero [1,8,13]. In the literature it was suggested that inherited factors govern the processes leading to cell division [13] and it was convincingly demonstrated in colony size studies after subculturing of cell populations, that there is a epigenetic and genetic heritability reflected in growing cells that is transferred from mother to daughter [2]. The reports in the literature of negative or near zero values of r_{md} may be a trifle confusing if both epigenetic and genetic heritabilities are transferred from one generation to the next. It has been speculated whether there may be strong compensatory factors that modulate the r_{md} value towards zero – or even to a negative value [39].

In the present study, we examined coefficients of correlation between cousin cell pair IDTs (r_{cc}), to ascertain if they could shed further light upon the confusing mother-daughter correlations. Earlier, we analysed data from IDT pedigrees of a murine embryonal carcinoma cell line, published elsewhere [29]. Later we inserted the data into the computer program written for the (TSCM) [34]. The model includes three cell generations postulated by us to be necessary to give a correct picture of cell proliferation, viz. the cycle preceding and the cycle following the current cell cycle under study. The three coefficients of correlation r_{ss} , r_{md} and r_{cc} have in this report been estimated both from experiments and in the simulations.

1.2. Cell cycle model

The TSCM has been described and discussed in several papers [31,33,34,35]. The model divides the cell cycle into two 'sub-cycles' [17], one of which the 'DNA-division cycle' (DDC), spans the S phase and G_2-M phases, plus a pre-S phase when the cell is already committed to enter S phase, but is not yet incorporating thymidine – though synthesizing enzymes such as dihydrofolate reductase, thymidine kinase, thymidine synthetase and DNA-polymerase-alfa. These enzymes are reported to be activated by the "cyclin-D1-cdk4/6 retinoblastoma protein-E2F pathway" in the mid-G1 phase [11,42]. The second sub-cycle i.e. the 'cell-growth cycle' (CGC), reflects the increase in cell mass. Completion of CGC implies a doubling of cell mass that is usually assumed to occur in close association with mitosis to ensure coordination between doubling of the genome and a correct monitoring of cell size. The dissociation reported between DDC and CGC [18] leads us to believe that CGC is most frequently initiated in one cell cycle, but is completed in the G1 phase of the subsequent daughter cells, thus representing an alternative picture of the first part of G1 phase and explaining how the cell attains its 'critical cell size' [33]. In some reports, the growth rate of cells in G1 has been assumed to be determined in the preceding cell cycle [10].

1.3. Checkpoints

The retinoblastoma protein (Rb) regulates transcription of a range of S-phase specific genes by repressing the transcription factor E2F which regulates the activity of RNA polymerase II. E2F is released by cyclin-D1-cdk4/6 dephosphorylation. Recent reports tentatively suggest that the Rb also suppresses the expression of genes transcribed by the two nuclear RNA polymerases, pol I (ribosomal rRNA) and pol III (small RNAs and transfer tRNA) . This makes Rb the only presently known suppressor of all three RNA polymerases in the cell [3,40], thus indicating an emerging role for Rb to synchronize the monitoring of both cell growth and DNA-synthesis. Overexpression of D1 cyclins in rodent fibroblasts accelerated their transit through G1 and the resulting cells were smaller than their normal counterparts [27].

We would suggest that a candidate, such as the cyclin-D1-cdk4/6-Rb-polymerase I and III inhibition-activation pathway is involved in initiating and regulating CGC and thus creating a point of growth rate regulation ('PGRR') in mid-G1, as postulated by us in the presentation of the model [33]. Signal transducer cascades, triggered by growth factors via tyrosine kinase receptors, by estradiol via estrogen receptors, and by cAMP-elevating agents via G protein coupled thyrotropin receptors, all converge and require cyclin D-cdk activity in order to cause progression of the cell cycle [16]. Recently reported experiments have shown that different sites on the Rb protein are necessary to inhibit different Rb activities [12]. Thus cyclin D1-cdk4/6-Rb activity may play an emerging part in creating a 'point of growth rate regulation' (PGRR) to determine the growth rate of the approaching CGC, provided that the pathway is intact and not mutated which could generate transformed cells. However, in view of the growth rate achieved at 'start', we conclude that completion of CGC usually takes place in the next G1 period, sometimes closely associated with mitosis and on some other occasion during the G2 period prior to the initiation of mitotis promoting factors [22,25] resulting in another round of DNA synthesis. Mechanisms have been identified which are necessary to help the cell to decide whether it is in G1 or G2 [23].

1.4. Cell mass and DNA synthesis

The reason for dividing the cell cycle into two 'subcycles' is that the DDC and the CGC have been found to be only loosely related and to some extent uncoupled to each other. Even when the DDC is blocked the cell continues to grow, forming a huge mass several times its ordinary size at division [7]. When the block is released the cell will return to its normal size several generations later. But if the cell is deprived of growth factors after passing a certain restriction point in G1, DNA synthesis will commence and the cell will divide whilst very small [24].

When the S period in a Chinese hamster cell line was extended by applying $10\mu g$ hydroxyurea, G1 was shortened without altering the IDT [36]. This finding gives us cause to regard DDC and CGC as two somewhat independent events in the cell cycle, though checking each other at certain time points to maintain the cell's balanced growth. In evolutionary terms the DDC (represented by the nucleus) is a latecomer in the cytoplasm, not appearing until about 500 million years ago, initially perhaps as an RNA virus without a nuclear membrane (prokaryote), whereas the cell cytoplasm has existed as a separate entity for three to four billion years. One recently reported cloning experiment involving a ewe highlights the loose relation between cell nucleus and cytoplasm, as the nucleus of an egg from a Scottish Blackface ewe could be replaced by a nucleus from the udder of a Finn Dorset ewe and become accepted by the egg cytoplasm, leading to the birth of a healthy Finn Dorset lamb [41]. The relation suggested by us between DDC and CGC is illustrated in a flowchart in Figure 1. The checkpoints are included in the figure caption.

§2. Data Analysis

2.1. Analysing experimental data

The origin of the PCC4azal cell line, culture conditions and TV-video time-lapse technique are described elsewhere [29,30,31]. The data collected were a sample from seven TV-video time-lapse experiments including 178 cell generation times with a variation coefficient of 2.7% between the experiments, the two extreme values being excluded.

The IDT correlations found in the PCC4azal cells between sister cells, mother-daughter cell pairs and cousin pairs are illustrated graphically in Figure 2, together with the results of the simulation. The r_{ss} proved to be significantly positive ($r_{ss} = 0.92$), while the r_{md} value was close to zero ($r_{md} = 0.07$). A significantly positive correlation coefficient for cousin cell pairs was found ($r_{cc} = 0.72$). (See Table 1).

2.2. Comparisons with published data

Coefficients of correlations between cousin cell generation times are rarely reported in the literature, but from pedigrees included in published papers one can calculate the values. We have extracted data listed in Table 2 from

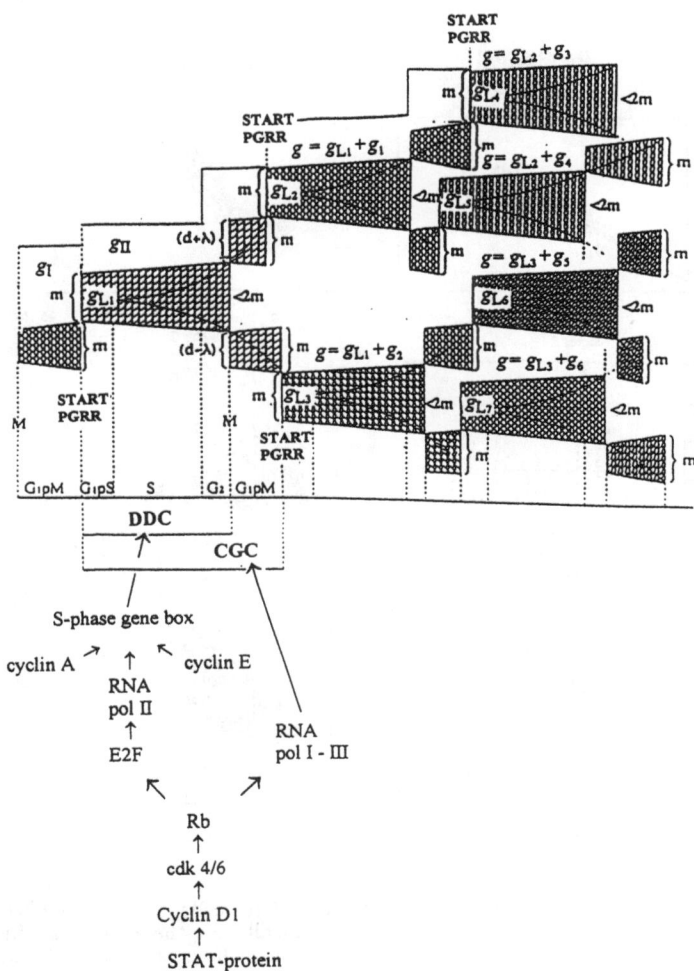

Fig. 1. A flowchart is shown for simulation experiments over several generations. The CGC (cell growth cycle) extends mitosis in the figure, generating a G1pM subcompartment before reaching the 'critical' mass ($\underline{m}$) needed to complete CGC. The lines drawn from the 'latent growth rates' (g_{L_n}) within the figure reflect the epigenetic and genetic inheritance transferred from the mother cell and expressed equally in the sister cells. At START, a new 'latent growth rate' is selected and stored until the next START-event in the sister cells. A growth rate 'g' is also selected, different in each sister cell at START. Therefore the growth rate between two START events is $g = g_{L_n} + g_n$. The molecular regulation of both CGC and DDC over the retinoblastoma protein (Rb) is shown (see main text). The position for the activation of cyclin A and cyclin E in comparition to cyclin D1 is postulated by the arrows in the figure.

PCC4azal   Simulation

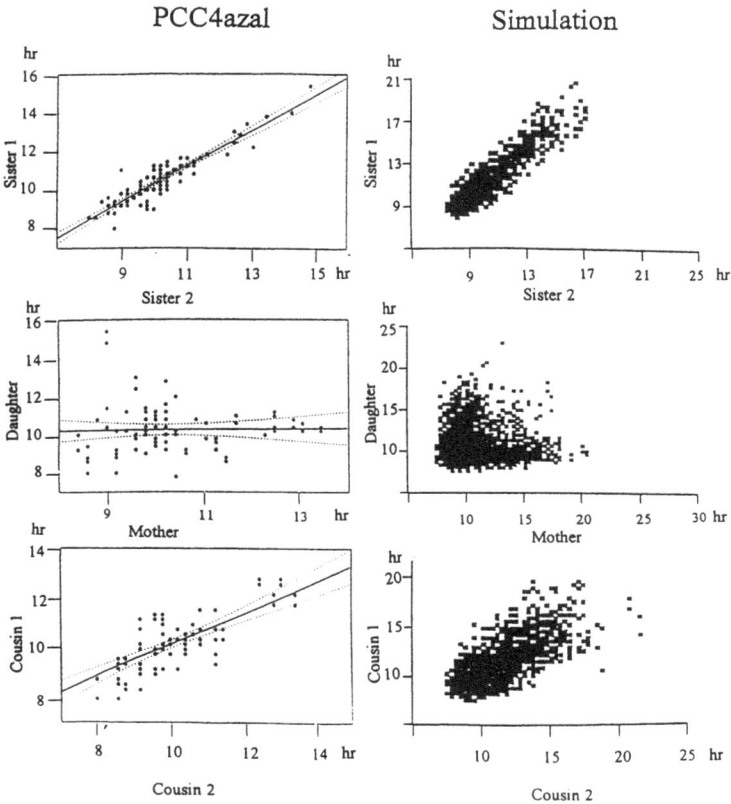

Fig. 2. The correlations between IDTs of sister cells, mother-daughter cells and cousin cell pairs are shown graphically for the PCC4azal line and together with the results of the simulations, where experimental data were inserted into the computer program.The values obtained are shown in Table 1.

two papers from the 1960s that analysed E.coli [13] and HelaS cells [8], and two reports from the 1980s analysing EMT6 and PCC3 cells [30,37]. The mean values for r_{ss}, r_{md} and r_{cc} were 0.84, 0.35 and 0.72 respectively, when comparing results from all five reports. The r_{md} was significantly positive in only one case [37], while r_{ss} and r_{cc} were significantly positive in all reports (Table 2). To summarize: There is rarely any correlation between IDTs of mother-daughter cell pairs, whereas there is a significantly positive correlation between sister cell pairs and cousin cell pairs.

Table 1: Experimental Data and Numerical Results

Coefficients of correlation		r_{ss}		r_{md}		r_{cc}
No. of pairs	$\underline{n}$		$\underline{n}$		$\underline{n}$	
Experiment on PCC4azal	86	**0.92** sign.	84	**0.07** ns.	83	**0.72** sign.
Simulations	2034	**0.90** sign.	4068	**0.03** ns.	4068	**0.68** sign.

Tab. 1. Coefficient of intermitotic time correlations between sister cells (r_{ss}), mother-daughter cells (r_{md}), and cousin cell pairs (r_{cc}) from experiments on PCC4azal cells are compared with results obtained from the literature over several decades. The references are given in the square brackets.

Table 2: Cell Cycle Time Correlations

	E.coli Kubitshek 1962 [13]	HelaS Froese 1964 [8]	EMT6 Staudte 1984 [37]	PCC3 Sennerstam 1988 [30]	PCC4 Sennerstam 1997
s-s mean=0.84	**0.95** sign.	**0.95** sign.	**0.80** sign.	**0.95** sign.	**0.95** sign.
M-d mean=0.24	**0.11** ns.	**0.12** ns.	**0.50** ns.	**0.41** ns.	**0.08** ns.
c-c mean=0.72	**0.68** sign.	**0.83** sign.	**0.59** sign.	**0.77** sign.	**0.72** sign.

Tab. 2. Coefficients of correlations in intermitotic times comparing sister cell pairs (r_{ss}), mother-daughter cells (r_{md}) and cousin cell pairs (r_{cc}), are shown from the experiments performed on the PCC4azal line and from the simulation with the parameters in Table 3 inserted into the computer program. The results are very similar, showing no significant differences. The r_{ss} values were significantly positive ($\underline{p} < 0.001$), as were the r_{cc} values ($\underline{p} < 0.001$) both experimentally and in the simulations and the r_{md} values were close to zero.

Table 3: Parameters Stipulated in the Simulation Experiments

Parameters needed to start the first cell

Maximum number of generations	12
Upper time limit (h)	700
Critical cell size (rel. size units)	8.3
DDC (h)	8
SD of DDC	0
First growth rate g_I	0.07
Second growth rate g_{II}	0.06
Latent growth rate in parental cell g_{L_0}	0.07
Birth size (rel. size units)	5.36
Start time (h)	2.0

Parameters generating intermitotic time heterogeneity

Mean value of mass distribution between sisters (rel. size units)	0.42
SD of mass distribution between sisters	0.8
SD of growth rate distribution	0.01
Mean of first latent growth rate distribution $g_{L_{1a}}$	0.071
SD of first latent growth rate distribution	0.009
Probability of second latent growth rate distribution	0.1
Mean of second latent growth rate distribution $g_{L_{1b}}$	0.05
SD of second latent growth rate distribution	0.008

Tab. 3. Parameters inserted into the computer program. The first two set out the limits for the number of generations run and the time limit in hours. 'Critical size' and DDC are parameters obtained experimentally. No standard deviation was put on DDC found to be fairly constant in time. The first growth rate (g_I) represents the growth rate only in the first cell from mitosis to START. Increase in cell mass follows the equation e^{gt}, where g (growth rate) is given in the Table and t is time. The second growth rate (g_{II}) is growth rate in the first cell from START in the first cycle to START in the subsequent cycle. Birth size is determined automatically when start time (i.e. the interval from mitosis to START) is selected. The mean value of mass difference between sister cell pairs (0.42) is a relative value found experimentally. In the PCC4 line an intraclonal bimodal IDT distribution was observed [30] and the parameters selected for the two latent growth rates $(g_{L_{1ab}})$ and their standard deviations are chosen to fit the experimental data.

§3. Simulations

The computer program written for the TSCM was published in 1995 and simulations of experimental data have been reported [34,35]. The parameters inserted are listed in Table 3. The first two determine the scope of the simulation, viz. 1) *the number of generations required*, and 2) *the time frame for the experiment*. The number of generations is limited only by the capacity of the computers hard disc. We have run up to fifty thousand cells. Parameter 3) reflects *critical size*, i.e. the size of the cell at the end of the CGC initiated in the previous cycle. The next three parameters are needed only to define the first cell in the experiment, i.e. the components of its growth rate: 4) *first growth rate* = growth rate from mitosis to 'start' (g I), and 5) *second growth rate* = growth rate from 'start' to the next 'start event' (g II). This will affect the duration of entrance of CGC into the next G1 period (G1pM).

To reflect epigenetic and genetic inheritance influencing growth rate we have introduced a 'latent growth rate' having a Gaussian distribution and selected randomly in the mother cell and stored until PGRR in the two daughter cells in the next cell cycle [33].

The 'latent growth rate' (g_L) adds its effect to the 'growth rate' (g), differing in the two daughter cells, and chosen randomly from a Gaussian distribution at the PGRR. However, since the two growth rates initiated at PGRR are added ($g_L + g_n$), the latent growth rate only is given a mean value (Table 3). This is easier to handle in the computer program and gives the same result as adding mean values of two Gaussian-distributed parameters. The standard deviations inserted for the two different growth rates determine the degree of influence from each of the two.

Due to an intraclonal instability found in the embryonal carcinoma cell lines used when developing the model [29,30,31,32], we have introduced two 'latent growth rates' ($g_{L_{a,b}}$) that can be chosen at a certain level of probability, depending on what emanates from the experimental data used for simulations. This phenomenon is of particular interest when analysing embryonal cell [34]. As a rule, when simulating experimental data, only one 'latent growth rate' is needed.

The computer program runs like Markov processes. All parameters given a mean and standard deviation have a Gaussian distribution. They are selected randomly at certain time points. Cell mass is set to increase exponentially. The duration of the DDC is found experimentally, as is critical size [31]. The mean difference in size between newborn sister cells is obtained from a cell line originating from the same mouse embryo and thus closely related to the line used for IDT analysis in this report [34]. The intraclonal instability found in these EC cell lines is presented in this simulation as two 'latent growth rates' with the probability of 0.1 for the slower growing subvariant (Table 3). Growth rate and 'latent growth rate' and their standard deviations are selected to fit the distribution of experimental data (Figure 3).

The parameters selected in the simulation rendered cell loss negligible. This is a very favourable situation, compared with experiments using time-lapse filming of living cells, where cell loss from the visual field and cell crowding sometimes make it impossible to trace individual cells. The correlation coefficients obtained in the simulations (r_{ss}, r_{md} and r_{cc}) were compared with the experimental results and showed that no significant differences had arisen (Table 1 and Figure 2).

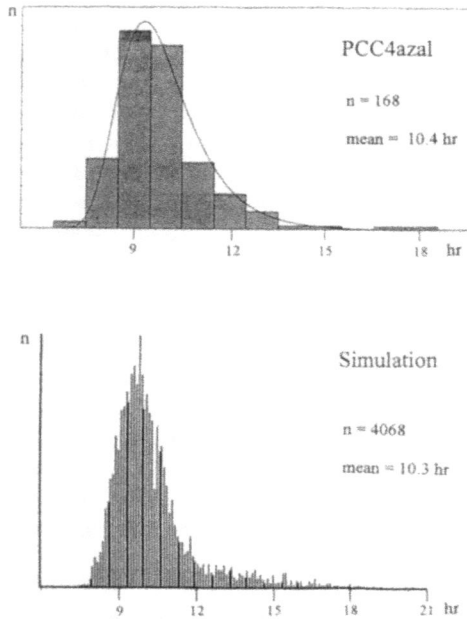

Fig. 3. Distributions of intermitotic times are shown from experimental data of the PCC4azal line and from the simulations based on the parameters in Table 3. A log-normal curve is put on the histogram generated from experimental data representing a good fit.

§4. Discussion

This report shows that experimental data analysed and inserted into the computer program created for the TSCM, considering a factor of epigenetic and genetic inheritance, could still allow the mother-daughter cell coefficient of correlation to approximate zero, as was found experimentally. This will resolve the conflict between models of inherited properties [15]. Furthermore the model includes a size control in G1 phase, but a near-zero r_{md} nevertheless appeared [38]. We thereby overcame the postulated negative r_{md} assumed to appear in the case of a size control model.

By modifying the idea of the relation between growth in cell size (CGC) and DNA synthesis (DDC) as is done in the TSCM, where the start and end of the two processes do not completely overlap each other (Figure 1), the positive r_{cc} found in this work and in published reports cited (Table 2) is given a plausible explanation. The effect of epigenetic and genetic inheritance is exerted first in the cousin-cell generation due to the relation suggested between DDC and CGC. The strength of the positive correlation between cousin-cell pairs reflects the power of the epigenetic and genetic inheritance upon growth rate in the population. This is a logical consequence of the theory presented. *Hence the epigenetic and genetic inheritance may well be transferred from mother to daughters - and all knowledge in cell biology speaks in favour of this - yet there is no correlation between their IDTs. It appears first in the cousin-cell generation.*

The G1 checkpoint uses the P53 gene product to impel DNA-damaged cells to apoptosis [14]. The recently reported RNA polymerase-inhibition ability governed by retinoblastoma protein – which may monitor cell size to control all three RNA polymerases (pol I-III) – can form a 'checkpoint' and 'start event' for growth in size, i.e. a 'cell-growth cycle', and thus include a point of growth rate regulation (PGRR) prior to and in close association with initiation of the 'DNA-division cycle' (DDC). The presence of certain signal transducer and activator (STAT) family of proteins [5,28], following the cyclin-D1-cdk4/6 retinoblastoma protein pathway might also be involved in controlling the increase in cell mass. We want to postulate this point in the cell cycle (PGRR+START) as the restriction point (R) as postulated by Pardee [24]. When running several experiments without altering the parameters in the computer program we have found some values of r_{md} to be positive and others negative, but all close to zero [33]. When reducing the number of generations run in the simulation experiments more closely to what is experimentally possible (six to seven generations), the gap between the highest positive r_{md} value and the lowest negative r_{md} value widened considerably, up to tenfold.

We suggest that the near-zero r_{md} is found when the checkpoints in G1 are intact. When for example the P53 or Rb genes are mutated, we feel that it is possible for the r_{md} to be significantly positive (or negative), *since the G1 checkpoints (PGRR) are set out of sequence, thus putting the point of growth rate regulation out of order.*

The cell line analysed in this work was a murine embryonal carcinoma cell line. The term 'carcinoma' denotes in general a transformation and therefore we should not have a zero value for r_{md}. Yet, cells from these lines derived from mouse embryos have proved capable of (when reintroduced into a mouse embryo) being incorporated and taking part in normal embryonic development. Thus, the transformation in this case is more a matter of being in the wrong place.

To summarize, this report presents a model that offers alternative solutions to questions such as 1) how does the cell maintain balanced growth and constant size over several cell generations; 2) how and why does the cell reach a 'critical size' in mid-G1 phase; 3) why does the sister cell IDT coefficient of correlation have a significantly positive value, yet 4) there can be a near-zero mother-daughter IDT correlation coefficient; and 5) why is the cousin cell IDT coefficient of correlation significantly positive despite a zero mother-daughter cell correlation? Size control is evidently active in the model without generating a negative mother-daughter cell cycle time correlation. Finally, we postulate the size control in G2 to be negative in character, i.e. the cell mass may not grow too large to avoid entering another S-phase.

Acknowledgments. This work was supported by grants from the funds of Karolinska Institute, Stockholm, Sweden.

References

1. Absher, M. and V. J. Cristofalo, Analysis of cell division by time-lapse cinematographic studies on hydrocortisone-treated embryonic lung fibroblasts, J. Cell. Physiol. **119** (1984), 315–319.

2. Axelrod, D.E., Y. Gusev and T. Kuczek, Persistence of cell cycle times over many generations as determined by heritability of colony sizes of ras oncogene transformed and nontransformed cells, Cell Prolif. **26** (1993), 235–249.

3. Cavanaugh, A. H., W. M. Hempel, L. J. Taylor, V. Roglasky, G. Todorov and L.I.Rothblum, Activity of RNA polymerase I transcription factor UBF blocked by Rb gene product, Nature **374** (1995), 177–180.

4. Collyn-d'Hooghe, M., A. J. Valleron and E. P. Malaise, Time-lapse cinematography studies of cell cycle and mitosis duration, Exp.Cell Res. **106**(2) (1977), 405–407.

5. Darnell, J. E., J. M. Kerr and G. R. Stark, Jak-STAT pathways and transcriptional activation in response to IFNs and other extracellular signaling proteins, Science **264** (1994), 1415–1421.

6. Dawson, K.B., H. Madoc-Jones and E. O. Field, Variation in the generation times of a strain of rat sarcoma cells in culture, Exp.Cell Res. **38** (1965), 75–84.

7. Forsburg, S. L. and P. Nurse, Cell cycle regulation in the yeast Saccharomyces cerevisiae and Schizosaccharomyces pombe, Ann. Rev. Cell Biol. **50** (1991), 213–219.

8. Froese, G., The distribution and interdependence of generation times of HeLa cells, Exp. Cell Res. **35** (1964), 415–419.

9. Hartwell, L. H. and T. A. Weinert, Checkpoints: controls that ensure the order of cell cycle events, Science **246** (1989), 629–634.

10. Hola, M. and P. A. Riley, The relative significance of growth rate and interdivision time in the size control of cultured mammalian cells, J. Cell Science **88** (1987), 73–80.

11. Ikeda, M.-A., L. Jakoi and J. R. Nevins, A unique role for the Rb protein in controlling E2F accumulation during cell growth and differentiation, Proc. Natl. Acad. Sci. USA, **93** (1996), 3215–3220.

12. Knudsen, E.S. and J. Y. J. Wang, Differential regulation of retinoblastoma protein function by specific Cdk phosphorylation sites, J. Biol.Chem. **271** (1996), 8313–8320.

13. Kubitschek, H. E., Normal distribution of cell generation rate, Exp.Cell Res. **26** (1962), 439–450.

14. Lane, D. P., P53, guardian of the genome, Nature **358** (1992), 15–17.

15. Lebowitz, J. L. and A. Rubinov, A theory for the age and generation time distribution of a microbial population, J. Math. Biol. **1** (1974), 17–36.

16. Lukas, J., J. Bartkova and J. Bartek, Convergence of mitogenic signalling cascades from diverse classes of receptors on the cyclin D/cdk-Rb-controlled G1 checkpoint, Mol.Cell Biol. **16**(12) (1996), 6917–6925.

17. Mazia, D., The cell cycle, Sci. Am. **230** (1974), 54–64.

18. Mitchison, J. M., *Biology of the Cell Cycle*, Cambridge University Press, Cambridge, 1971.

19. Murray, A. W., Creative blocks: Cell cycle checkpoints and feedback control, Nature **359** (1992), 559–604.

20. Murray, A. W., Cell cycle checkpoints, Curr. Opin. Cell Biol. **6**(6) (1994), 872–876.

21. Murray, A. W., Genetics of cell cycle checkpoints, Curr. Opin. Genet. Dev. **5**(1) (1995), 5–11.

22. Nurse, P., Universal control mechanism regulating onset of M-phase, Nature **344** (1990), 503–508.

23. O'Connell, M. J. and P. Nurse, How cells know they are in G1 or G2, Curr. Opin. Cell Biol. **6**(6) (1994), 867–871.

24. Pardee, A. B., G1 events and regulation of cell proliferation, Science bf 246 (1989), 603–605.

25. Parker, L.L. and H. Piwnica-Worms, Inactivation of the p34cdc/cyclinB complex by the human WEE1 tyrosine kinase, Science **257** (1992), 1955–1957.

26. Plank, L.D. and J.D. Harvey, Generation time statistics of Escherichia coli B measured by synchronous culture techniques, J. Gen. Microbiol. **115** (1979), 69–77.

27. Quelle, D. E., R. A. Ashmun, S. A. Shurtleff, J. Y. Kato, D. Bar-Sagi, M. F. Roussel and C. J. Sherr, Overexpression of mouse D-type cyclins accelerates G1 phase in rodent fibroblasts, Genes Dev. **7**(8) (1993), 1559–1571.

28. Schindler, C. and J. E. Darnell, Transcriptional responses to polypeptide ligands: The JAK-STAT pathway, Annu. Rev. Biochem. **64** (1995), 621–651.

29. Sennerstam, R. and J.-O. Strömberg, A comparative study of cell cycles of nullipotent and multipotent embryonal carcinoma cell lines during exponential growth, Dev. Biol. **103** (1984), 221–229.

30. Sennerstam, R. and J.-O. Strömberg, Evidence for a random shift between two types of cell cycle times in an embryonal carcinoma cell line, J. Theor. Biol. **131** (1988), 151–162.

31. Sennerstam, R. and J.-O. Strömberg, Dissociation of cell growth and DNA synthesis and alteration of the nucleo-cytoplasmic ratio in growing embryonal carcinoma cells, Dev. Growth & Diff. **33**(4) (1991), 353–363.

32. Sennerstam, R., The Two-subcycle Cell Cycle Model, in *Mathematical Population Dynamics. Proceedings of the Second International Confer-*

ence, Arino, O., D. E. Axelrod and M. Kimmel (eds), M. Dekker, Inc. 40, 1991, 609–621.

33. Sennerstam, R. and J.-O. Strömberg, Cell cycle progression: Computer simulation of uncoupled subcycles of DNA replication and cell growth, J. Theor. Biol. **175** (1995), 177–189.

34. Sennerstam, R. and J.-O. Strömberg, Embryonic cell commitment by a simultaneous alteration in nucleo/cytoplasmic ratio in sibling cells between subsequent cell cycles, Dev. Growth & Diff. **38** (1996), 653–662.

35. Sennerstam, R. and J.-O. Strömberg, Exponential growth, random transitions and progress through the G1 phase: Computer simulation of experimental data, Cell Prolif. **29** (1996), 609–622.

36. Stancel, G. M., Prescott, D. M. and R. M. Liskay, Most of the G1 period in hamster cells is eliminated by lengthening the S period, Proc. Natl. Acad. Sci. U.S. **78**(10) (1981), 6295–6298.

37. Staudte, R.G., M. Guiguet and M. C. dHooghe, Additive models for dependent cell populations, J. Theor. Biol. **109**(1) (1984), 127–146.

38. Tyson, J. and K. Hannsgen, The distribution of cell size and generation time in a model of the cell cycle incorporating size control and random transitions, J. Theor. Biol. **113** (1985), 29–62.

39. van Wijk, R. and K. W. van der Poll, Variability of cell generation times in a hepatoma cell pedigree, Cell Tissue Kinet. **12** (1979), 659–663.

40. White, R. J., D. Trouche, K. Martin, S. P. Jackson and T. Koutzarides, Repression of RNA polymerase III transcription by the retinoblastoma protein, Nature **382** (1996), 88–90.

41. Wilmut, I., A. E. Schnieke, J. McWhir, A. J. Kind and K. H. Campbell, Viable offspring derived from fetal and adult mammalian cells, Nature **385** (1997), 810–813.

42. Zhu, X., M. Ohtsubo, R. M. Böhmer, J. M. Roberts and R. K. Assician, Adhesion-dependent cell cycle progression linked to the expression of cyclin D1, activation of cyclin E-cdk2, and phosphorylation of the retinoblastoma protein, J. Cell Biol. **133** (1996), 391–403.

Roland Sennerstam
Division of Cell and Molecular Analysis
Department of Oncology and Pathology
Karolinska Institute and Hospital
S-171 76 Stockholm
Sweden
roland.sennerstam@haninge.mail.telia.com

Jan-Olof Strömberg
Institute of Mathematical and Physical Sciences
University of Tromsø
Norway

Some State Space Models of HIV Pathogenesis

Wai-Yuan Tan and Zhihua Xiang

Abstract. In this paper we have developed a state space model for the HIV pathogenesis at the cellular level involving free HIV (i.e., HIV not in cells or tissues) and different types of CD4$^+$ T cells. In this state space model, the stochastic system model is the stochastic model of the HIV pathogenesis developed by Tan and Wu [14], whereas the observation model is a statistic model based on the log of observed total numbers of CD4$^+$ T-cell counts at different times. This is a continuous time-discrete time nonlinear Kalman filter model. For this model, we have developed procedures for estimating and predicting the numbers of different types of CD4$^+$ T cells and free HIV through the extended Kalman filter method. As an illustration, we have applied the method of this paper to the data of a hemophilia patient from NCI/NIH with observed CD4$^+$ T-cell counts at 16 occasions. For this individual, it is shown that there is an acute infectivity phase during which there are high levels of infected CD4$^+$ T cells and free HIV.

§1. Introduction

Recent studies by Ho et al. [6] and Wei et al. [19] have shown that the HIV pathogenesis is a highly dynamic process. The turnover of free HIV is both rapid and continuous as both free HIV and actively HIV-infected CD4$^+$ T cells are short lived [10]. It follows that free HIV are continuously being removed and replenished by the death of actively HIV-infected CD4$^+$ T cells. For in-depth understanding of the HIV pathogenesis, it is therefore important to develop mathematical models of the HIV pathogenesis at the cellular level in HIV-infected individuals. To this end, some deterministic models have been developed by Kirschner et al. [8], Perelson et al. [9], Schenzle [12] and Philip [11], among others. Because the HIV pathogenesis is basically a stochastic process, to assess how randomness of the state variables would affect the HIV progression, Tan and Wu [13, 14] have attempted to develop a stochastic model at the cellular level in HIV-infected individuals.

In this paper we will proceed to develop some state space models for the HIV pathogenesis at the cellular level in HIV-infected individuals. In these

Mathematical Models in Medical and Health Sciences
Mary Ann Horn, Gieri Simonett, and Glenn Webb (eds.), pp. 351–368.

state space models, the stochastic system model is the stochastic model of the HIV pathogenesis at the cellular level in HIV-infected individuals involving free HIV and different types of CD4$^+$ T cells (HIV- infected as well as uninfected CD4$^+$ T cells); the observation model of the state space model is a statistical model based on the total number of CD4$^+$ T-cell counts at different times, since this type of data is usually available. (The observation model will also include the number of RNA virus load at different times if such data are available.) As such, state space models are advantageous over both the corresponding stochastic models and statistical models as they combine information and advantages from both of these models. As shown in [15, 17], state space models have an additional advantage over other models in that they permit updating of the model by new data which may become available in the future.

In Section 2, we will describe how to derive stochastic models for the HIV pathogenesis at the cellular level in HIV-infected individuals by taking into account basic mechanisms of the HIV pathogenesis. In Section 3, by using results from Section 2, we will derive some state space models for HIV pathogenesis at the cellular level in HIV-infected individuals using data from CD4$^+$ T-cell counts. As an application of our models, in Section 4 we will apply the results of our model to the data of a hemophilia patient from the NCI/NIH hemophilia studies. In Section 5, we will generate some Monte Carlo studies to assess the efficiency and usefulness of the Kalman filter methods. Finally, in Section 6, we will draw some conclusions and discuss some relevant issues regarding state space models.

§2. A Stochastic Model of the HIV Pathogenesis

Consider a HIV-infected individual. For the HIV pathogenesis in this individual, we anticipate four types of cells in the blood: The normal uninfected CD4$^+$ T cells (to be denoted as T_1 cells), the latently HIV-infected CD4$^+$ T cells (to be denoted as T_2 cells), the actively HIV-infected CD4$^+$ T cells (to be denoted as T_3 cells) and the free HIV. Then we may describe the life cycle of free HIV and the stochastic dynamic of the HIV pathogenesis briefly as follows: Free HIV can infect T_1 cells as well as the precursor stem cells in the bone marrow and thymus; see Remark 1. When a resting T_1 cell is infected by a free HIV, it becomes a T_2 cell which may either revert back to a T_1 cell or be activated at some time to become a T_3 cell. On the other hand, when a dividing T_1 cell is infected by a free HIV, it becomes a T_3 cell which will release free HIV when it dies. T_2 cells will not release free HIV until being activated to become T_3 cells. Further, T_1 cells are generated by precursor stem cells in the bone marrow and mature in the thymus; the matured T_1 cells then move to the blood stream.

Remark 1. Although it is not clear how it happened, Essunger and Perelson [2] and Fauci [3] have provided evidence to indicate that precursor stem cells can be infected by free HIV. (For biological evidence, we refer the readers to Fauci [3] and the references therein.) These observations have then been incorporated into HIV pathogenesis models in [8, 9]. In fact, as noted by Perelson and Kirschner [8, 9] and by Tan and Wu [14], the term involving infection of precursor stem cells by free HIV is essential for the model to yield results which fit observed clinical data in HIV progression.

Let $T_i(t)$, $i = 1, 2, 3$, and $V(t)$ be the numbers of T_i, $i = 1, 2, 3$, cells and free HIV in the blood at time t, respectively. Then $\boldsymbol{X}(t) = \{T_i(t), i = 1, 2, 3, V(t)\}$ is a 4-dimensional stochastic process. To model this dynamic stochastic process, consider the time interval $[t, t + \triangle t)$ and define the following variables.

$S(t)$ =Number of T_1 cells generated stochastically by the precursor
 stem cells in the bone marrow and thymus during $[t, t + \triangle t)$;

$G_1(t)$ =Number of T_1 cells generated by stochastic logistic growth
 of T_1 cells during $[t, t + \triangle t)$ through stimulation by free HIV
 and existing antigens;

$F_1(t)$ =Number of T_1 cells infected by free HIV during $[t, t + \triangle t)$;

$G_2(t)$ =Number of T_2 cells among the HIV-infected T_1 cells during
 $[t, t + \triangle t)$;

$F_2(t)$ =Number of T_2 cells which become T_3 cells during $[t, t + \triangle t)$;

$D_i(t)$ =Number of deaths of T_i cells during $[t, t + \triangle t)$, $i = 1, 2, 3$;

$D_V(t)$ =Number of free HIV which have lost infectivity, or die, or
 have been removed during $[t, t + \triangle t)$;

$N(t)$ =Average number of free HIV released by a T_3 cell when it dies
 at time t.

Then, we have

$$T_1(t + \triangle t) = T_1(t) + S(t) + G_1(t) - F_1(t) - D_1(t), \tag{1}$$
$$T_2(t + \triangle t) = T_2(t) + G_2(t) - F_2(t) - D_2(t), \tag{2}$$
$$T_3(t + \triangle t) = T_3(t) + [F_1(t) - G_2(t)] + F_2(t) - D_3(t), \tag{3}$$
$$V(t + \triangle t) = V(t) + N(t)D_3(t) - F_1(t) - D_V(t), \tag{4}$$

In the above equations, the variables on the right side are random variables which specify the random transition during the time interval $[t, t + \triangle t)$ from elements of $\boldsymbol{X}(t)$ to elements of $\boldsymbol{X}(t + \triangle t)$. Let k_1 be the HIV infection rate of T_1 cells, k_2 the rate of T_2 cells being activated, $\mu_i(i = 1, 2, 3)$ the death rate of T_i cells (i=1,2,3) and μ_V the rate by which free HIV are being removed, die, or have lost infectivity. Let γ be the rate of proliferation of T_1 cells by stimulation by HIV and antigens, $\omega(t)$ the probability that an infected T_1 cell is a T_2 cell at time t and $s(t)$ the rate by which T_1 cells are generated by precursor stem cells in the bone marrow and thymus at time t. (Following [8, 9], we assume $s(t) = s\theta/[\theta + V(t)]$.) Then the conditional probability distributions of the above variables given $\boldsymbol{X}(t)$ can be specified as follows:

- $S(t) \mid V(t) \sim$Poisson with mean $s(t)\triangle t$;
- $G(t) \mid T_1(t) \sim$Binomial$[T_1(t); \lambda(t)\triangle t]$;
- $[F_1(t), D_V(t)] \mid [V(t), T_1(t)] \sim$Multinomial$[V(t); k_1 T_1(t)\triangle t, \mu_V \triangle t]$;
- $[F_2(t), D_2(t)] \mid T_2(t) \sim$ Multinomial $[T_2(t); k_2\triangle t, \mu_2\triangle t]$;
- $G_2(t) \mid F_1(t) \sim$ Binomial $[F_1(t); \omega(t)]$;
- $D_1(t) \mid [T_1(t), F_1(t)] \sim$ Binomial $[T_1(t) - F_1(t); \mu_1\triangle t]$;
- $D_3(t) \mid T_3(t) \sim$ Binomial $[T_3(t); \mu_3\triangle t]$;

where $\lambda(t) = \gamma[1 - \sum_{j=1}^{3} T_j(t)/T_{\max}]$.

Given $\boldsymbol{X}(t)$, conditionally $S(t)$, $G(t)$, $[F_1(t), D_V(t)]$, $[F_2(t), D_2(t)]$, and $D_3(t)$ are independently distributed of one another; given $F_1(t)$, conditionally $G_2(t)$ is independently distributed of other variables. Let $\varepsilon_i(t)$, $i = 1, 2, 3, 4$, be defined by

$$\begin{aligned}
\varepsilon_1(t)\triangle t &= [S(t) - s(t)\triangle t] + [G_1(t) - \lambda(t)T_1(t)\triangle t] \\
&\quad - [F_1(t) - k_1 T_1(t)V(t)\triangle t] - [D_1(t) - \mu_1 T_1(t)\triangle t], \\
\varepsilon_2(t)\triangle t &= [G_2(t) - \omega(t)k_1 V(t)T_1(t)\triangle t] - [F_2(t) - k_2 T_2(t)\triangle t] \\
&\quad - [D_2(t) - \mu_2 T_2(t)\triangle t], \\
\varepsilon_3(t)\triangle t &= \{[F_1(t) - k_1 T_1(t)V(t)\triangle t] - [G_2(t) - \omega(t)k_1 T_1(t)V(t)\triangle t]\} \\
&\quad + [F_2(t) - k_2 T_2(t)\triangle t] - [D_3(t) - \mu_3(t)T_3(t)\triangle t], \\
\varepsilon_4(t)\triangle t &= N(t)[D_3(t) - T_3(t)\mu_3\triangle t] - [F_1(t) - k_1 T_1(t)V(t)\triangle t] \\
&\quad - [D_V(t) - \mu_V V(t)\triangle t].
\end{aligned}$$

Then, in terms of mean square error, equations (1)-(4) lead to the following stochastic differential equations for $T_i(t), i = 1, 2, 3, V(t)$:

$$\frac{dT_1(t)}{dt} = s(t) + \lambda(t)T_1(t) - \mu_1 T_1(t) - k_1 V(t)T_1(t) + \varepsilon_1(t), \qquad (5)$$

$$\frac{dT_2(t)}{dt} = \omega(t)k_1 V(t)T_1(t) - \mu_2 T_2(t) - k_2 T_2(t) + \varepsilon_2(t), \qquad (6)$$

$$\frac{dT_3(t)}{dt} = [1 - \omega(t)]k_1 V(t)T_1(t) + k_2 T_2(t) - \mu_3 T_3(t) + \varepsilon_3(t), \qquad (7)$$

$$\frac{dV(t)}{dt} = N(t)\mu_3 T_3(t) - k_1 V(t)T_1(t) - \mu_V V(t) + \varepsilon_4(t). \qquad (8)$$

In equations (5)-(8), the random noises $\varepsilon_j(t), j = 1, 2, 3, 4$ have expectation zero. The variances and covariances of these random variables are easily obtained as

$$Q_{11}(t) = \text{VAR}[\varepsilon_1(t)] = \text{E}\{s(t) + \lambda(t)T_1(t) + [\mu_1 + k_1 V(t)]T_1(t)\},$$

$$Q_{12}(t) = \text{COV}[\varepsilon_1(t), \varepsilon_2(t)] = -k_1 \omega(t)\text{E}[V(t)T_1(t)],$$

$$Q_{13}(t) = \text{COV}[\varepsilon_1(t), \varepsilon_3(t)] = -k_1[1 - \omega(t)]\text{E}[V(t)T_1(t)],$$

$$Q_{14}(t) = \text{COV}[\varepsilon_1(t), \varepsilon_4(t)] = k_1\text{E}[V(t)T_1(t)],$$

$$Q_{22}(t) = \text{VAR}[\varepsilon_2(t)] = \text{E}[k_1\omega(t)V(t)T_1(t) + (\mu_2 + k_2)T_2(t)],$$

$Q_{23}(t) = \text{COV}[\varepsilon_2(t), \varepsilon_3(t)] = -\text{E}\{\omega(t)[1 - \omega(t)]k_1 V(t)T_1(t) + k_2 T_2(t)\},$

$Q_{24}(t) = \text{COV}[\varepsilon_2(t), \varepsilon_4(t)] = -k_1\omega(t)\text{E}[V(t)T_1(t)],$

$Q_{33}(t) = \text{VAR}[\varepsilon_3(t)] = \text{E}\{[1 - \omega(t)]k_1 V(t)T_1(t) + k_2 T_2(t) + \mu_3 T_3(t)\},$

$Q_{34}(t) = \text{COV}[\varepsilon_3(t), \varepsilon_4(t)] = -[1 - \omega(t)]k_1\text{E}[V(t)T_1(t)] - N(t)\mu_3\text{E}T_3(t),$

$Q_{44}(t) = \text{VAR}[\varepsilon_4(t)] = \text{E}\{N^2(t)\mu_3 T_3(t) + [\mu_V + k_1 T_1(t)]V(t)\}.$

By using the formula

$$Cov(X, Y) = E\{Cov[(X, Y)|Z]\} + Cov[E(X|Z), E(Y|Z)],$$

it can be easily shown that the random noises $\varepsilon_j(t)$ are uncorrelated with the state variables $T_i(t), i = 1, 2, 3$ and $V(t)$. Since the random noises $\varepsilon_j(t)$ are random variables associated with the random transitions during the interval $[t, t + \triangle t)$, one may also assume that the random noises $\varepsilon_j(t)$ are uncorrelated with the random noises $\varepsilon_l(\tau)$ for all j and l if $t \neq \tau$.

§3. A State Space Model for HIV Pathogenesis

The state space model consists of a stochastic system model which is the stochastic model of the system and an observation model which is a statistical model to relate the observed data to the system. Thus, the state space model can be superior to both the stochastic model and the statistical model since it combines information from both models.

For the state space model of the HIV pathogenesis in the absence of treatment, the stochastic system model is the stochastic model given by the stochastic equations (1)-(4) of the previous section. Let y_j be the log of the observed total number of CD4$^+$ T-cell counts at time t_j. Then the observation model, based on the CD4$^+$ T-cell counts, is given by

$$y_j = \log(\sum_{i=1}^{3} T_i(t_j)) + e_j, \quad j = 1, \ldots, n, \tag{9}$$

where e_j is the random error associated with measuring y_j.

In equation (9), one may assume that e_j has expected value 0 and variance σ_j^2 and is uncorrelated with the random noises of equations (1)-(4) of the previous section. From [1], one may also assume that e_j is uncorrelated with e_u if the absolute value of $t_j - t_u$ is greater than 6 months. For the example in Section 4, we will thus assume that the e_j are uncorrelated with the e_u for all $j \neq u$.

The above state space model has continuous time for the stochastic system model, but has discrete time for the observation model. Further, both the system model and the observation model are nonlinear. For these models, it has been shown by Wu and Tan [20] through Monte Carlo studies that results from the extended Kalman filter method provide very close approximations to the computer-generated data; see also Section 5. (Since the infection rate is very small, this is not surprising.) In this paper we will thus use the extended Kalman filter method to derive the estimates and the predicted numbers of the state variables.

To illustrate, write equations (1)-(4) and (5), respectively, as

$$\frac{d}{dt}X(t) = f[X(t)] + \epsilon(t)$$

for $t_j \leq t < t_{j+1}, j = 0, 1, \cdots, n;$

$$y_j = h[X(t_j)] + e_j, \quad j = 1, \cdots, n.$$

Let $\hat{X}(t)$ be an estimator of $X(t)$ with estimated residual $\hat{\epsilon}(t) = \hat{X}(t) - X(t)$ and define $\hat{X}(t)$ as an unbiased estimator of $X(t)$ if $E\hat{\epsilon}(t) = 0$. Suppose that $\hat{X}(0)$ is unbiased for $X(0)$ with covariance matrix $P(0)$. Then, starting with $\hat{X}(0)$, the procedures given in the following two subsection provide close approximations to some optimal methods for estimating and predicting $X(t)$. The proof of these procedures can be found in Tan and Xiang [16].

3.1. Estimation of $X(t)$ given $y_u, u = 1, \cdots, j$ $(j \leq n)$.

Let $\hat{X}(t|t_j)$ be an estimator (or predictor) of $X(t)$ given data $y_u, u = 1, \cdots, j$ with estimated residual $\hat{\epsilon}(t|t_j) = \hat{X}(t) - X(t)$. Denote the covariance matrix of $\hat{\epsilon}(t|t_j)$ by $Q(t|t_j)$ and write $\hat{X}(0) = \hat{u}(0|0)$, $\hat{u}(j|j) = \hat{X}(t_j|t_j) = \lim_{t \to t_j} \hat{X}(t|t_j)$, $P(0) = P(0|0)$ and $P(j|j) = \lim_{t \to t_j} Q(t|t_j) = Q(t_j|t_j)$. Then, starting with $\hat{X}(0) = \hat{u}(0|0)$ with $P(0) = P(0|0)$, the linear, unbiased and minimum varianced estimators of $X(t)$ corresponding to given data $y_u, u = 1, \cdots, j$ $(j \leq n)$ are closely approximated by the following recursive equations:

(i) For $t_j \leq t < t_{j+1}$, $j = 0, 1, \cdots, n$ $(t_0 = 0, t_{n+1} = \infty)$, $\hat{X}(t|t_j)$ satisfies the following equations with boundary conditions

$$\lim_{t \to t_j} \hat{X}(t|t_j) = \hat{X}(t_j|t_j) = \hat{u}(j|j),$$

where $\hat{u}(j|j)$ is given in (iii):

$$\frac{d}{dt}\hat{X}(t|t_j) = f[\hat{X}(t|t_j)] \quad t_j \leq t < t_{j+1}, j = 0, 1, \cdots, n;$$

(ii) For $t_j \leq t < t_{j+1}$, $j = 0, 1, \cdots, n$, the covariance matrix $Q(t|t_j)$ satisfies the following equations with boundary conditions

$$\lim_{t \to t_j} Q(t|t_j) = Q(t_j|t_j) = P(j|j),$$

where $P(j|j)$ is given in (iii):

$$\frac{d}{dt}Q(t|t_j) = F(t|t_j)Q(t|t_j) + Q(t|t_j)F^T(t|t_j) + V_X(t),$$

for $t_j \leq t < t_{j+1}, j = 0, 1, \cdots, n$, where $F(t|t_j) = (\frac{\partial}{\partial \boldsymbol{X}^T} \boldsymbol{f}(\boldsymbol{X}))_{\boldsymbol{X}=\hat{\boldsymbol{X}}(t|t_j)}$. and where $V_X(t)$ is the covariance matrix of the random noises $\{\varepsilon_j(t), j = 1, 2, 3, 4\}$.

(iii) Denote by $\hat{\boldsymbol{u}}(j + 1|j) = \lim_{t \to t_{j+1}} \hat{\boldsymbol{X}}(t|t_j)$ from (i) and $P(j + 1|j) = \lim_{t \to t_{j+1}} Q(t|t_j)$ from (ii). Then $\hat{\boldsymbol{u}}(j + 1 \,|\, j + 1)$ and $P(j + 1|j + 1)$ are given respectively by

$$\hat{\boldsymbol{u}}(j + 1 \,|\, j + 1) = \hat{\boldsymbol{u}}(j + 1 \,|\, j) + K_{j+1}\{Y_{j+1} - h[\hat{\boldsymbol{u}}(j + 1|j)]\},$$

and

$$P(j + 1|j + 1) = [I - K_{j+1}H_{j+1}]P(j + 1 \,|\, j),$$

where

$$H_{j+1} = [\frac{\partial}{\partial \boldsymbol{X}} h(\boldsymbol{X})]_{\boldsymbol{X}=\hat{\boldsymbol{u}}(j+1|j)}$$

and

$$K_{j+1} = P(j + 1 \,|\, j)H_{j+1}[H_{j+1}^T P(j + 1| j)H_{j+1} + \sigma_j^2]^{-1}.$$

To implement the above procedure, one starts with $\hat{\boldsymbol{X}}(0) = \hat{\boldsymbol{u}}(0|0)$ and $P(0) = P(0|0)$. Then by (i) and (ii), one derives $\hat{X}(t|t_0)$ and $Q(t|t_0)$ for $t_0 \leq t \leq t_1$ and derives $\hat{\boldsymbol{u}}(1|1)$ and $P(1|1)$ by (iii). Repeating these procedures one may derive $\hat{X}(t|t_j)$ and $Q(t|t_j)$ for $t_j \leq t < t_{j+1}$, $j = 0, 1, \cdots, n$. These procedures are referred to as forward filtering procedures (see [4]).

3.2. Estimation of $X(t)$ given $y_1, \cdots, y_n$ and $t_j \leq t < t_{j+1}$.

Let $\hat{X}(t|n)$ be an estimator of $X(t)$ given data $y_j, j = 1, \cdots, n$. Let $Q(t|n)$ be the covariance matrix of $\hat{\boldsymbol{\epsilon}}(t|n) = \hat{\boldsymbol{X}}(t|n) - \boldsymbol{X}(t)$. Denote by $\hat{\boldsymbol{u}}(j|n) = \hat{\boldsymbol{X}}(t_j|n)$ and $P(j|n) = Q(t_j|n)$. Then, starting with $\hat{\boldsymbol{X}}(0) = \hat{\boldsymbol{u}}(0|0)$ and $P(0) = P(0|0)$, the linear, unbiased and minimum varianced estimators of $X(t)$ given data $(y_j, j = 1, \cdots, n)$ are closely approximated by the following recursive equations:

(i) For $t_j \leq t < t_{j+1}$, $j = 0, 1, \cdots, n$, $\hat{X}(t|n)$ satisfies the following equations with boundary conditions $\lim_{t \to t_j} \hat{\boldsymbol{X}}(t|n) = \hat{\boldsymbol{u}}(j|n)$, where $\hat{\boldsymbol{u}}(j|n)$ is given in (iii):

$$\frac{d}{dt}\hat{\boldsymbol{X}}(t|n) = \boldsymbol{f}[\hat{\boldsymbol{X}}(t|n)]$$

for $t_j \leq t < t_{j+1}, j = 0, 1, \cdots, n$.

(ii) For $t_j \leq t < t_{j+1}$, $j = 0, 1, \cdots, n$, $Q(t|n)$ satisfies the following equations with boundary condition

$$\lim_{t \to t_j} Q(t|n) = P(j|n),$$

where $P(j|n)$ is given in (iii):

$$\frac{d}{dt}Q(t|n) = F(t|n)Q(|n) + Q(t|n)F^T(t|n) + V_X(t),$$

for $t_j \le t < t_{j+1}, j = 0, 1, \cdots, n,$ where $F(t|n) = (\frac{\partial}{\partial X^T} f(X))_{X = \hat{X}(t|n)}.$

(iii) $\hat{u}(j|n)$ and $P(j|n)$ for $j = 1, \cdots, n-1$ are given by the following recursive equations:

$$\hat{u}(j|n) = \hat{u}(j|j) + A_j\{\hat{u}(j+1|n) - \hat{u}(j+1|j)\}$$

and

$$P(j|n) = P(j|j) - A_j\{P(j+1|j) - P(j+1|n)\}A_j^T,$$

where

$$A_j = P(j|j)F^T(t_{j+1}|t_j)P^{-1}(j+1|j).$$

To implement the above procedure to derive $\hat{X}(t|n)$ for given initial distribution of $\hat{X}(t)$ at t_0, one first derives results by using formulas in Section (3.1) (forward filtering). Then one goes backward from n to 1 by using formulas in Section 3.2. (This is the backward filtering; see [4]).

§4. An Illustrative Example

As an application of the above results, we consider a hemophilia patient from NCI/NIH Multi-Center Hemophilia Cohort Studies. This patient contracted HIV at age 11 through a blood transfusion. The CD4$^+$ T-Cell counts for this patient were taken at 16 occasions and are given in Table 1 ($|t_j - t_u| > 6$ months for $j \ne u$, see Table 1). We will use this patient as an example to illustrate the theories of this paper; see Remark 2. Note that different people are expected to have different parameter values, owing to genetic differences and differences in health status. Thus, to monitor the HIV progression of an HIV-infected individual, it is desirable to estimate the parameter values from data of that particular individual. For the patient described above, the estimates of the parameters are : $s = 10/\text{day}/mm^3$, $\theta = 0.7571/\text{day}/mm^3$, $\gamma = 0.03/\text{day}/mm^3$, $\mu_1 = \mu_2 = 0.02/\text{day}$, $\mu_3 = 0.3/\text{day}$, $\mu_V = 4.6/\text{day}$, $T_{\max} = 1656.16/\text{day}/mm^3$, $N_0 = .3351$, $\beta_1 = 0.794378E - 05$, $\beta_2 = 49.9061E + 03/$, $k_1 = 1.3162 \times 10^{-6}/\text{day}/mm^3$, $k_2 = 7.9873 \times 10^{-3}/\text{day}/mm^3$, $\omega = 0.2$, where $N(t) = N_0 \exp(-\beta_1 t) + \beta_2(1 - \exp(-\beta_1 t))$. In these estimates the values of the parameters $s, \gamma, \mu_i, i = 1, 2, 3, \mu_V, \omega$ were taken from literature ([6, 9]) (see Remark 2) but the values of the parameters $k_1, k_2, N_0, \beta_1, \beta_2, \theta, T_{\max}$ were estimated by nonlinear least square procedures (see [13,14]).

Remark 2. Because of genetic differences and differences in health status, different individuals are expected to have different parameter values. (For example, slow HIV progressors and fast HIV progressors are expected to have different infection rates (k_1 values).) The recent discovery of the CCR-5 receptor gene for HIV infection has further confirmed this; for more details, see Hill and Littman [5]. Thus, the model should be applied to a single individual. It is applicalbe to a cohort only if the same model is applicable to all individuals of the cohort. To determine which parameters may be fairly constant and which parameters may vary between HIV-infected individuals, in [18] we have applied the above model to 200 individuals from the NCI hemophilia data set and have estimated the parameter values for each of these 200 individuals. Our results show that the estimates of the parameters $\{s, \gamma, \mu_i, i = 1, 2, 3, \mu_V, \omega\}$ are fairly constant (standard error less than 10%), but the other parameters, especially $\{N_0, \beta_1, \beta_2, k_1\}$, may vary considerably between individuals.

Tab. 1. The Observed Total Numbers of CD4$^+$ T Cells of an HIV Infected Patient.

Days After Infection	T Cell Counts (mm^3)	Days After Infection	T Cell Counts (mm^3)
1152	1254	2952	686
1404	1005	3096	357
1692	1022	3312	440
1872	1105	3456	584
2124	372	3708	508
2376	432	3852	583
2592	520	4032	328
2736	660	4212	345

Using these estimates and the methods given in previous sections, we have estimated the number of free HIV, the total number of CD4$^+$ T cells and the numbers of T_i cells ($i = 1, 2, 3$) at different times. Plotted in Figure 1 are the estimated total number of CD4$^+$ T-cell counts together with the observed CD4$^+$ T-cell counts. Plotted in Figures 2 and 3 are the estimated numbers of infected CD4$^+$ T cells and free HIV, respectively.

From Figure 1, we observed that the Kalman filter estimates tried to trace the observed numbers. On the other hand, if we ignore the random variations and simply use the deterministic model to fit the data, then the fitted numbers would draw a smooth line between the observed numbers. This is not surprising since the deterministic model would yield continuous solutions.

From Figures 2 and 3, we observed that prior to the 2,800th day after initial HIV infection, the estimated numbers of the HIV infected T cells and free HIV are very small (almost zero) by both the Kalman filter methods and the deterministic model. Beyond the 2,800th day of HIV infection, however, there are significant differences between the Kalman filtering estimates and the estimates by the deterministic model. It appears that for the Kalman filter estimates, both the numbers of the HIV-infected CD4$^+$ T cells and free

Total Number of CD4 $^+$ T Cell Counts

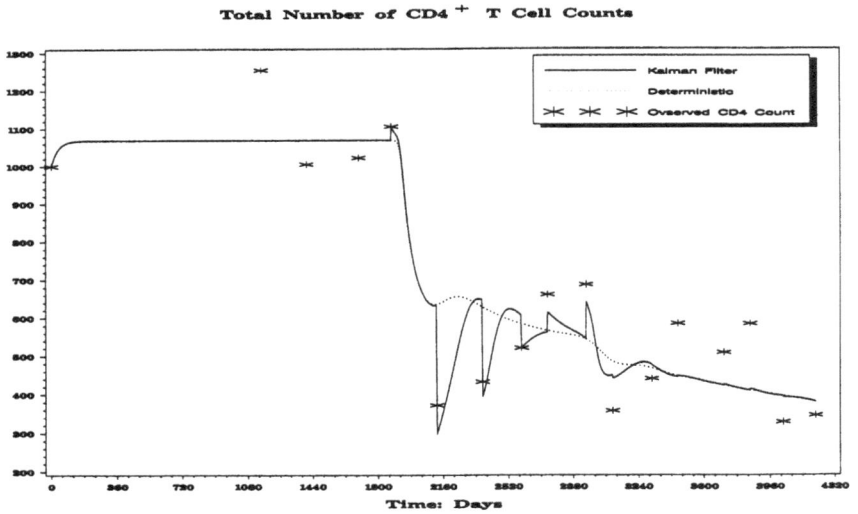

Fig. 1. Plots showing the observed total number of CD4 T cell counts and the estimates by the Kalman filter method and by the deterministic model.

Number of Latently Infected and Actively Infected CD4 $^+$ T Cells

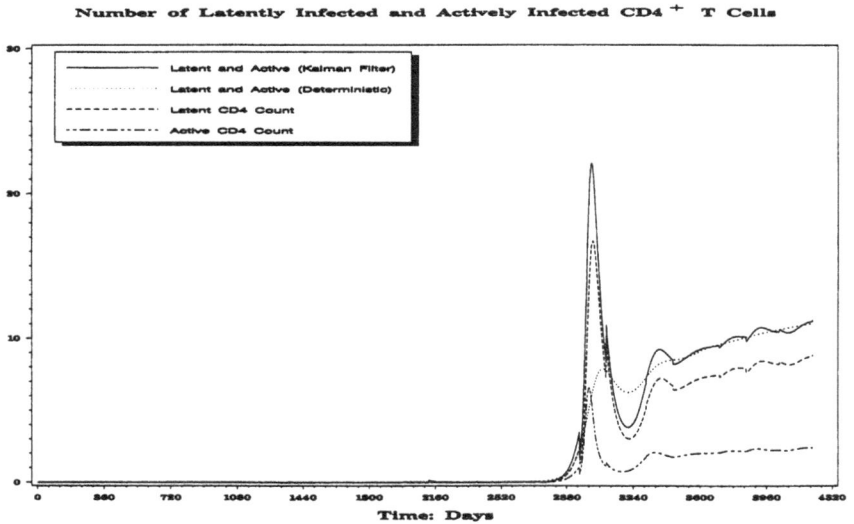

Fig. 2. Plots showing the Kalman filter estimates of the numbers of HIV infected T cells and the estimates by the deterministic model.

Number of Free HIV

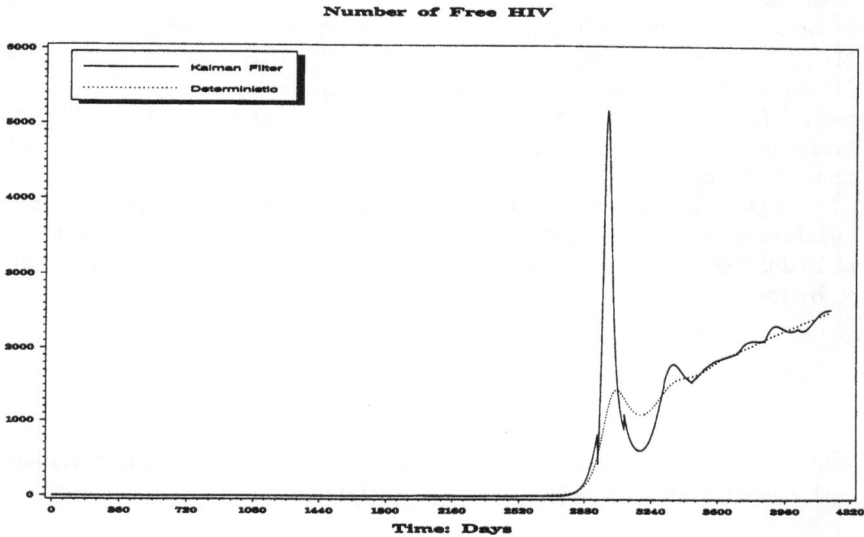

Fig. 3. Plots showing the Kalman filter estimates of the number of free HIV together with the estimates by the deterministic model.

HIV first increase very sharply, reach a maximum about 3,000 days after initial HIV infection and then decrease to a very lower level around day 3,240; after that the curves increase steadily. These results appear to be consistent with the observation by Phillips [11], suggesting an acute infectivity phase early on. On the other hand, the deterministic results show only moderately increasing curves without an initial high peak; also no decreasing pattern has been observed. From Figures 2 and 3, we also observe that the estimated curves of the infected T cells and free HIV show similar patterns, suggesting a positive correlation between infected CD4$^+$ T cells and free HIV. This is not surprising since free HIV are released mainly from the death of T_3 cells.

§5. Monte-Carlo Methods

To justify and confirm the usefulness of the extended Kalman filter method for the state space model given in Section 3, in this section we generate some Monte Carlo studies through computer by using the models in Sections 2 and 3. The parameter values of these models were taken from those of the estimates of the numerical example in Section 4 above.

To generate the numbers of T_i cells (i=1,2,3) and the number of free HIV by computer for the model in Section 2, we use the distribution theories given in Section 2. Thus, we use a Poisson generator with mean $s(t)\triangle t$ to generate $S(t)$ and use a binomial generator to generate $G_1(t)$ by assuming $G_1(t) \sim \mathrm{B}[T_1(t); \lambda(t)\triangle t]$; we generate $[F_1(t), D_V(t)]$ from the multinomial distribution, $\mathrm{MULT}[V_1(t); k_1 T_1(t)\triangle t, \mu_V \triangle t]$. Given $F_1(t)$, $D_1(t)$ is generated

from the binomial distribution, $B[T_1(t) - F_1(t); \mu_1 \triangle t]$ and $G_2(t)$ from the
binomial distribution, $B[F_1(t); \omega(t)]$. Similarly, we generate $[F_2(t), D_2(t)]$ from
$MULT[T_2(t); k_2 \triangle t, \mu_2 \triangle t]$ and $D_3(t)$ from $B[T_3(t); \mu_3 \triangle t]$. Then equations (1)-
(4) are used to generate $T_1(t + \triangle t)$, $T_2(t + \triangle t)$, $T_3(t + \triangle t)$ and $V(t + \triangle t)$
from $X(t)$. All the random generators are taken from the IMSL [7] library
functions. The time unit for generating these random numbers is taken as 2.4
hours or 0.1 day.

To generate the observation model, we add some Gaussian noises to the
log of the generated total number of CD4$^+$ T-cell counts to produce $y_j = Y(t_j)$
at 16 different times, as given in the example of Section 4. That is, we generate
y_j by the equation

$$y_j = \log(\sum_{i=1}^{3} T_i(t_j)) + e_j, \quad j = 1, \dots, n,$$

where e_j is assumed as independently distributed normal random variables
with mean 0 and variance $\pi(1 - \pi) \sum_{i=1}^{3} T_i(t_j)$ with $\pi = 0.1$.

Tab. 2. Computer Generated Total Numbers of CD4$^+$ T Cells at 16 Time Points.

Time (days)	y_j	Time (days)	y_j
1152	1064	2952	547
1404	1056	3096	495
1692	1055	3312	468
1872	1082	3456	448
2124	634	3708	421
2376	634	3852	411
2592	558	4032	386
2736	550	4212	395

Given the above setup with the parameter values as above, one can readily
generate the observed y_j's. Table 2 contains one set of the generated $y_j = Y(t_j)$. We have repeated the experiments 200 times. We now illustrate the
results with the generated data in Table 2. Similar results have been obtained
by using other generated data sets.

Given in Figure 4 are the fitted curves by using the observed total number
of CD4$^+$ T-cell counts. Given in Figures 5-7 are the extended Kalman filter
estimates of the numbers of latently infected CD4$^+$ T cells, actively infected
CD4$^+$ T cells and free HIV, respectively. To illustrate the usefulness of the
state space model and the impacts of ignoring the random variation of the
variables and the observation model, we have also plotted the curves of the
Monte Carlo generated numbers and of the estimates by the deterministic
model in these figures along with the Kalman filter estimates. From these
Monte Carlo studies, we have observed the following results.

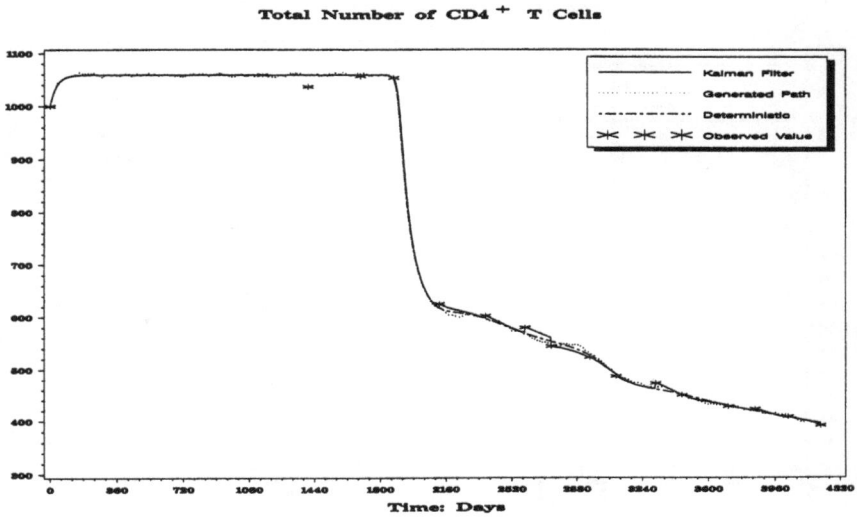

Fig. 4. Plots showing the generated number of CD4 T cell counts together with the Kalman filter estimates of these cell numbers and the estimates by the deterministic model.

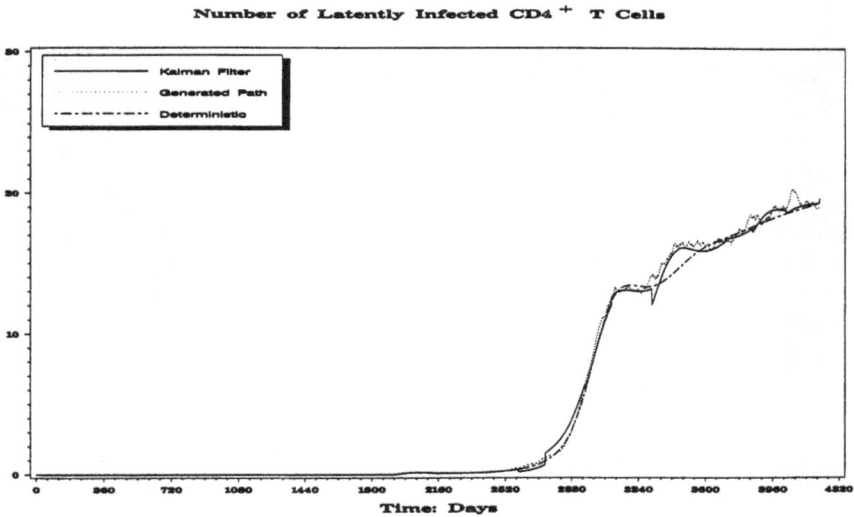

Fig. 5. Plots showing the generated numbers of latently infected T cells together with the Kalman filter estimates and the estimates by the deterministic model.

Number of Actively Infected CD4 $^+$ T Cells

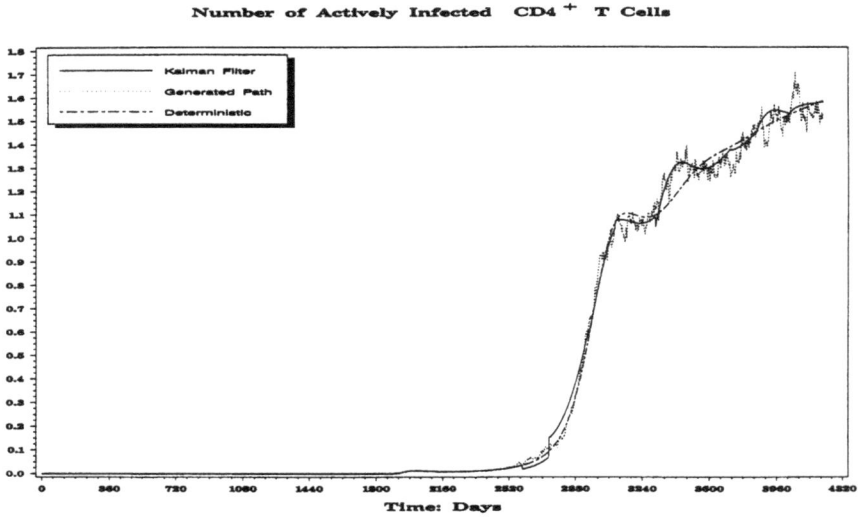

Fig. 6. Plots showing the generated numbers of actively infected T cells together with the Kalman filter estimates and the estimates by the deterministic model.

Number of Free HIV

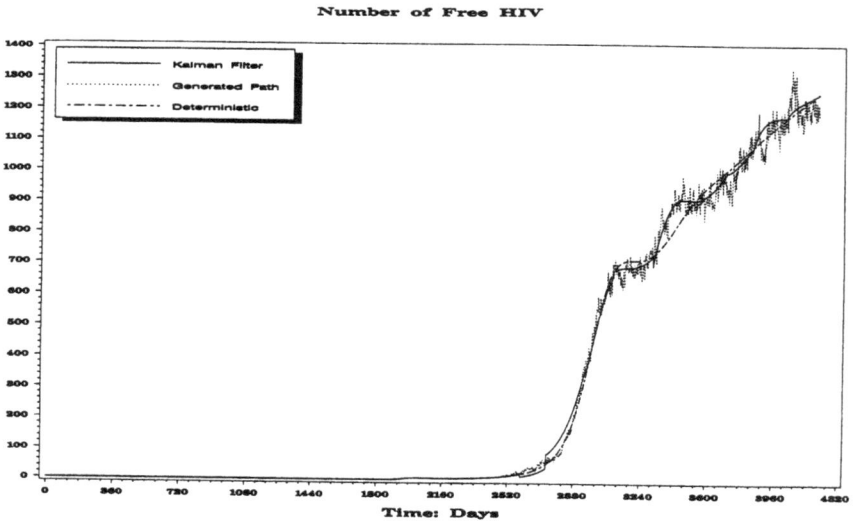

Fig. 7. Plots showing the generated numbers of free HIV together with the Kalman filter estimates and the estimates by the deterministic model.

(1) For the numbers of T_i cells ($i = 1, 2, 3$) and free HIV, the results in Figures 5-7 show clearly that the estimates obtained by using the extended Kalman filter method can trace the generated numbers very closely. These results suggest that in estimating the number of T_i cells ($i = 1, 2, 3$) and free HIV, one may in fact use the extended Kalman filter method as described in Section 3. Similar results have also been obtained by Wu and Tan [20]. Note that the Kalman filter estimates can trace the variation of the generated data very closely in most of the cases.

(2) As shown in Figures 5-7, the estimates obtained by using the deterministic model seem to draw a smooth line through the generated numbers and hence can not trace the variation of the generated data as did the Kalman filter estimates. This result suggests that in deriving estimates of the numbers of T cells and free HIV, it is important to take into account the random variation of the variables. These results are expected because the numbers of infected CD4$^+$ T cells (T_2 and T_3 cells) are quite small so that randomness of the variables have an important impact on the estimates. On the other hand, as has been demonstrated in [14], one would expect that deterministic models are still useful in revealing trends and behavior of the HIV progression in HIV infected individuals; for more detail see [14] and Remark 3.

Remark 3. Extensive Monte Carlo studies by Tan and Wu [14] have shown that the HIV progression in HIV-infected individual can be classified by three phases: The infection period, the transition period, and the steady-state period. It was observed in [14] that after the infection period (the first 2 to 3 years since infection), the numbers of T_i cells ($i = 1, 2, 3$) and free HIV are very large, in which case the equations of the conditional mean numbers are approximately the same as the corresponding equations defining the deterministic model. This may help to explain why after the middle stage and at the late stage of HIV infection, the HIV progression in HIV-infected individuals may be closely simulated by simply using the deterministic model. However, it is important to note that this result is conditional on the assumption that the HIV infection is not extinct. Furthermore, as illustrated in [14] and [18], the probability of extinction by random chance and the future pattern of HIV progression in HIV-infected individuals depend heavily on the early stochastic behavior of the HIV pathogenesis; for more details, see [14] and [18]. This may help to explain why it is necessary and important to use stochastic models.

§6. Conclusions and Discussion

In this paper we have developed a state space model for the HIV pathogenesis in the absence of treatment by antiviral drugs. In this state space model, the stochastic system model is the stochastic model developed by Tan and Wu [13, 14], whereas the observation model is a statistical model based on the observed total number of CD4$^+$ T-cell counts. This model is a nonlinear model with continuous-time system equations and discrete-time observation equations. General theories for such models are still non-existent. By using the extended Kalman filter as an approximation, in this paper we have developed some efficient procedures to estimate the numbers of different T cells and the number of free HIV.

To illustrate the application of the state space model given in Section 3, we have applied the model to the data of a hemophilia patient from the NCI/NIH hemophilia data set. This patient contracted HIV at age 11 through a blood transfusion and had the total number of $CD4^+$ T-cell counts taken at 16 occasions. By using this data set we have developed a state space model for this patient and have obtained Kalman filter estimates of the numbers of different types of $CD4^+$ T cells and free HIV. Our Kalman filter estimates showed clearly that both the numbers of HIV-infected $CD4^+$ T cells and free HIV had reached the maximum at about 3,000 days after HIV infection and then decreased to a much lower level around 3240 days after infection; after that the curves increase steadily. These results suggest an acute infectivity phase early on. Such a pattern of initial high level was not revealed by results of the deterministic model, however.

To assess the efficiency and usefulness of the Kalman filter methods, in this paper we have also generated some Monte Carlo studies by using the model in Section 3. Our numerical results have clearly shown that the estimates by the extended Kalman filter method can trace the generated numbers very closely in most of the cases. These results suggest that the extended Kalman filter estimates would provide very close approximations to the true numbers, due presumably to the fact that the HIV infection rate is usually very small. On the other hand, results by the deterministic model appear to draw a smooth line across the generated numbers, suggesting that there are significant differences between results of state space models and results of deterministic model. It is to be noted, however, that results of deterministic models are still useful in monitoring the trend and behavior of the HIV progression in HIV infected individuals; for more details, see Remark 3.

From the above demonstration, it is apparent that the state space model provides a powerful tool for in-depth understanding of the HIV pathogenesis and for linking the stochastic model to the observed data of $CD4^+$ T-cell counts to validate the model. To broaden its application, more research is needed to extend the model to more complex situations and to include treatment by antiviral drugs. These will be topics of our future research.

Acknowledgments. The research of this paper was partially supported by a research grant from National Institute of Allergy and Infections Diseases/NIH, Grant Nō: RO1 AI31869. The authors wish to thank the referee for smoothing the English language.

References

1. DeGruttola, V., N. Lange and U. Dafni, Modeling the progression of HIV infection, Jour. Amer. Stat. Assoc. **86** (1991), 569–677.

2. Essunger, P. and A. S. Perelson, Modeling HIV infection of CD4+ T-cell subpopulations, J. Theor. Biol. **170** (1994), 367–391.

3. Fauci, A. S., Immunopathogenic mechanisms in human immunodeficiency virus (HIV), Annals of Internal Medicine **114** (1993), 678-693.

4. Gelb, A., *Applied Optimal Estimation*, M.I.T. Press, Cambridge, MA, 1974.

5. Hill, C. M. and D. R. Littman, Natural resistance to HIV, Nature **382** (1996), 668-669.

6. Ho, D. D., A. U. Neumann, A. S. Perelson, W. Chen, J. M. Leonard and M. Markowitz, Rapid turnover of plasma virus and CD4 lymphocytes in HIV-1 infection, Nature **373** (1995), 123-126.

7. IMSL, *MATH/LIBRARY User's Manual*, IMSL, Houston, Texas, 1989.

8. Kirschner, D. E. and A. S. Perelson, A Model for the Immune System Response to HIV: AZT Treatment Studies, in *Mathematical Population Dynamics: Analysis of Heterogeneity, Vol.1, Theory of Epidemics*, O. Arino, D. Axelrod, M. Kimmel and M. Langlais (eds.), Marcel Dekker, New York, 1995, 295-310.

9. Perelson, A. S., D. E. Kirschner and R. D. Boer, Dynamics of HIV Infection of CD4$^+$ T Cells, Math. Biosciences **114** (1993), 81-125.

10. Perelson, A. S., A. U. Neumann, M. Markowitz, J. M. Leonard and D. D. Ho, HIV-1 dynamics in vivo: Virion clearance rate, infected cell life-span, and viral generation time, Science **271** (1996), 1582-1586.

11. Phillips, A. N., Reduction of HIV Concentration During Acute Infection: Independence from a Specific Immune Response, Science **271** (1996), 497-499.

12. Schenzle, D., A Model for AIDS Pathogenesis, Statistics in Medicine **13** (1994), 2067-2079.

13. Tan, W. Y. and H. Wu, A stochastic model for the pathogenesis of HIV at the cellular level and some Monte Carlo studies, in *Simulation in the Medical Sciences,* J. G. Anderson and M. Katzper (eds.), Society for Computer Simulation, San Diego, 1997, 78-88.

14. Tan, W. Y. and H. Wu, Stochastic modeling of the dynamics of CD4$^+$ T cells by HIV infection and some Monte Carlo studies, Math. Biosciences **147** (1998), 173-205.

15. Tan, W. Y. and Z. Xiang, A stochastic model for the HIV epidemic in homosexual populations: Estimation of parameters and validation of the model, in *Simulation in the Medical Sciences,* J. G. Anderson and M. Katzper (eds.), Society for Computer Simulation, San Diego, 1996, 77-88.

16. Tan, W. Y and Z. Xiang, A state space model of the HIV pathogenesis under treatment by an anti-viral drug, Invited paper at the International Conference on Deterministic and Stochastic Modeling of Biointeraction, August 28-September 1, 1997, Sofia, Bulgaria, Math. Biosciences, to appear.

17. Tan, W. Y. and Z. Xiang, State space models for the HIV epidemic in homosexual populations and some applications, Math. Biosciences, to appear, 1998.

18. Tan, W. Y. and Z. Ye, Assessing effects of different types of HIV and macrophage on HIV pathogenesis by stochastic models of HIV pathogenesis in HIV-infected individuals, Invited paper at the Fifth International Conference on Mathematical Population Dynamic, June 21-June 26, 1998, Zapokane, Poland.

19. Wei, X., S. K. Ghosh, M. E. Taylor, V. A. Johnson, E. A. Emini, P. Deutsch, J. D. Lifson, S. Bonhoeffer, M. A. Nowak, B. H. Hahn, M. S. Saag and G. M. Shaw, Viral dynamics in human immunodeficiency virus type 1 infection, Nature **373** (1995), 117–122.

20. Wu, H. and W. Y. Tan, Modeling and Monitoring the Progression of HIV Infection Using Nonlinear Kalman Filter, paper presented at the 1996 Annual Statistical Meeting in Chicago, August 4-8, 1996.

Wai-Yuan Tan and Zhihua Xiang
Department of Mathematical Sciences
The University of Memphis
Memphis, TN 38152
tanwy@msci.memphis.edu

Cell Cycle Checkpoints and the
Overall Dynamics of Cell Cycle Control

C. D. Thron

Abstract. The cycle of cell division is thought to be driven by an oscillatory biochemical system, but unlike simple chemical oscillators the cell cycle consists of a sequence of distinct stages, such as DNA replication and mitosis. Some stage transitions are known as "checkpoints" because there appear to be mechanisms that halt progress if the cell is not ready to enter the next stage. It has been proposed that checkpoints and other stage transitions are controlled by bistable subsystems that switch by saddle-node bifurcation. The relation of these subsystem saddle-node bifurcations to the bifurcation of the whole system between cycling and non-cycling behavior is discussed.

§1. Introduction

Experimental evidence has indicated that repetitive cell division is driven by an oscillatory biochemical system, and several simple mathematical models (cited in [30, 31]) have been proposed. More realistic models [17–22] are more complicated, and it has usually been necessary to reduce them to simpler models in order to understand the dynamics qualitatively. A special feature of the cycle of cell division is that it consists of a sequence of distinct stages, such as DNA replication and the several events of mitosis; and each stage must be entered decisively, fully, and irrevocably. Several of these transition points are known as "checkpoints" [15, 25], because there appear to be surveillance systems that monitor cellular processes such as DNA replication or repair, and halt progress through the cell cycle if the cell is not ready to enter the next stage. The cell cycle can therefore be arrested at any of several points, and this makes it appear quite different from the usual simple oscillatory system with one fixed point whose stability changes by Hopf bifurcation.

It has been suggested [19, 31–34] that biochemically a cell cycle checkpoint is controlled by a bistable subsystem which switches by saddle-node bifurcation in an all-or-none and locally irrevocable manner. When the switching

Mathematical Models in Medical and Health Sciences
Mary Ann Horn, Gieri Simonett, and Glenn Webb (eds.), pp. 369–380.
Copyright © 1998 by Vanderbilt University Press, Nashville, TN.
ISBN 0-8265-1310-7.

of a checkpoint initiates repetitive cell cycling, the subsystem saddle-node bifurcation evidently coincides with a bifurcation of the whole system. On the other hand, subsystem bifurcation may occur during the course of the cell cycle without bifurcation of the whole system. For example, there may appear to be a temporary arrest at a checkpoint, with resumption of progress when the surveillance system indicates readiness to proceed. The temporary arrest would correspond to a quasi-steady state of the bistable subsystem, and it would be terminated when continuing changes in other state variables bring about a saddle-node bifurcation of the subsystem, with no bifurcation of the whole system.

The following example illustrates, for a simple system, the relation between the subsystem saddle-node bifurcation at a checkpoint and the bifurcation which changes overall cell cycle behavior from non-cycling to cycling.

§2. A Bistable Biochemical Switch Model

In the mitotic switch model previously proposed [31] the active enzyme M which initiates mitosis is formed from an inactive precursor P by an effectively autocatalytic process at a rate F (defined below), and is reconverted to P by a first-order process at a rate $R = wM$, where w is constant and italic M denotes the concentration of M. There is also a protein which binds and inhibits M, so that the autocatalysis depends only on the concentration M_f of M unbound to inhibitor. Finally there is a relatively slow non-autocatalytic formation of M from P. The total concentration Q of M and P is assumed constant, so that $P = Q - M$. The equations for this switch model are

$$\frac{dM}{dt} = F - R = F - wM, \tag{1}$$

$$F = \left[e + (f - e)\frac{K_D M_f}{1 + K_D M_f} \right] D(Q - M), \tag{2}$$

$$M_f = \frac{-(B - M + K) + \sqrt{(B - M + K)^2 + 4KM}}{2}, \tag{3}$$

where e, f, K_D, D, B, and K are constant. Further explanation of equations (2) and (3) have been given elsewhere [31]. Here we note only that F can be written as the sum of non-autocatalytic and autocatalytic terms, and M_f is an increasing function of M with a more or less sharp break where M comes to exceed the concentration of inhibitor.

The operation of this switch model is shown in Figure 1, where the rate F of formation of M and the rate R of reconversion of M to P are plotted as functions of M. R increases linearly with M. Over a certain range, F also increases with M, because of the autocatalysis; but the autocatalysis is very weak at low M because of inhibitor binding. As M approaches 0, F approaches a low but finite non-autocatalytic rate; and as M approaches Q, F approaches 0 because of the factor $Q - M$. The sigmoid curvature in F gives rise to three intersections with R, i.e. three steady states or fixed points. These are shown

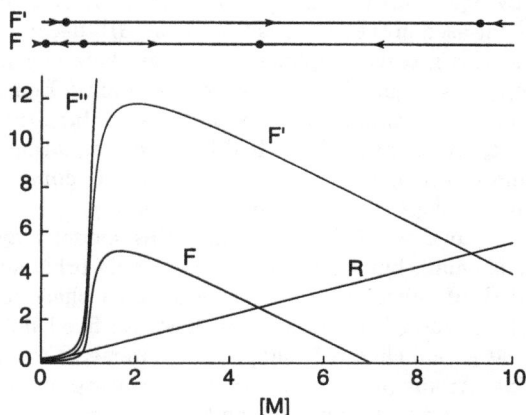

Fig. 1. Rates of formation F (equation (2)) and deactivation $(R = wM)$ of M. $e = 0.01, f = 1.1, K = 10^{-3}, K_D = 10, B = 1, D = 1, w = 0.55, Q = 7\ (F), 13.7451\ (F'), 20\ (F'')$.

as dots in the "phase portrait" ([7], pp. 10 ff.) labeled F above the graph. The direction of spontaneous change depends on the magnitude of F relative to R, and is shown by the arrows in the phase portrait. The two outer fixed points are stable, and the middle fixed point is unstable.

Switching of this bistable system occurs by a parameter change which shifts the relative positions of curves F and R. Increasing the parameter Q causes curve F to rise and break contact (at low M) with curve R (curves F' and F'', Figure 1). When the formation and removal rate curves are just tangent (curve F'), the left-hand fixed point in the phase portrait is nonhyperbolic. This is a bifurcation of the saddle-node type ([7], pp. 25 ff.). Such saddle-node bifurcations, produced by increased Q or some other parameter change, obliterate the steady state with low M and cause an abrupt shift to a steady state with high M. This has been proposed to be the mechanism for abrupt full activation of the enzyme which initiates mitosis [31, 32]. The activation is locally irrevocable, in that reversing the change in the bifurcation parameter does not destabilize the high-activity steady state and does not cause return to the low-activity steady state.

§3. Bifurcations of an Oscillatory Model

The above switch model becomes a component of an oscillatory model by assuming that M is formed at a constant rate i and removed by a first-order process at a rate gM. The equations for the oscillatory model are

$$\frac{dM}{dt} = i + F - (w + g)M, \tag{4}$$

$$\frac{dQ}{dt} = i - gM, \tag{5}$$

with F given by equations (2) and (3). Equation (5) is used instead of the equation for dP/dt used in the previous treatment [31], because dQ/dt depends only on M, and this greatly simplifies the phase plane analysis, since the Q nullcline is simply a straight line parallel to the Q axis. Equation (4) defines a subsystem which is a bistable switch with Q as a bifurcation parameter (F is a function of Q by equation (2)). It differs from equation (1) only in the parameters i and g, which change Figure 1 by shifting curve F up a distance i and increasing the slope of curve R by an amount g.

The previous analysis [31] showed that this model may have a stable fixed point if i is small, but on increasing i a stable orbit appears, followed by a subcritical Hopf bifurcation. Figure 2A shows a phase plane plot of this system with i large enough to produce an unstable fixed point and a stable closed orbit. The M nullcline is N-shaped and intersects the Q nullcline at a single fixed point. At any point on the orbit, the corresponding phase portrait of the switch subsystem (equation (4)) can be constructed by drawing through the state point a line parallel to the M axis. The values of M where this line intersects the M nullcline are the fixed points of the switch subsystem (two stable and one unstable); and the direction of spontaneous change in the subsystem (shown by arrows in Figure 2A) depends on whether the M nullcline lies above or below the phase portrait. As the state point moves around the orbit, the corresponding subsystem phase portrait is carried with it and changes; and when Q rises past the level of the maximum of the M nullcline, the left-hand stable fixed point and the unstable fixed point merge and are extinguished in a saddle-node bifurcation. Another saddle-node bifurcation occurs when Q falls below the minimum of the M nullcline. Q acts as a bifurcation parameter for the switch subsystem, and the motion of the state point around the orbit drives the subsystem to switch back and forth in an all-or-none manner. The bifurcations are in the subsystem only and do not correspond to bifurcations of the whole system.

In Figure 2B i has been reduced, and the fixed point is stable. To the right of the Q nullcline the direction of change of Q is downward; therefore if an orbit crosses the Q nullcline from left to right (above the M nullcline) at a level below the maximum of the M nullcline, that orbit will not rise to the level of the M nullcline maximum, and will not carry the subsystem phase portrait through the corresponding bifurcation; and the system consequently comes to rest at a steady state with low M.

The qualitative change between Figs. 2A and 2B is due to a Hopf bifurcation [31]. Hopf bifurcation occurs where the trace of the Jacobian matrix of equations (4) and (5) is zero, i.e. where $\partial F/\partial M - (w + g) = 0$, at the fixed point. This condition is met only at the extrema of the M nullcline, as can be seen by differentiation of the M nullcline (equation (4) with $dM/dt = 0$) which gives

$$0 = \frac{\partial F}{\partial M} + \frac{\partial F}{\partial Q}\frac{dQ}{dM} - (w + g). \tag{6}$$

The condition for Hopf bifurcation is met only where $dQ/dM = 0$. Therefore a Hopf bifurcation can occur only at i such that the Q nullcline intersects the

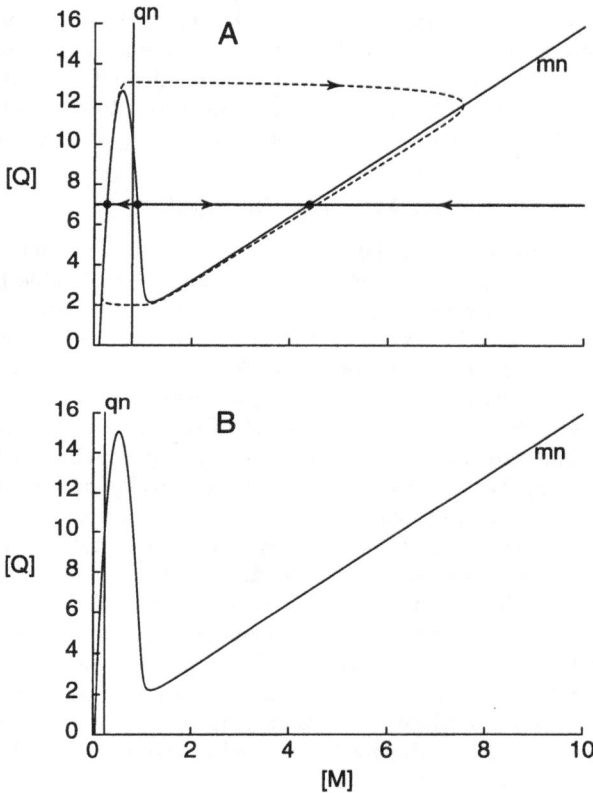

Fig. 2. Phase plane plot of equations (4) and (5), with (2) and (3). qn: Q nullcline. mn: M nullcline. Parameters: $g = 0.1$; other parameters as in Figure 1. A. $i = 0.0779451$: stable orbit (dashed line). B. $i = 0.0237461$: stable fixed point.

M nullcline at one of the extrema of the latter. There is in fact a second Hopf bifurcation (in addition to the one between Figs. 2A and 2B) when the Q null-cline intersects the minimum of the M nullcline; and at high i the fixed point is again stable. As noted above, the extrema of the M nullcline correspond to saddle-node bifurcations of the switch subsystem (equation (4)); therefore Hopf bifurcations of the full system coincide with saddle-node bifurcations of the switch subsystem.

This is an oversimplified model of the cell cycle, but it has the advantage that one can visualize in Figure 2 all the important dynamical features: the changing subsystem phase portrait, the variable Q that acts as a bifurcation parameter for the subsystem, the orbit, and the Hopf bifurcation parameter i. In a more realistic and more complicated cell cycle model, Novak and Tyson [18] have shown, at several points in the cell cycle, the two-dimensional phase portrait of a two-component bistable subsystem with all other system state variables held constant. In the course of the cell cycle this phase portrait is carried through two saddle-node bifurcations, without any bifurcation of the whole system. However the model is quite complicated, so it is not easy to see the exact relation of these subsystem bifurcations to those bifurcations of the whole system which switch it between non-cycling and cycling behavior.

§4. Multiple Checkpoints

The above bistable switch model was designed to control the activation of P to M, but it also controls the reconversion of M to P in a bistable manner. The oscillatory model therefore has, in effect, two potential checkpoints. These correspond to Hopf bifurcations at the two extrema of the M nullcline (Figure 2). Despite the multiple potential checkpoints the system never has more than one fixed point with a given set of parameter values. Two checkpoints arise because as parameters are changed the fixed point moves about in state space, and there are two distinct regions of state space where it is stable.

In principle, there might be more than two checkpoints if there are more than two distinct regions of state space where the fixed point is stable. In that case, opening a checkpoint, though it may be due to a saddle-node bifurcation in a subsystem, would cause Hopf bifurcation of the whole system. It seems likely that Hopf bifurcation in the cell cycle would be subcritical (as it is in the model of Figure 2), because the all-or-none character of cell cycle events seems inconsistent with low- or intermediate-amplitude oscillations.

However in a cell with two or more checkpoints a bifurcation destabilizing one checkpoint may produce progress only up to a later checkpoint, without producing cycling. This behavior is obtained in the model of Figure 2 if P as well as M is assumed to be removed:

$$\frac{dQ}{dt} = i - gM - hP = i - (g - h)M - hQ. \tag{7}$$

This changes the Q nullcline (Figure 3) so that an increase in i produces a saddle-node bifurcation rather than a Hopf bifurcation. On destabilization of the low-activity stable steady state the system evolves only as far as the high-activity stable steady state, and does not commence cycling. Similar switching from one checkpoint to another may presumably occur in systems with more than two stable fixed points.

Finally saddle-node bifurcation as well as Hopf bifurcation can in principle cause switching to a stable closed orbit. This can be either saddle-node bifurcation on a loop (Figure 4), or plain saddle-node bifurcation when the remaining attractor is a stable orbit (Figure 5 from B to A). In the latter case there is hysteresis, in that reversal of the saddle-node bifurcation re-establishes a stable fixed point but does not destabilize the orbit. Destabilization of the orbit can occur by elementary homoclinic loop bifurcation (Figure 5 from B to C to D). With either of these mechanisms, multiple checkpoints would correspond to distinct fixed points which arise and disappear by saddle-node

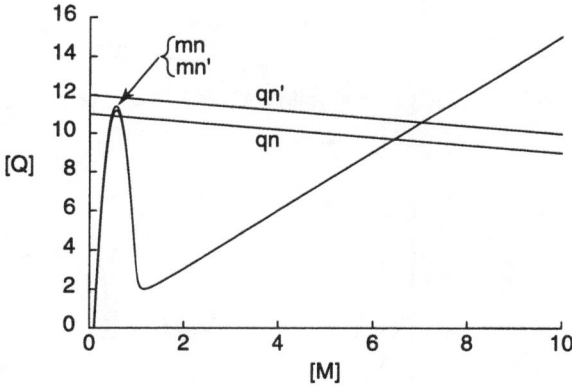

Fig. 3. Phase plane plot of equations (4) and (7), with (2) and (3). mn, mn′, qn, qn′: M and Q nullclines. Parameters as in Figure 2A except $g = 0.006$, $h = 0.005$, $i = 0.055$ (mn, qn), 0.06 (mn′, qn′).

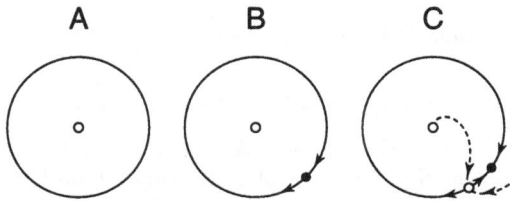

Fig. 4. Saddle-node bifurcation on a loop. Dashed lines are the stable manifold.

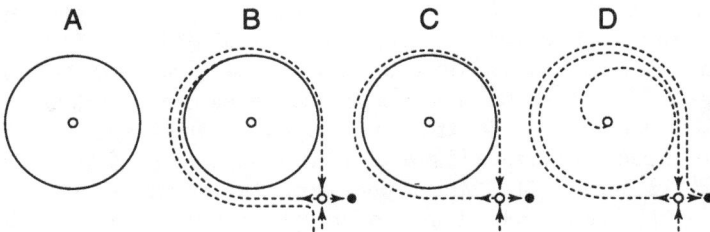

Fig. 5. Saddle-node and elementary homoclinic loop bifurcations.

bifurcation. This is in contrast to the above concept of a single fixed point with Hopf bifurcations in different locations in state space. It is not currently known which (if any) of these mechanisms switches cells with multiple checkpoints between non-cycling and cycling behavior.

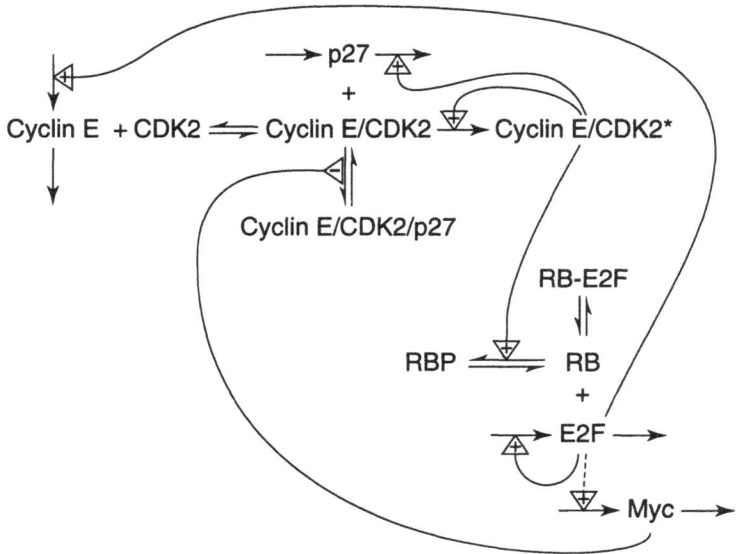

Fig. 6. Reactions involved in the transition from G1 to S phase.

§5. The G1-S Transition in Mammalian Cells

As an example of a checkpoint we may consider the transition to the phase of DNA replication (S phase) from the preceding phase (G1 phase) of the cell cycle (Figure 6). This is a rather complicated example, but it is also a very important example, because it is usually considered to be the start of the process of cell division.

There are two factors, E2F and Myc, which promote the transcription of several cell cycle genes and can drive quiescent cells all the way through G1 phase into S phase [37]. However evidence suggests that the key factor in initiating S phase is the enzyme cyclin E/CDK2 [1, 3, 12]. That this enzyme is in a bistable subsystem and is activated by saddle-node bifurcation is suggested by the fact that it exerts positive feedback on its own formation by several pathways. First, it activates its own activating enzyme CDC25A [9]. Second, it phosphorylates and promotes the disappearance of its own inhibitor p27$^{\mathrm{Kip1}}$ [13, 14, 28, 35]. Third, it phosphorylates the retinoblastoma protein RB [2, 4, 36]. The retinoblastoma protein [8] binds E2F and thereby inhibits it; and there is also evidence that complexes of RB with E2F are active repressors of gene transcription [11, 16, 27, 38]. Phosphorylation of RB liberates E2F, which promotes transcription of the gene for cyclin E [6, 23], which tends to increase cyclin E/CDK2, completing a positive feedback loop. Within this loop, E2F promotes transcription of its own gene [10, 11, 16], forming another positive-feedback loop. E2F also appears to promote transcription of the gene for Myc [24], which stimulates transcription of the gene for cyclin E [26], inhibits the binding of p27 to cyclin E/CDK2 [14, 26], and activates transcription of the gene for CDC25A [5] (perhaps only weakly [26]). Myc may also create positive feedback through the enzyme cyclin D/CDK4, which (like cyclin E/CDK2) phosphorylates RB. Myc apparently does not stimulate transcription of the cyclin D gene, but it can increase cyclin D1-associated enzyme activity without increasing the amount of cyclinD1/CDK4 [29].

This information comes from the work of many different investigators working with different material and different methods, and there are some differences in interpretation of the relative importance of the several factors and reactions involved. Research in this area is very active, and it is to be expected that new findings will change the picture. Here a number of factors and reactions have been omitted, in order to focus on the positive-feedback loops; but the system remains quite complicated, and further simplification would be very desirable for understanding the dynamics. At present it is not known which, if any, of the feedback loops creates bistability. In the case of autocatalysis, bistability is produced only if in some range of concentrations the reaction order for autocatalysis is greater than the reaction order for substrate removal [31]. Bistability also requires factors or reactions (like the inhibitor in the above bistable switch model) that counteract the autocatalysis at the stable steady states; and little is known about these factors in the reactions in Figure 6. It seems likely that the most important positive-feedback loops for switching cyclin E/CDK2 are those involving its activation of CDC25A and its inactivation of p27. The function of seemingly redundant positive feedback loops may be related to making the switch dependent on a number of different conditions or signals. This redundancy may frustrate attempts to stop repetitive cell division by inhibiting specific processes.

§6. Conclusion

The term "checkpoint" emphasizes the halting of progress through the cell cycle. However bistable mechanisms may play an essential role in promoting cell cycling. It has been suggested elsewhere [30] that inhibition of enzyme activation in the period before mitosis may be necessary in order to allow accumulation of sufficient enzyme precursor to produce a large pulse of active enzyme on activation. In addition the bistability of a checkpoint mechanism drives the cell cycle: the biochemical mechanism in the switch of equations (1–3) is essentially the same mechanism that causes instability of the fixed point in the oscillatory model of equations (4–5). The effect of disabling a checkpoint may not be to permit cell cycling to go forward but rather to abolish cell cycling.

A great deal of biological research is now being focused on checkpoints and other cell cycle transitions, and as more biological information is acquired it will become possible to understand these transitions mathematically much better. However the subsystems effecting these transitions are driven through their bifurcations by other components of the whole system, and a full understanding of cell cycle dynamics will undoubtedly require that we understand not only the subsystem dynamics but the interactions of the subsystems.

References

1. Alevizopoulos, A., J. Vlach, S. Hennecke and B. Amati, Cyclin E and c-Myc promote cell proliferation in the presence of p16^{INK4a} and of hypophosphorylated retinoblastoma family proteins, EMBO J. **17** (1997), 5322–5333.

2. Chow, K. N. B., P. Starostik and D. C. Dean, The Rb family contains a conserved cyclin-dependent kinase-regulated transcriptional repressor motif, Mol. Cell. Biol. **16** (1996), 7173–7181.

3. Duronio, R. J., A. Brook, N. Dyson and P. H. O'Farrell, E2F-induced S phase requires *cyclin E*, Genes Devel. **10** (1996), 2505–2513.

4. Dynlacht, D., O. Flores, J.A. Lees and E. Harlow, Differential regulation of E2F *trans*-activation by cyclin/cdk2 complexes, Genes Devel. **8** (1994), 1772–1786.

5. Galaktionov, K., X. Chen and D. Beach, Cdc25 cell-cycle phosphatase as a target of c-myc, Nature **382** (1996), 511–517.

6. Geng, Y., E. N. Eaton, M. Picón, J. M. Roberts, A. S. Lundberg, A. Gifford, C. Sardet and R. A. Weinberg, Regulation of cyclin E transcription by E2Fs and retinoblastoma protein, Oncogene **12** (1996), 1173–1180.

7. Hale, J. K. and H. Koçak, *Dynamics and Bifurcations*, Springer-Verlag, New York, 1991.

8. Herwig, S. and M. Strauss, The retinoblastoma protein: a master regulator of cell cycle, differentiation and apoptosis, Eur. J. Biochem. **246** (1997), 581–601.

9. Hoffmann, I., G. Draetta and E. Karsenti, Activation of the phosphatase activity of human cdc25A by a cdk2-cyclin E dependent phosphorylation at the G_1/S transition, EMBO J. **13** (1995), 4302–4310.

10. Hsiao, K.-M., S. L. McMahon and P. J. Farnham, Multiple DNA elements are required for the growth regulation of the mouse *E2F1* promoter, Genes Devel. **8** (1994), 1526–1537.

11. Johnson, D. G., K. Ohtani and J. R. Nevins, Autoregulatory control of *E2F1* expression in response to positive and negative regulators of cell cycle progression, Genes Devel. **8** (1994), 1514–1525.

12. Lukas, J., T. Herzinger, K. Hansen, M. C. Moroni, D. Resnitzky, K. Helin, S. I. Reed and J. Bartek, Cyclin E-induced S phase without activation of the pRb/E2F pathway, Genes Devel. **11** (1997), 1479–1492.

13. Morisaki, H., A. Fujimoto, A. Ando, Y. Nagata, K. Ikeda and M. Nakanishi, Cell cycle-dependent phosphorylation of p27 cyclin-dependent kinase (Cdk) inhibitor by cyclin E/Cdk2, Biochem. Biophys. Res. Commun. **240** (1997), 386–390.

14. Müller, D., C. Bouchard, B. Rudolph, P. Steiner, I. Stuckmann, R. Saffrich, W. Ansorge, W. Huttner and M. Eilers, Cdk2-dependent phosphorylation of p27 facilitates its Myc-induced release from cyclin E/cdk2 complexes, Oncogene **15** (1997), 2561–2576.

15. Murray, A. W., Cell cycle checkpoints, Curr. Opin. Cell Biol. **6** (1994), 872–876.

16. Neuman, E., E. K. Flemington, W. R. Sellers and W. G. Kaelin, Jr., Transcription of the E2F-1 gene is rendered cell cycle dependent by E2F DNA-binding sites within its promoter, Mol. Cell. Biol. **14** (1994) 6607–6615. [Correction *ibid.* **15** (1995), 4660.]

17. Novak, B. and J. J. Tyson, Modeling the cell division cycle: M-phase trigger, oscillations, and size control, J. theor. Biol. **165** (1993), 101–134.

18. Novak, B. and J. J. Tyson, Quantitative analysis of a molecular model of mitotic control in fission yeast, J. theor. Biol. **173** (1995), 283–305.

19. Novak, B. and J. J. Tyson, Modeling the control of DNA replication in fission yeast, Proc. Natl. Acad. Sci. USA **94** (1997), 9147–9152.

20. Obeyesekere, M. N., S. L. Tucker and S. O. Zimmerman, A model for regulation of the cell cycle incorporating cyclin A, cyclin B and their complexes, Cell Prolif. **27** (1994), 105–113.

21. Obeyesekere, M. N., J. R. Herbert and S. O. Zimmerman, A model of the G1 phase of the cell cycle incorporating cyclin E/cdk2 complex and retinoblastoma protein, Oncogene **11** (1995), 1199–1205.

22. Obeyesekere, M. N., E. S. Knudsen, J. Y. J. Wang and S. O. Zimmerman, A mathematical model of the regulation of the G1 phase of Rb+/+ and Rb−/− mouse embryonic fibroblasts and an osteosarcoma cell line, Cell Prolif. **30** (1997), 171–194.

23. Ohtani, K., J. DeGregori and J. R. Nevins, Regulation of the cyclin E gene by transcription factor E2F1, Proc. Natl. Acad. Sci. USA **92** (1995), 12146–12150.

24. Oswald, F., H. Lovec, T. Möröy and M. Lipp, E2F-dependent regulation of human MYC: *trans*-activation by cyclins D1 and A overrides tumour suppressor functions, Oncogene **9** (1994),S 2029–2036.

25. Paulovitch, A. G., D. P. Toczyski and L. H. Hartwell, When checkpoints fail, Cell **88** (1997), 315–321.

26. Pérez-Roger, I., D. L. C. Solomon, A. Sewing and H. Land, Myc activation of cyclin E/Cdk2 kinase involves induction of *cyclin E* gene transcription and inhibition of p27^{Kip1} binding to newly formed complexes, Oncogene **14** (1997), 2373–2381.

27. Qin, X.-Q., D. M. Livingstone, M. Ewen, W. R. Sellers, Z. Arany, and W. G. Kaelin, Jr., The transcription factor E2F-1 is a downstream target of RB action, Mol. Cell. Biol. **15** (1994), 742–755.

28. Sheaff, R. J., M. Groudine, M. Gordon, J. M. Roberts and B. E. Clurman, Cyclin E-CDK2 is a regulator of p27^{Kip1}, Genes Devel. **11** (1997), 1464–1478.

29. Steiner, P., A. Philipp, J. Lukas, D. Godden-Kent, M. Pagano, S. Mittnacht, J. Bartek and M. Eilers, Identification of a Myc-dependent step

during the formation of active G_1 cyclin-cdk complexes, EMBO J. **14** (1995), 4814–4826.

30. Thron, C. D., Theoretical dynamics of the cyclin B-MPF system: a possible role for p13^{suc1}, BioSystems **32** (1994), 97–109.

31. Thron, C. D., A model for a bistable trigger of mitosis, Biophys. Chem. **57** (1996), 239–251.

32. Thron, C. D., Bistable biochemical switching and the control of the events of the cell cycle, Oncogene **15** (1997), 317–325.

33. Tyson, J. J., B. Novak, K. Chen and J. Val, Checkpoints in the cell cycle from a modeler's perspective, in *Progress in Cell Cycle Research*, L. Meijer, S. Guidet and H. Y. L. Tung (eds.), Plenum Press, New York, 1995. 1–8.

34. Tyson, J. J., B. Novak, G. M. Odell, K. Chen and C. D. Thron, Chemical kinetic theory: understanding cell-cycle regulation, Trends Biochem. Sci. **21** (1996), 89–96.

35. Vlach, J., S. Hennecke and B. Amati, Phosphorylation-dependent degradation of the cyclin-dependent kinase inhibitor p27^{Kip1}, EMBO J. **16** (1997), 5334–5344.

36. Weinberg, R. A., The retinoblastoma protein and cell cycle control, Cell **81** (1995), 323–330.

37. Weinberg, R. A., E2F and cell proliferation: a world turned upside down, Cell **85** (1996), 457–459.

38. Zacksenhaus, E., Z. Jiang, R. A. Phillips and B. L. Gallie, Dual mechanisms of repression of E2F1 activity by the retinoblastoma gene product, EMBO J. **15** (1996), 5917–5927.

C. D. Thron
5 Barrymore Road
Hanover, NH 03755
dennis.thron@valley.net

Modeling the Probability of Tumor Cure after Fractionated Radiotherapy

Susan L. Tucker

Abstract. Mathematical modeling plays an important role in the design of improved treatment schedules for the clinical radiotherapy of cancer. The most widely used model of tumor cure is known in radiobiology as the Poisson model. However, recent studies have shown that the Poisson model consistently underestimates the probability of tumor cure when tumor-cell proliferation occurs during treatment. In some cases, the error can be fully 100%, with the Poisson model predicting a cure rate of 0% when the true cure rate is 100%. Several alternative, empirical models are described that are considerably more accurate than the Poisson model, though still subject to considerable error in some settings. In addition, a new model of tumor cure is derived, based on mechanistic assumptions regarding the distribution of cell cycle times, the rate of tumor-cell differentiation, and the cell loss rate.

§1. Introduction

Radiation has been used for the treatment of cancer since shortly after the discovery of X-rays by Roentgen in 1895 [7]. In principal, every tumor can be cured by exposing it to a dose of radiation high enough to kill every malignant cell in the tumor. In practice, however, radiation doses to patients must be limited in order to avoid severe, potentially life-threatening injury to normal tissues included in the treatment field. For example, treatment of lung cancer leads to exposure of normal lung and sometimes heart or esophagus, while radiotherapy for prostate cancer leads to exposure of the rectal wall.

Clinical radiotherapy for the treatment of cancer is given as sequence of small radiation doses, called dose fractions, separated by intervals that allow normal tissues time to repair some of the radiation-induced damage. Tumor and normal-tissue responses to radiotherapy depend markedly on the length of the time interval between dose fractions, as well as on other treatment-related factors such as total dose, size of dose per fraction, and type of radiation. As a consequence, there is continual interest in altering these parameters to

Mathematical Models in Medical and Health Sciences
Mary Ann Horn, Gieri Simonett, and Glenn Webb (eds.), pp. 381–396.
Copyright © 1998 by Vanderbilt University Press, Nashville, TN.
ISBN 0-8265-1310-7.

obtain new radiotherapy regimens that improve the therapeutic ratio, i.e., that increase the probability of tumor control while minimizing the risk of serious complications to normal tissue. At present, the most commonly used radiotherapy schedule in the United States consists of dose fractions of size 2 Gray (Gy) given once per day, five days per week, for a period of 5 to 7 weeks [6].

Mathematical models of tumor cure probability have played an important role in the effort to design improved radiotherapy schedules. They are frequently used to estimate the cure rate after altered fractionation schedules or are fitted to data to obtain estimates of clinically relevant parameters such as tissue repair halftimes or tumor dose-response characteristics. The most widely used tumor-cure model is known in radiobiology as the Poisson model because of its connection with Poisson statistics, as described in section 3 below. The purpose of this manuscript is to illustrate that the Poisson model does not accurately predict the tumor cure rate after fractionated radiotherapy when proliferation of tumor cells occurs during treatment. Several alternative models of tumor cure are presented that have been shown to be considerably more accurate than the Poisson model, though still subject to considerable error in some settings. In addition, a more general, improved model of tumor cure probability is derived.

§2. Clonogens and Tumor Cure

Tumors may contain many different types of cells, including normal, non-malignant cells such as macrophages. To achieve local tumor control, it is clearly not necessary to kill all cells in the tumor mass, but simply to eradicate the clonogenic cells, where tumor clonogens are defined operationally to be the cells capable of tumor regeneration. The probability of tumor cure after a particular treatment therefore depends ultimately on only three factors: the number of clonogens in the tumor at the start of treatment, the number of clonogens killed during treatment, and the number of new clonogens produced during treatment via cell proliferation.

§3. The Poisson Model

Consider a tumor containing N_0 clonogenic cells, each having precisely the same probability, S, of surviving a dose D of radiation. The probability of tumor cure after the single dose D is given by binomial statistics. Specifically,

$$\text{Prob}(k \text{ clonogens survive}) = \binom{N_0}{k} = S^k (1 - S)^{N_0 - k},$$

so in particular,

$$\text{Prob(tumor cure)} = \text{Prob(no clonogens survive)} = (1 - S)^{N_0}. \tag{1}$$

Using the well-known approximation of the binomial distribution by the Poisson distribution, the expression in equation (1) can be rewritten as

$$\text{Prob(tumor cure)} \approx \exp(-\lambda) = \exp(-S \cdot N_0), \tag{2}$$

where $\lambda = S \cdot N_0$ is the expected number of clonogens surviving irradiation. The Poisson approximation to the binomial is known to be highly accurate for cases in which S is small and N_0 is large, a condition that is easily met in the present setting. Clinically detectable tumors are estimated to contain at least $N_0 = 10^5$ clonogenic cells (ranging up to perhaps 10^9 clonogens), and in the dose range where cures are occurring ($\lambda < 1$), it follows that $S < 10^{-5}$.

Although the Poisson model of tumor cure was originally proposed only for large single doses of radiation [8], it has become commonplace to use the model for fractionated treatments as well, with the quantity λ in equation (2) replaced by various mechanistic models representing the average number of surviving clonogens per tumor at the end of treatment. For example, Bentzen et al. [2] fitted a version of equation (2) with

$$\lambda = c_1 \cdot h^{c_2} \cdot \exp(-D(\alpha + \beta d)) \cdot \exp(k_1 T)$$

to clinical data from patients with malignant melanoma. In this model, h is the mean tumor diameter, and the initial clonogen number is assumed to be a power function of the average tumor diameter: $N_0 = c_1 \cdot h^{c_2}$, with unknown parameters c_1 and c_2. The expression $\exp(-D(\alpha + \beta d))$ represents the fraction of surviving clonogens after exposure to total dose D given in a fractionated course of radiotherapy with dose per fraction d; this is the well-known LQ (for 'linear-quadratic') model of cell survival in radiation biology, with unknown parameters α and β [9]. The remaining factor, $\exp(k_1 T)$, is a simple growth model representing an exponential increase in clonogen number during treatment; here, T is the overall treatment time and k_1 is an unknown parameter representing the clonogen growth rate. In the study of Bentzen et al., a second growth model was also considered, in which simple exponential growth was replaced by an exponential model having a 28-day lag period, i.e. the growth factor was set identically equal to 1 for the first 28 days of treatment, and equal to $\exp(k_2(T - 28))$ for $T > 28$ days. The results of the analysis indicated no significant effect of overall treatment time using either of the clonogen growth models. The key finding of the analysis was that the ratio of the LQ parameters, α/β, is much smaller for malignant melanoma ($\alpha/\beta = 0.6$ Gy, with 95% confidence limits -1.1 Gy to 2.5 Gy) than the value found for most tumors (≈ 10 Gy). A small α/β ratio for melanoma suggests that radiotherapy for malignant melanoma could be significantly improved by the use of much larger-than-conventional doses per fraction, perhaps in the range of 6 Gy per fraction.

As a second example, Tucker and Chan [10] used the Poisson model with

$$\lambda = \begin{cases} N_0 \cdot \exp(-2n/D_0) \cdot \exp(\ln 2 \cdot T/60), & \text{if } T \leq 30 \text{ days,} \\ N_0 \cdot \exp(-2n/D_0) \cdot \exp(\ln 2 \cdot T/T_D), & \text{if } T > 30 \text{ days,} \end{cases}$$

to calculate the predicted cure rates among heterogeneous groups of tumors treated with various radiotherapy schedules. Here, D_0 is a tumor dose-response parameter related to the surviving fraction of cells at 2 Gy (SF2) by $D_0 = -2/\ln \text{SF2}$, n is the number of dose fractions, and T_D is the clonogen doubling time, which is assumed to be fixed at 60 days during the first 30 days of treatment (slow tumor growth phase), but could be much shorter thereafter (rapid growth phase). Intertumor heterogeneity was introduced by assuming that the parameters D_0 and T_D are distributed lognormally from tumor to tumor, and the aim of the paper was to determine how much the overall cure rate in the patient population could be improved if the treatment of each individual patient was based on his or her tumor characteristics (D_0 and T_D). The main finding of the study was that individualization of treatment based on tumor-cell kinetics (T_D) is unlikely to lead to detectable improvements in local tumor control unless differences in tumor radiosensitivity (D_0) are taken into account.

As a final example, Brenner et al. [3] carried out a mathematical modeling study using the Poisson model with

$$\lambda = N_0 \cdot \exp(-\alpha D - \beta G D^2)$$

to describe the responses of both normal tissues and tumors. The quantity D again represents the total radiation dose, α and β are the parameters of the LQ model of cell survival, and G (the generalized Lea-Catcheside function) is an expression depending on the particular fractionation pattern with which dose D is delivered to the patient and on the rate of repair of sublethal radiation damage repair for the tumor or normal tissue in question. The aim of this modeling study was to design optimal treatment protocols for brachytherapy, a technique in which radiotherapy is performed by implanting low-dose-rate radiation sources in the body. Two optimized protocols were identified, based on assumed differences in the repair rates between tumors and dose-limiting normal tissues.

The examples described above are but three of the many, many instances in the literature in which the Poisson model has been used in theoretical studies to predict tumor response or in data analyses to obtain estimates of clinically relevant biological parameters.

§4. Inaccuracy of the Poisson Model

In recent studies [11,12], it has been shown that the Poisson model does not accurately predict the probability of tumor control after fractionated radiotherapy when proliferation of tumor clonogens occurs during treatment. This is illustrated in Figure 1, which shows the true probability of cure as a function of dose (solid curve) for a hypothetical tumor treated with daily 2-Gy fractions and having a clonogen doubling time of approximately 2 days, compared with the predictions of the Poisson model (dashed curve) based on exact knowledge of the initial clonogen number, extent of cell killing during treatment, and proliferation kinetics. The absolute error in the Poisson model, which is represented by the vertical distance between the dashed and solid curves, ranges up to about 15% in this example.

The explanation for the inaccuracy of the Poisson model is as follows. Let p be the probability that a clonogen *initially present in the tumor* either

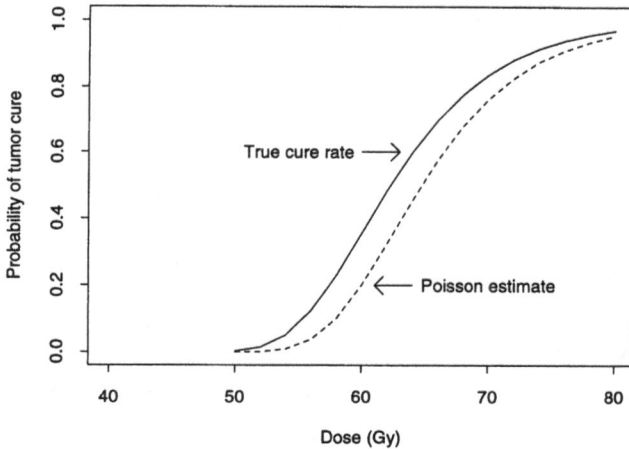

Fig. 1. Error in the Poisson model.

survives treatment itself or has one or more clonogenic progeny that are still surviving at the end of treatment. Then $p \cdot N_0$ is the expected number of *initial* clonogens per tumor that survive treatment in this extended sense, and the probability of tumor cure is given accurately by $\exp(-p \cdot N_0)$ [5]. In the standard Poisson model, however, the expression substituted in place of λ in equation (2) represents the expected number of surviving clonogens per tumor at the *end of treatment*. When clonogen proliferation occurs during treatment, the quantity λ will be greater than $p \cdot N_0$. To see this, note that every initial clonogen surviving in the extended sense has, by definition, at least one surviving offspring, and some will have more than one. Thus the number of offspring from a surviving *initial* clonogen is, on average, greater than one. Hence $\lambda > p \cdot N_0$ and therefore $\exp(-\lambda) \leq \exp(-p \cdot N_0)$, i.e., the Poisson model underestimates the true probability of tumor cure. The amount of error in the Poisson model clearly depends on the extent to which the average number of offspring of each initial clonogen differs from 1. In general, the extent of the error will increase with the rate of clonogen proliferation during treatment.

Another problematic feature of the Poisson model is illustrated in Figure 2, where the Poisson model was used to compute the predicted probability of cure as a function of dose for a hypothetical tumor treated with 2 Gy per fraction once every 3 days. The proliferation rate was assumed to be low during the first month of treatment (30-day clonogen doubling time) but much faster thereafter (2-day clonogen doubling time). The Poisson model makes the nonsensical prediction that the cure rate will be lower after a dose of 120 Gy (0%) than after a dose of 20 Gy (100%). The problem here is that the expression for the average number of clonogens per tumor (λ) decreases monotonely for doses up to 20 Gy (10 fractions), then begins to increase for

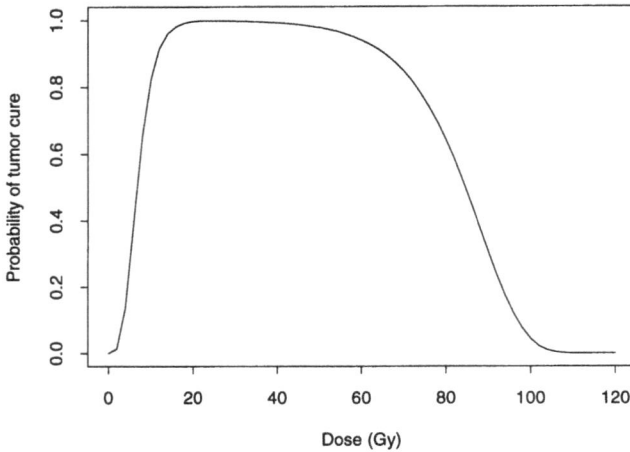

Fig. 2. Nonsensical dose-response curve predicted by the Poisson model.

larger doses, when the assumed rate of cell proliferation begins to exceed the
rate of cell killing. Since the Poisson estimate of the cure rate is based only
on the average number of clonogens per tumor, it does not take into account
tumors that are cured during treatment, and therefore allows them to become
effectively 'uncured' after subsequent dose fractions. In view of the fact that
the Poisson model always underestimates the true tumor cure rate, this example also illustrates that the Poisson model can have an absolute error of
fully 100%, predicting a cure rate of 0% when the true cure rate is 100%.

§5. Alternative Tumor-Cure Models

Yakovlev [15] provided an exact model for the probability of tumor cure in
the special case in which every cell in the tumor has the same radiosensitivity,
s, and the same probability, p_{div}, of dividing to produce two daughter cells
during each fractionation interval. The model of Yakovlev is based on the
theory of probability generating functions (p.g.f.s), as follows.

Suppose X is a random variable that assumes non-negative integer values
$0, 1, 2, \ldots$. The p.g.f. for X is defined to be the function

$$f_X(x) = \mathrm{E}[x^X] = \sum_{i=0}^{\infty} p_i x^i = p_0 + p_1 x + p_2 x^2 + \cdots,$$

where $\mathrm{E}[\cdot]$ denotes the expected value and $p_i = \mathrm{Prob}(X = i)$. If X is the
random variable representing the number of surviving cells after irradiation
of a single cell with survival probability s, then $X = 1$ with probability s and
$X = 0$ with probability $1 - s$, so the p.g.f. associated with X is

$$f_X(x) = 1 - s + s \cdot x. \tag{3}$$

Similarly, consider a clonogen that survives the ith dose of radiation during a fractionated treatment, and let Y_i be the random variable representing the number of cells present just prior to the $(i+1)$st dose, at the end of the ith fractionation interval. Under the assumption that the cell divides ($Y_i = 2$) with probability p_{div} and remains undivided ($Y_i = 1$) with probability $1 - p_{\mathrm{div}}$, the p.g.f. corresponding to Y_i is

$$g_{Y_i}(x) = (1 - p_{\mathrm{div}}) \cdot x + p_{\mathrm{div}} \cdot x^2. \tag{4}$$

According to the theory of probability generating functions, the random variable Z representing the number of cells present at the end of a fractionated treatment, given that we start with a single cell, and assuming that the processes of cell killing and cell division are independent, is

$$f_Z(x) = f_X \circ g_{Y_1} \circ f_X \circ \cdots \circ g_{Y_{(n-1)}} \circ f_X(x), \tag{5}$$

where n is the number of dose fractions. Finally, the p.g.f. for the number of cells present at the end of treatment, assuming that we start with N_0 clonogens, is $f_Z^{N_0}(x)$. The model of Yakovlev is obtained by setting $x = 0$, i.e.,

$$\text{Prob(tumor cure)} = f_Z^{N_0}(0) = [f_X \circ g_{Y_1} \circ f_X \circ \cdots \circ g_{Y_{(n-1)}} \circ f_X(0)]^{N_0}, \tag{6}$$

where f_X and g_{Y_i} are the functions given in equations (3) and (4), respectively.

Although the Yakovlev model provides a significant improvement to the Poisson model of tumor cure in some settings, it too has certain limitations. First, the tumor response characteristics (cell radiosensitivity and growth kinetics) may change during treatment, although this limitation is easily addressed by allowing the functions f_X and g_Y in equation (6) to change during the course of treatment, if necessary. Second, there may be heterogeneity among tumor cells with respect to cell radiosensitivity and kinetics, although this limitation can in principle be addressed by integrating over the appropriate distributions. Third, model (6) ignores the cell cycle structure. That is, cell division is not a probabilistic event in the sense suggested by equation (4), since a cell divides only at the end of its cell cycle, after it has completed the biochemical events necessary for cell division. Furthermore, cell radiosensitivity may depend on the position of the cell in the cell cycle, and radiation can induce delays in cell-cycle progression. These considerations indicate that the processes of cell killing and division are not actually independent, and therefore the p.g.f. formulation given in equation (5) is not strictly correct. Fourth, the p.g.f. for proliferation given in equation (4) limits each cell to at most one cell division during a fractionation interval. In practice, however, cells may easily undergo two or more divisions during the fractionation intervals used in clinical radiotherapy.

Some of the limitations to the Yakovlev model listed above are of only minor significance for clinical radiotherapy. For example, cell radiosensitivity depends only slightly on cell-cycle position at the small doses per fraction

($\approx$ 2 Gy) used clinically. In the clinical setting, the greatest limitation of the Yakovlev model is the restriction that each clonogenic cell is assumed to divide at most once during any fractionation interval. In reality, a tumor cell with a cycle time of approximately 24 hours will divide at least twice and possibly three times during the three-day weekend intervals (Friday morning to Monday morning) typical of conventional radiotherapy. Even more cell divisions will be expected during the much longer treatment breaks (two weeks or more) introduced into the middle of radiotherapy by split-course regimens.

To address this limitation, a number of alternative models have been proposed having the same basic structure as the Yakovlev model, but allowing for increased amounts of cell proliferation during treatment [11]. In each of these models, some other expression is substituted in place of the function $g_{Y_i}(x)$ in the Yakovlev model. In the GS (for 'geometric-stochastic') model, the function g_{Y_i} in equation (6) is replaced by

$$g_{Y_i}(x) = \frac{x \cdot \exp[-(\Delta t_i/T_{D_i}) \cdot \ln 2]}{1 - x(1 - \exp[-(\Delta t_i/T_{D_i}) \cdot \ln 2])}, \tag{7}$$

where Δt_i is the duration of the ith fractionation interval and T_{D_i} is the clonogen doubling time during that interval. The expression in equation (7) is the p.g.f. for a geometric probability distribution with mean $\mu = 2^{(\Delta t_i/T_{D_i})}$ and variance $\mu \cdot (\mu - 1)$. In the PS (for 'Poisson-stochastic') model, the function g_{Y_i} is replaced by the p.g.f. for the random variable $Y = 1 + X$, where X has a Poisson distribution with mean $1 - 2^{(\Delta t_i/T_{D_i})}$:

$$g_{Y_i}(x) = x \cdot \exp\{(1 - x)(1 - \exp((\Delta t_i/T_{D_i}) \cdot \ln 2))\}.$$

The random variable Y has mean $2^{(\Delta t_i/T_{D_i})}$ and variance $2^{(\Delta t_i/T_{D_i})} - 1$. A third model, the DS (for 'deterministic-stochastic') model, replaces the function g_{Y_i} in equation (6) by

$$g_{Y_i}(x) = x^{\exp[(\ln 2) \cdot (\Delta t_i/T_{D_i})]}. \tag{8}$$

Equation (8) is the p.g.f. for a constant random variable representing a deterministic growth process that does not, in general, correspond to an integer number of cells. In each of the GS, PS, and DS models, then, the function $g_{Y_i}(x)$ in the Yakovlev model is replaced by the p.g.f. for a random variable representing exponential cell growth with doubling time T_{D_i} during the ith fractionation interval, and having varying amounts of assumed variability in the proliferative process.

Previous studies based on computer simulations of tumor response to radiotherapy [11] suggest that when clonogen proliferation occurs during treatment, the GS, PS, and DS models models are all significantly more accurate than the Poisson model in predicting cure rates based on the biological characteristics of the tumor (initial clonogen number, radiosensitivity, and growth rate). Of these, the DS model is markedly inferior to the other two. In other words, the assumption of variability in cell proliferation built into the

GS and PS models improves their accuracy considerably compared with the DS model, which incorporates variability in the cell killing component of the model (equation 3) but not in the proliferation component (equation 8). The greater accuracy of the GS and PS models occurs despite the fact that the variability in cell proliferation in these models is not based on any mechanistic modeling, but simply on the use of standard, computationally convenient probability distributions.

Although the GS and PS models are considerable more accurate than the Poisson model, these alternative models are still subject to substantial error in some circumstances [11]. In the present paper, therefore, we develop a more general model for the probability of tumor cure. Unlike the GS, PS, and DS models, this new model is based on mechanistic assumptions concerning the proliferation of tumor cells during treatment.

§6. A General Model Incorporating Cell Loss and Differentiation

In this section we derive the p.g.f. corresponding to a mechanistic model for cell proliferation during radiotherapy fractionation intervals, assuming that the clonogenic cells are subject not only to cell division, but also to cell loss and differentiation.

Consider a population of clonogenic cells in which the distribution of cell cycle times, τ, among newborn cells has density function $\phi(\tau)$. A clonogenic cell divides at the end of its cycle time, producing two daughter cells. Each daughter cell is assumed to have probability ρ of being clonogenic and probability $1 - \rho$ of proceeding instead up the differentiation pathway toward becoming a mature, non-proliferative cell. Cell differentiation therefore represents a way in which newborn cells are lost from the clonogenic compartment. A second cell loss mechanism is also assumed, in which cells may be lost from the population at any point in the cell cycle, for example via apoptosis. This second loss process is assumed to occur at rate μ.

Let $n(a, \tau, t)$ represent the density of clonogenic cells at time t having chronological age a (i.e., time elapsed since division of the mother cell) and cell-cycle length τ. The density $n(a, \tau, t)$ satisfies the balance equation

$$\frac{\partial}{\partial a} n(a, \tau, t) + \frac{\partial}{\partial t} n(a, \tau, t) = -\mu \cdot n(a, \tau, t),$$

with birth condition

$$n(0, \tau, t) = 2\rho \cdot \phi(\tau) \int_0^\infty n(a, a, t) \, da.$$

Here, we are assuming that the cell cycle times of newborn clonogens are assigned at random from the cycle-time distribution, so in particular there is no correlation between the cycle times of mother cells and daughter cells or between sister cells.

It is a well-known phenomenon that every population of cells, no matter how synchronous or homogeneous at time zero, will converge rapidly to a stable asynchronous distribution if allowed to grow in unrestricted conditions [1,13]. That is, the cell population grows exponentially in number but maintains a stable, characteristic distribution with respect to virtually any measurable cell feature such as age, size, cycle time, DNA content, etc. For the present model, the stable solution has the form $n(a, \tau, t) = N_0 \cdot w(a, \tau) \cdot \exp(\gamma t)$, where N_0 is the initial number of cells in the population, $w(a, \tau)$ is the stable age- and cycle-time-distribution, and γ is the population growth rate.

We solve for $w(a, \tau)$ by plugging the stable solution into the balance equation to obtain

$$\frac{d}{da} w(a, \tau) + \gamma \cdot w(a, \tau) = -\mu \cdot w(a, \tau)$$

for each τ, with solution

$$w(a, \tau) = w(0, \tau) \cdot \exp(-(\mu + \gamma)a).$$

Substituting this expression into the birth equation, we find that $w(0, \tau) = 2\rho \cdot \phi(\tau) \cdot c$, where $c = \int_0^\infty w(0, a) \cdot \exp(-(\mu + \gamma)a)\, da$. We use the fact that $w(a, \tau)$ integrates to 1 to evaluate c. Specifically, c satisfies the equation

$$1 = \int_0^\infty \int_0^\tau w(a, \tau)da\, d\tau = \frac{2\rho c}{\mu + \gamma} \left[1 - \int_0^\infty \phi(\tau)\, e^{-(\mu+\gamma)\tau}\, d\tau \right].$$

Therefore

$$w(a, \tau) = \begin{cases} \frac{\phi(\tau) \cdot (\mu+\gamma) \cdot e^{-(\mu+\gamma)a}}{1 - \int_0^\infty \phi(\tau)\, e^{-(\mu+\gamma)\tau}\, d\tau} & \text{for } a \leq \tau, \\ 0 & \text{for } a > \tau. \end{cases} \tag{9}$$

The population growth rate, γ, is determined by the rate of cell division (i.e., the distribution of cell cycle times), the probability that newborn cells are retained in the clonogenic compartment, and the cell loss rate via

$$\gamma = -\mu + (2\rho - 1) \int_0^\infty w(a, a)\, da.$$

Simplifying this expression using equation (9), we find that γ, ρ, and μ satisfy the relation

$$1 = 2\rho \int_0^\infty \phi(a) \cdot e^{-(\gamma+\mu)a}\, da. \tag{10}$$

Now consider a cell selected at random at time $t = 0$ from the stable distribution described above (equation 9), and let $Y(t)$ be the random variable representing the number of cells descended from the initial cell at time t. We wish to determine the p.g.f. associated with $Y(t)$, i.e. $g_{Y(t)}(y; t) = \mathrm{E}[y^{Y(t)}]$. However, we first consider the case in which the selected cell happens to have age $a = 0$ at time $t = 0$, i.e., the cell is a newborn clonogen. We therefore first wish to find the conditional expectation

$$h(y; t) = \mathrm{E}[y^{Y(t)} | \text{ the initial cell has age zero}]. \tag{11}$$

Let τ be the cycle time of the randomly-selected newborn cell. For $t < \tau$, the initial cell will not yet have divided, and in fact may have been lost from the population through the cell loss process, with probability $1 - \exp(-\mu t)$. Hence, the conditional expectation is

$$E[y^{Y(t)} | \text{ cell age } = 0, \text{ cycle time } = \tau, \text{ and } t < \tau] = 1 - e^{-\mu t} + e^{-\mu t} y. \quad (12)$$

For $t \geq \tau$, there are four possible fates for the cell:
(i) The initial cell is lost from the population prior to the end of its division cycle; this occurs with probability $1 - \exp(-\mu\tau)$.
(ii) The initial cell survives in the population until division, but has no clonogenic offspring; this occurs with probability $(1 - \rho)^2 \cdot \exp(-\mu\tau)$.
(iii) The initial cell survives to mitosis and has exactly one clonogenic daughter; this occurs with probability $2\rho(1 - \rho) \cdot \exp(-\mu\tau)$.
(iv) The initial cell survives to mitosis and both daughter cells are clonogenic; this occurs with probability $\rho^2 \cdot \exp(-\mu\tau)$.
It then follows that

$$E[y^{Y(t)} | \text{ age } = 0, \text{ cycle time } = \tau, t \geq \tau]$$
$$= 1 - e^{-\mu\tau} + (1 - \rho)^2 \cdot e^{-\mu\tau} + 2\rho(1 - \rho) \cdot e^{-\mu\tau} \cdot h(y; t - \tau) \quad (13)$$
$$+ \rho^2 \cdot e^{-\mu\tau} \cdot h^2(y; t - \tau),$$

where $h(y; t)$ is the p.g.f. defined in equation (11). Averaging (12) and (13) over the distribution of cell cycle times, we obtain

$$h(y; t) = (1 - e^{-\mu t} + e^{-\mu t} \cdot y) \cdot (1 - \Phi(t))$$
$$+ \int_0^t \left[1 - e^{-\mu\tau} + (1 - \rho)^2 \cdot e^{-\mu\tau} + 2\rho(1 - \rho) \cdot e^{-\mu\tau} \cdot h(y; t - \tau) \right.$$
$$\left. + \rho^2 e^{-\mu\tau} \cdot h^2(y; t - \tau) \right] \cdot \phi(\tau) d\tau, \quad (14)$$

where $\Phi(t)$ is the cumulative distribution corresponding to ϕ.

We now impose the hypothesis that $\phi(\tau) \equiv 0$ for $\tau \in [0, T]$, i.e., there is some minimum cell cycle time, T. Biologically, this is an appropriate assumption since there are certain biochemical events such as DNA replication that must take place before a newly-formed clonogenic cell can divide to produce two daughter cells. Mathematically, the assumption of a minimum cell cycle time allows us to solve for $h(y; t)$ iteratively on intervals of length T. Specifically, letting $h_i(y; t)$ denote the function $h(y; t)$ on the interval $[iT, (i + 1)T]$, we find that for $t \in [0, T]$, equation (14) reduces to

$$h_0(y; t) = (1 - e^{-\mu t} + e^{-\mu t} \cdot y),$$

and for $t \in [T, 2T]$, we have

$$h_1(y; t) = (1 - e^{-\mu t} + e^{-\mu t} \cdot y) \cdot (1 - \Phi(t))$$
$$+ \int_T^t (1 - e^{-\mu\tau} + (1 - \rho)^2 \cdot e^{-\mu\tau}) \cdot \phi(\tau) d\tau$$
$$+ \int_0^{t-T} e^{-\mu(t-s)} \cdot \phi(t - s) \cdot [2\rho(1 - \rho) \cdot h_0(y; s) + \rho^2 \cdot h_0^2(s)] \, ds.$$

In general, for $t \in [nT, (n+1)T]$, $n = 0, 1, 2, \ldots$, we have

$$
\begin{aligned}
h_n(y;t) = {}& (1 - e^{-\mu t} + e^{-\mu t} \cdot y) \cdot (1 - \Phi(t)) \\
& + \int_T^{\max[T,t]} (1 - e^{-\mu\tau} + (1-\rho)^2 \cdot e^{-\mu\tau}) \cdot \phi(\tau) d\tau \\
& + \sum_{i=0}^{n-1} \left[\int_{iT}^{(i+1)T} e^{-\mu(t-s)} \cdot \phi(t-s) \right. \\
& \left. \qquad\qquad \times \left[2\rho(1-\rho) \cdot h_i(y;s) + \rho^2 \cdot h_i^2(y;s) \right] ds \right]. \quad (15)
\end{aligned}
$$

Next, consider a cell selected at random from the entire stable age and cycle-time distribution (equation 9). Let a denote the age and τ the cycle time of the selected cell. For $t < \tau - a$ the initial cell will not yet have divided, and therefore the conditional expectation is

$$
E[y^{Y(t)}|\text{age } = a, \text{ cycle time } = \tau, \text{ and } t < \tau - a] = 1 - e^{-\mu t} + e^{-\mu t} \cdot y.
$$

For $t \geq \tau - a$, there are four possible fates for the cell, analogous to those listed in points (i)–(iv) above. Therefore, the conditional expectation is

$$
\begin{aligned}
E[y^{Y(t)}|& \text{ age } = a, \text{ cycle time } = \tau, \ t \geq \tau - a] \\
& = 1 - e^{-\mu(\tau - a)} + (1-\rho)^2 \cdot e^{-\mu(\tau - a)} \\
& \quad + 2\rho(1-\rho) \cdot e^{-\mu(\tau - a)} \cdot h(y; t - (\tau - a)) \\
& \quad + \rho^2 \cdot e^{-\mu(\tau - a)} \cdot h^2(y; t - (\tau - a))
\end{aligned}
$$

where, again, $h(y;t)$ is the p.g.f. defined in equation (11). Averaging over the stable distribution of cell ages and cycle times, we get

$$
\begin{aligned}
g_{Y_i}(y;t) = {}& \int_{\max[T,t]}^{\infty} \int_0^{\tau - t} (1 - e^{-\mu t} + e^{-\mu t} \cdot y) \cdot w(a,\tau)\, da d\tau \\
& + \int_T^{\infty} \int_{\max[0,\tau - t]}^{\tau} \left[1 - e^{-\mu(\tau - a)} + (1-\rho)^2 \cdot e^{-\mu(\tau - a)} \right. \\
& \qquad + e^{-\mu(\tau - a)} \cdot \left(2\rho(1-\rho) \cdot h(y;, t - (\tau - a)) \right. \\
& \qquad\qquad \left. \left. + \rho^2 \cdot h^2(y; t - (\tau - a)) \right) \right] w(a,\tau)\, da d\tau. \quad (16)
\end{aligned}
$$

Written in terms of the functions $h_i(y;t)$, the solution given in equation (16) is, for $nT \leq t \leq (n+1)T$, $n = 0, 1, 2, \ldots$,

$$g_{Y_i}(y;t) = \int_{\max[T,t]}^{\infty} \int_0^{\tau-t} (1 - e^{-\mu t} + e^{-\mu t} \cdot y) \cdot w(a,\tau)\,da\,d\tau$$

$$+ \int_T^{\infty} \int_{\max[0,\tau-t]}^{\tau} \left[1 - e^{-\mu(\tau-a)} + (1-\rho)^2 \cdot e^{-\mu(\tau-a)}\right] w(a,\tau)\,da\,d\tau$$

$$+ \int_{\max[T,t]}^{\infty} \sum_{i=0}^n \int_{\tau-(t-iT)}^{\min[\tau-(t-(i+1)T),\tau]} e^{-\mu(\tau-a)}$$

$$\times \left[2\rho(1-\rho) \cdot h_i(y; t - (\tau - a))\right.$$

$$\left. + \rho^2 h_i^2(y; t - (\tau - a))\right] w(a,\tau)\,da\,d\tau$$

$$+ \sum_{i=1}^n \sum_{j=i-1}^n \int_{\max[T,t-iT]}^{t-(i+1)T} \int_{\max[0,\tau-(t-jT)]}^{\min[\tau-(t-(j+1)T),\tau]} e^{-\mu(\tau-a)}$$

$$\times \left[2\rho(1-\rho) \cdot h_j(y;, t - (\tau - a))\right.$$

$$\left. + \rho^2 \cdot h_j^2(y; t - (\tau - a))\right] w(a,\tau)\,da\,d\tau. \qquad (17)$$

Our new model for the probability of tumor cure after fractionated radiother-apy is given by equation (6), with the same p.g.f. for cell killing, f_X, as in the model of Yakovlev (equation 3) but the p.g.f. for proliferation during the ith fractionation interval replaced by the function g_{Y_i} given in equation (17), where the functions h_i, $i = 0, 1, 2, \ldots$, are defined iteratively as in equation (15), $w(a, \tau)$ is given by equation (9), and the constants γ, ρ, and μ satisfy the relationship given in equation (10).

§7. Discussion

We have developed a new model (equations 3, 6, and 17) for the probability of tumor cure during fractionated radiotherapy, based on mechanistic assump-tions regarding the distribution of cell cycle times, the rate of differentiation of tumor clonogens, and the rate at which cells are lost from the clonogenic compartment through mechanisms other than differentiation. Like other al-ternatives to the Poisson model proposed thus far (the Yakovlev model, plus the GS, PS, and DS models; see section 5), the new model takes into account stochastic variability in the number of cells killed by a fractional radiation dose and/or variability in the number of offspring produced by a clonogenic cell during a fractionation interval. Like the GS, PS, and DS models, but unlike the Yakovlev model, the new model allows for the possibility of more than one division per cell during each interval. The new model improves upon the GS, PS, and DS models in that the variability in the number of offspring per clonogenic cell per fractionation interval is based on mechanistic assump-tions regarding the proliferative process, rather than upon computationally convenient expressions for variability drawn from standard probability distributions.

A test of the accuracy of the new tumor-cure model presented here would require comparing the predictions of the model with true tumor cure rates under conditions not incorporated into the model, for example, in situations in which there is a substantial correlation in the cycle times of mother and daughter cells, or between sister cells. These sorts of calculations are beyond the scope of this paper. Similarly, comparisons between the new model and existing models such as the Poisson and GS models would require calculation of the cure rate under a range of tumor-response assumptions, and that too is beyond the scope of the present study. The new model is expected to be considerably more accurate than existing models simply because it allows the incorporation of much more specific assumptions regarding tumor response to radiation than do the previous models.

The use of the new tumor-cure model requires that explicit assumptions be made regarding the distribution of cell cycle times ($\phi(\tau)$), the differentiation rate $(1 - \rho)$, and the cell loss rate (μ). Alternatively, if the overall clonogen growth rate is known (γ), one can solve for either ρ or μ using equation (10). Depending on the form of $\phi(\tau)$, numerical integrations may be required when evaluating the functions $h_n(y; t)$ and $g_{Y_i}(y; t)$ given in equations (15) and (17), respectively. However, a reasonable choice for $\phi(\tau)$ that allows these expressions to be computed in closed form is a gamma distribution with a lag of length T introduced to model the minimum cell-cycle time,

$$
\phi(\tau) = \begin{cases} 0, & \text{for } \tau < T, \\ \frac{1}{\Gamma(m+1)} \cdot \theta^{m+1} \cdot (\tau - T)^m \cdot e^{-\theta(\tau - T)}, & \text{for } \tau \geq T, \end{cases}
$$

where $\Gamma[\cdot]$ is the well-known Euler gamma function ($\Gamma(u) = \int_0^\infty e^{-z} z^{u-1} dz$) and m, θ are parameters with $m > -1$ and $\theta > 0$. Equations (15) and (16) can then be calculated for the necessary number of time intervals $[nT, (n + 1)T]$ (depending on the length of the maximum fractionation interval), for example using a computer program such as Maple [4] or Mathematica [14] that performs symbolic manipulation. Values of $m \geq 2$ are especially appealing because they correspond to a density function $\phi(\tau)$ that is continuously differentiable for all $t \geq 0$.

The computational complexity of the new model obviously limits its routine use, but the degree of inaccuracy in the simpler models mandates the use of a more complex model in some settings. In particular, it is of considerable interest that the details of cell proliferation (differentiation rate, cell loss rate, and distribution of cell cycle times) influence the tumor cure probability, which is therefore not determined simply by the overall clonogen growth rate. Further studies are underway to investigate the relative extent to which each of the factors contributing to the clonogen growth rate influences tumor cure.

References

1. Bell, G. I. and E. C. Anderson, Cell growth and division I. A mathematical model with applications to cell volume distributions in mammalian cell cultures, Biophysical Journal **7** (1967), 329–351.

2. Bentzen, S. M., J. Overgaard, H. D. Thames, M. Overgaard, P. Vejby Hansen, H. von der Maase and J. Meder, Clinical radiobiology of malignant melanoma, Radiotherapy and Oncology **16** (1989), 169–182.

3. Brenner, D. J., E. J. Hall, Y. Huang and R. K. Sachs, Optimizing the time course of brachytherapy and other accelerated radiotherapeutic protocols, International Journal of Radiation Oncology Biology Physics **29** (1994), 893–901.

4. Char, B. W., K. O. Geddes, G. H. Gonnet, B. L. Leong, M. B. Monagan and S. M. Watt, *First Leaves: A Tutorial Introduction to Maple V*, Springer-Verlag, New York, 1992.

5. Deasy, J., Letter to the editor: Poisson models for tumor control probability with clonogen proliferation, Radiation Research **145** (1996), 382–384.

6. Fletcher, G. H., *Textbook of Radiotherapy* (3rd edition), Lea & Febinger, Philadelphia, 1980.

7. Kogelnik, H. D., Inauguration of radiotherapy as a new scientific speciality by Leopold Freund 100 years ago, Radiotherapy and Oncology **42** (1997), 203–11.

8. Porter, E. H., The statistics of dose/cure relationships for irradiated tumours, British Journal of Radiology **53** (1980), 210–227.

9. Thames, H. D. and J. H. Hendry, *Fractionation in Radiotherapy*, Taylor & Francis, New York, 1987.

10. Tucker, S. L. and K.-S. Chan, The selection of patients for accelerated radiotherapy on the basis of tumor kinetics and intrinsic radiosensitivity, Radiotherapy and Oncology **18** (1990), 197–211.

11. Tucker, S. L. and J. M. G. Taylor, Improved models of tumour cure, International Journal of Radiation Biology, **70** (1996), 539–553.

12. Tucker, S. L., H. D. Thames and J. M. G. Taylor, How well is the probability of tumor cure after fractionated irradiation described by Poisson statistics? Radiation Research **124** (1990), 273–282.

13. Webb, G. F., An operator-theoretic formulation of asynchronous exponential growth, Transactions of the American Mathematical Society **303** (1987), 751–763.

14. Wolfram, S., *The Mathematica Book* (3rd edition), Cambridge University Press, New York, 1996.

15. Yakovlev, A. Yu., Letter to the editor: Comments on the distribution of clonogens in irradiated tumors, Radiation Research **134** (1993), 117–120.

Susan L. Tucker
Department of Biomathematics, Box 237
The Univ. of Texas M. D. Anderson Cancer Center
1515 Holcombe Blvd.
Houston, Texas 77030
tucker@odin.mdacc.tmc.edu

www.ingramcontent.com/pod-product-compliance
Lightning Source LLC
Chambersburg PA
CBHW021428180326
41458CB00001B/179